Medical Microbiology and Infection

Lecture Notes

Edited by

Tom Elliott BM BS BMedSci PhD DSc MRCP FRCPath
Consultant Medical Microbiologist
The Queen Elizabeth Hospital
University Hospitals Birmingham NHS Foundation Trust
Birmingham, UK

Anna Casey BSc PhD
Clinical Research Scientist
Department of Clinical Microbiology
The Queen Elizabeth Hospital
University Hospitals Birmingham NHS Foundation Trust
Birmingham, UK

Peter Lambert BSc PhD DSc
Professor of Microbiology
School of Life and Health Sciences
Aston University
Birmingham, UK

Jonathan Sandoe Mb ChB PhD FRCPath
Consultant Microbiologist and Honorary Senior Lecturer
Department of Microbiology
Leeds Teaching Hospitals NHS Trust and University of Leeds
Leeds, UK

Fifth Edition

WILEY-BLACKWELL

A John Wiley & Sons, Ltd., Publication

Registered office: John Wiley & Sons, Ltd, The Atrium, Southern Gate, Chichester, West Sussex, PO19 8SQ, UK

Editorial offices:
9600 Garsington Road, Oxford, OX4 2DQ, UK
The Atrium, Southern Gate, Chichester, West Sussex, PO19 8SQ, UK
111 River Street, Hoboken, NJ 07030-5774, USA

For details of our global editorial offices, for customer services and for information about how to apply for permission to reuse the copyright material in this book please see our website at www.wiley.com/wiley-blackwell.

First published (As Lecture Notes on Bacteriology) 1967
First Edition 1975
Second Edition 1978
Reprinted 1979, 1983, 1986
Third Edition 1997
International edition 1997
Reprinted 2003, 2004
Fourth Edition 2007
Fifth Edition 2011

Library of Congress Cataloging-in-Publication Data

Lecture notes. Medical microbiology and infection / Tom Elliott . . . [et al.]. – 5th ed.
    p. ; cm.
  Medical microbiology and infection
  Includes bibliographical references and index.
  ISBN-13: 978-1-4443-3465-4 (pbk. : alk. paper)
  ISBN-10: 1-4443-3465-4 (pbk. : alk. paper) 1. Medical microbiology–Outlines, syllabi, etc. I. Elliott, Tom
(Thomas Stuart Jackson) II. Title: Medical microbiology and infection.
  [DNLM: 1. Microbiology. 2. Communicable Diseases–microbiology. QW 4]
  QR46.G49 2011
  616.9′041–dc22

                    2011012045

A catalogue record for this book is available from the British Library.

Set in 8.5pt/11pt Utopia font by Thomson Digital, Noida, India.
Printed and bound in Malaysia by Vivar Printing Sdn Bhd

1 2011

Contents

Self-assessment

Preface

The magnitude of recent changes in the field of medical microbiology has warranted this fifth edition of *Lecture Notes: Medical Microbiology and Infection*. While these changes have been encompassed in new chapters, this edition continues to maintain the well-received and user-friendly format of earlier editions, highlighting the pertinent key facts in medical microbiology and providing a sound foundation of knowledge which students can build on. The book for the first time is multi-authored, with chapters being written by recognised experts in their field.

This fifth edition is arranged into three main sections: basic microbiology, antimicrobial agents and infection. It covers all aspects of microbiology, including bacteriology, virology, mycology and parasitology. As in previous editions, the text is supported throughout with colour figures to illustrate the key points.

This book is written specifically for students in medicine, biomedicine, biology, dentistry, science and also pharmacology, who have an interest in medical microbiology at both undergraduate and postgraduate levels. In addition, this book will serve as a useful *aide memoire* for doctors sitting MRCS and MRCP examinations, as well as other healthcare professionals, for example biomedical scientists, working towards state registration.

Contributors

Erwin Brown Consultant Microbiologist, Department of Medical Microbiology, Frenchay Hospital, North Bristol NHS Trust, Bristol, UK

Anna Casey Clinical Research Scientist, Department of Clinical Microbiology, The Queen Elizabeth Hospital, University Hospitals Birmingham NHS Foundation Trust, Birmingham, UK

Chris Catchpole Consultant Microbiologist, Department of Clinical Microbiology, Worcestershire Royal Hospital, Worcestershire Acute Hospitals NHS Trust, Worcester, UK

John Cheesbrough Consultant Microbiologist, Department of Microbiology, Royal Preston Hospital, Lancashire Teaching Hospitals NHS Foundation Trust, Preston, Lancashire, UK

Peter Chiodini Consultant Parasitologist and Honorary Professor, The Hospital for Tropical Diseases and The London School of Hygiene and Tropical Medicine, London, UK

Barry Cookson Director of the Laboratory of Healthcare-associated Infection, Health Protection Agency, Microbiology Services, Colindale, London, UK

Rabih Darouiche VA Distinguished Service Professor, Departments of Medicine, Surgery and Physical Medicine & Rehabilitation and Director, Center for Prostheses Infection, Baylor College of Medicine, Houston, Texas, USA

Tom Elliott Consultant Microbiologist, The Queen Elizabeth Hospital, University Hospitals NHS Foundation Trust, Birmingham, UK

James Gray Consultant Microbiologist, Department of Medical Microbiology, Birmingham Children's Hospital NHS Foundation Trust, Birmingham, UK

Tariq Iqbal Consultant Physician and Gastroenterologist, Department of Gastrointestinal Medicine, The Queen Elizabeth Hospital, University Hospitals Birmingham NHS Foundation Trust, Birmingham, UK

Elizabeth Johnson Director of the Health Protection Agency Mycology Reference Laboratory, Bristol, UK

Shruti Khurana Specialist Registrar, Department of Respiratory Medicine, Manchester Royal Infirmary, Central Manchester University Hospitals NHS Foundation Trust, Manchester, UK

Peter Lambert Professor of Microbiology, School of Life and Health Sciences, Aston University, Birmingham, UK

David Livermore Director, Antibiotic Resistance Monitoring and Reference Laboratory, Health Protection Agency, Microbiology Services, Colindale, London, UK

Peter Mackie Consultant Clinical Scientist, Department of Microbiology, The General Infirmary at Leeds, Leeds Teaching Hospitals NHS Trust, Leeds, UK

Kaveh Manavi Consultant Physician HIV/ Genitourinary Medicine, Department of Genitourinary Medicine, The Queen Elizabeth Hospital, University Hospitals Birmingham NHS Foundation Trust, Birmingham, UK

Cliodna McNulty Consultant Microbiologist, Health Protection Agency, Microbiology Department, Gloucestershire Royal Hospital, Gloucestershire Hospitals NHS Trust, Gloucester, UK

David Mutimer Consultant Hepatologist, Department of Liver Medicine, The Queen Elizabeth Hospital, University Hospitals Birmingham NHS Foundation Trust, Birmingham, UK

Supriya Narasimhan Assistant Professor, Division of Infectious Diseases, Department of Medicine, Drexel University, Pittsburgh, USA

Eleni Nastouli Consultant Virologist and Honorary Consultant in Paediatric Infectious Diseases, Department of Virology, University College London Hospitals NHS Trust and Great Ormond Street Hospital for Children NHS Trust, London, UK

Susan O'Connell Consultant Microbiologist, Lyme Borreliosis Unit, Health Protection Agency Microbiology Laboratory, Southampton General Hospital, Southampton University Hospitals NHS Trust, Southampton, UK

Jonathan Sandoe Consultant Microbiologist and Honorary Senior Lecturer, Department of Micro-biology, Leeds Teaching Hospitals NHS Trust and University of Leeds, Leeds, UK

Sumeet Singhania Specialist Registrar, Depart-ment of Respiratory Medicine, Manchester Royal Infirmary, Central Manchester University Hospi-tals NHS Foundation Trust, Manchester, UK

Martin Skirrow Honorary Emeritus Consultant Microbiologist, Health Protection Agency, Micro-biology Department, Gloucestershire Royal Hospital, Gloucestershire Hospitals NHS Trust, Gloucester, UK

Richard Watkin Consultant Cardiologist, Good Hope Hospital, Heart of England NHS Foundation Trust, Sutton Coldfield, Birmingham, UK

Mark Woodhead Consultant in General and Respiratory Medicine and Honorary Senior Lecturer, Department of Respiratory Medicine, Manchester Royal Infirmary, Central Manchester University Hospitals NHS Foundation Trust and University of Manchester, Manchester, UK

Tony Worthington Senior Lecturer in Microbiol-ogy, School of Life and Health Sciences, Aston University, Birmingham, UK

Part 1

Basic microbiology

Basic bacteriology

Peter Lambert
Aston University, Birmingham, UK

Bacterial structure

Bacteria are single-celled prokaryotic microorganisms, and their DNA is not contained within a separate nucleus as in eukaryotic cells. They are approximately 0.1–10.0 μm in size (Figure 1.1) and exist in various shapes, including spheres (cocci), curves, spirals and rods (bacilli) (Figure 1.2). These characteristic shapes are used to classify and identify bacteria. The appearance of bacteria following the Gram stain is also used for identification. Bacteria which stain purple/blue are termed Gram-positive, whereas those that stain pink/red are termed Gram-negative. This difference in response to the Gram stain results from the composition of the cell envelope (wall) (Figure 1.3), which are described below.

Cell envelope

Cytoplasmic membrane

A cytoplasmic membrane surrounds the cytoplasm of all bacterial cells and are composed of protein and phospholipid; they resemble the membrane surrounding mammalian (eukaryotic) cells but lack sterols. The phospholipids form a bilayer into which proteins are embedded, some spanning the membrane. The membrane carries out many functions, including the synthesis and export of cell-wall components, respiration, secretion of extracellular enzymes and toxins, and the uptake of nutrients by active transport mechanisms.

Mesosomes are intracellular membrane structures, formed by folding of the cytoplasmic membrane. They occur more frequently in Gram-positive than in Gram-negative bacteria. Mesosomes present at the point of cell division of Gram-positive bacteria are involved in chromosomal separation; at other sites they may be associated with cellular respiration and metabolism.

Cell wall

Bacteria maintain their shape by a strong rigid outer cover, the cell wall (Figure 1.3).

Gram-positive bacteria have a relatively thick, uniform cell wall, largely composed of peptidoglycan, a complex molecule consisting of linear repeating sugar subunits cross-linked by peptide side chains (Figure 1.4a). Other cell-wall polymers, including teichoic acids, teichuronic acids and proteins, are also present.

Gram-negative bacteria have a thinner peptidoglycan layer and an additional outer membrane that differs in structure from the cytoplasmic membrane (Figure 1.4b). The outer membrane contains lipopolysaccharides on its outer face, phospholipids on its inner face, proteins and lipoproteins which anchor it to the peptidoglycan. Porins are a group of proteins that form channels through which small hydrophilic molecules, including nutrients, can cross the outer membrane. Lipopolysaccharides are

Medical Microbiology and Infection Lecture Notes, Fifth Edition. Edited by Tom Elliott, Anna Casey, Peter Lambert and Jonathan Sandoe.
© 2011 Blackwell Publishing Ltd. Published 2011 by Blackwell Publishing Ltd.

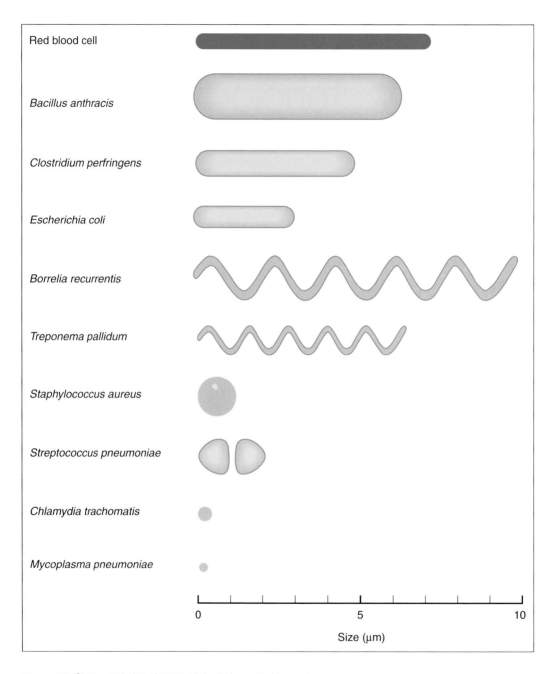

Red blood cell

Bacillus anthracis

Clostridium perfringens

Escherichia coli

Borrelia recurrentis

Treponema pallidum

Staphylococcus aureus

Streptococcus pneumoniae

Chlamydia trachomatis

Mycoplasma pneumoniae

0   5   10

Size (μm)

Figure 1.1 Shape and size of some clinically important bacteria.

a characteristic feature of Gram-negative bacteria and are also termed 'endotoxins' or 'pyrogen'. Endotoxins are released on cell lysis and have important biological activities involved in the pathogenesis of Gram-negative infections; they activate macrophages, clotting factors and complement, leading to disseminated intravascular coagulation and septic shock (Chapter 33).

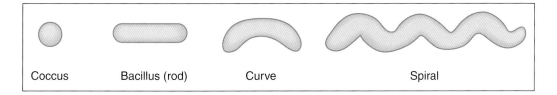

Figure 1.2 Some bacterial shapes.

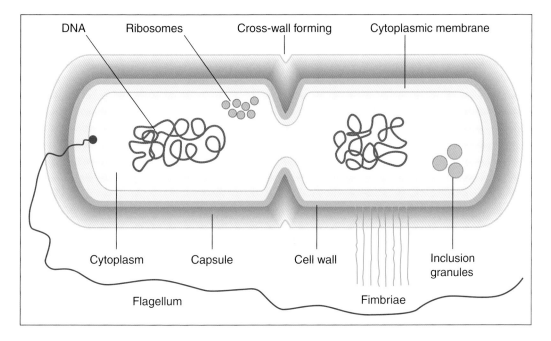

Figure 1.3 A section of a typical bacterial cell.

Mycobacteria have a distinctive cell wall structure and composition that differs from that of Gram-positive and Gram-negative bacteria. It contains peptidoglycan but has large amounts of high molecular weight lipids in the form of long chain length fatty acids (mycolic acids) attached to polysaccharides and proteins. This high lipid content gives the mycobacteria their acid fast properties (retaining a stain on heating in acid), which allows them to be distinguished from other bacteria (e.g. positive Ziehl-Neelsen stain).

The cell wall is important in protecting bacteria against external osmotic pressure. Bacteria with damaged cell walls, e.g. after exposure to β-lactam antibiotics such as penicillin, often rupture. However, in an osmotically balanced medium, bacteria deficient in cell walls may survive in a spherical form called protoplasts. Under certain conditions some protoplasts can multiply and are referred to as L-forms. Some bacteria, e.g. mycoplasmas, have no cell wall at any stage in their life cycle.

The cell wall is involved in bacterial division. After the nuclear material has replicated and separated, a cell wall (septum) forms at the equator of the parent cell. The septum grows in, produces a cross-wall and eventually the daughter cells may separate. In many species the cells can remain attached, forming groups, e.g. staphylococci form clusters and streptococci form long chains (Figure 1.5).

Capsules

Some bacteria have capsules external to their cell walls (Figure 1.3). These structures are bound

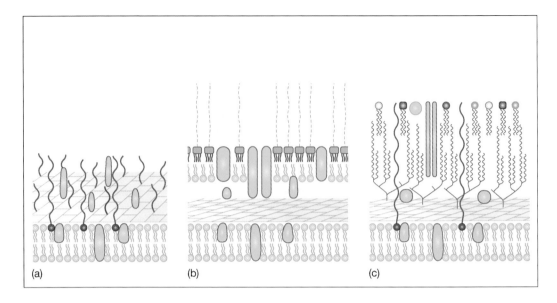

Figure 1.4 Cell wall and cytoplasmic membrane of (a) Gram-positive bacteria, (b) Gram-negative bacteria and (c) mycobacteria. The Gram-positive bacterial cell wall has a thick peptidoglycan layer with associated molecules (teichoic acids, teichuronic acids and proteins). The Gram-negative bacterial cell wall contains lipopolysaccharides, phospholipids and proteins in an outer membrane linked to a thin inner peptidoglycan layer. The mycobacterial cell wall contains long chain length fatty acids (mycolic acids).

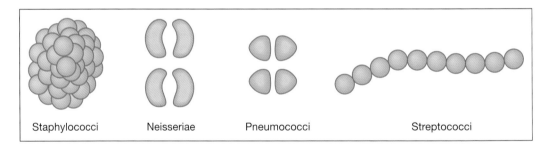

Figure 1.5 Some groups of bacteria.

to the bacterial cell and have a clearly defined boundary. They are usually polysaccharides with characteristic compositions that can be used to distinguish between microorganisms of the same species (e.g. in serotyping). Capsular antigens can be used to differentiate between strains of the same bacterial species, e.g. in the typing of *Streptococcus pneumoniae* for epidemiological purposes. The capsules are important virulence determinants in both Gram-positive and Gram-negative bacteria, because they may protect the bacteria from host defences and, in some bacteria, aid attachment to host cells.

Bacterial slime and biofilm

Extracellular slime layers are produced by some bacteria. They are more loosely bound to the cell surface than capsules and do not form a clearly defined surface boundary. The slime layer is composed predominantly of complex polysaccharides (glycocalyx), which acts as a virulence

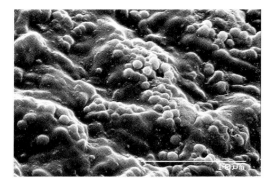

Figure 1.6 Scanning electronmicrograph of *Staphylococcus epidermidis* embedded in slime attached to a catheter.

factor through the formation of biofilm, e.g. by facilitating the attachment of *Staphylococcus epidermidis* onto artificial surfaces, such as intravascular cannulae (Figure 1.6), replacement joints and heart valves. Once formed, biofilms present a major problem for treatment and may require removal of the biomedical device.

Flagella

Bacterial flagella are spiral-shaped surface filaments consisting mainly of the protein, flagellin. They are attached to the cell envelope as single (monotrichous) or multiple (peritrichous) forms (Figure 1.7).

Flagella facilitate movement (motility) in bacteria by rapid rotation. They can be observed under the light microscope with special stains. Flagella are usually detected for diagnostic purposes by observing motility in a bacterial suspension or by spreading growth on solid media. The antigenic nature of the flagella may be used to differentiate between and identify strains of *Salmonella* spp.

Fimbriae

Fimbriae (also termed pili) are thin, hair-like appendages on the surface of many Gram-negative, and some Gram-positive, bacteria (Figure 1.3). They are approximately half the width of flagella, and are composed of proteins called pilins. In some bacteria they are distributed over the entire cell surface.

Fimbriae are virulence factors enabling bacteria to adhere to particular mammalian cell surfaces, an important initial step in colonisation of mucosal surfaces, e.g. *Neisseria gonorrhoeae* produce fimbriae that bind to specific receptors of cervical epithelial cells, whereas *Streptococcus pyogenes* have fimbriae containing 'M' protein, which facilitates adhesion to human cells in the pharynx.

Specialised fimbriae are involved in genetic material transfer between bacteria, a process called conjugation.

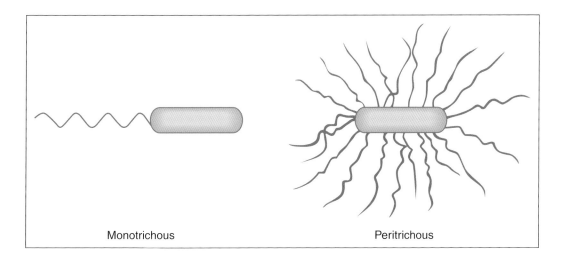

Monotrichous   Peritrichous

Figure 1.7 Arrangements of bacterial flagella.

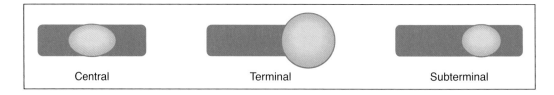

Central	Terminal	Subterminal

Figure 1.8 Size, shape and position of bacterial spores (from left to right): non-projecting, oval, central, e.g. *Bacillus anthracis*; projecting, spherical, terminal, e.g. *Clostridium tetani*; non-projecting, oval, subterminal, e.g. *C. perfringens*.

Intracellular structures

Nuclear material

The bacterial chromosome consists of a single circular molecule of double-stranded DNA, which is maintained in a compact form within the cell by supercoiling. When released from the cell and uncoiled the DNA would be about 1 mm long (10 to 100-times the length of the cell). Additional smaller extra-chromosomal DNA molecules, called plasmids, may also be present in bacteria. The chromosome usually codes for all the essential functions required by the cell; some plasmids control important phenotypic properties of pathogenic bacteria, including antibiotic resistance and toxin production. Extracellular nuclear material for encoding virulence and antibiotic resistance may also be transferred between bacteria and incorporated into the recipient's chromosome or plasmid. Transfer of genes encoding for virulence or antibiotic resistance may account for bacteria becoming resistant to antibiotics and for low-virulent bacteria becoming pathogenic.

Ribosomes

The cytoplasm has many ribosomes, which contain both ribonucleic acid (RNA) and proteins. Ribosomes are involved in protein synthesis.

Inclusion granules

Various cellular inclusions, which serve as energy and nutrient reserves, may be present in the bacterial cytoplasm. The size of these inclusions may increase in a favourable environment and decrease when conditions are adverse, e.g. *Corynebacterium diphtheriae* may contain high-energy phosphate reserves in inclusions termed 'volutin granules'.

Endospores

Endospores (spores) are small, metabolically dormant cells with a thick, multi-layered coat, formed intracellularly by members of the genera *Bacillus* and *Clostridium* (Figure 1.8). They are highly resistant to adverse environmental conditions and may survive desiccation, disinfectants or boiling water for several hours.

Spores are formed in response to limitations of nutrients by a complex process (sporulation) involving at least seven stages. When fully formed, they appear as oval or round cells within the vegetative cell. The location is variable, but is constant in any one bacterial species (Figure 1.9). Spores can remain dormant for long periods of time. However, they are able to revert to actively-growing cells (i.e. germinate) relatively rapidly in response to certain conditions such as the presence of specific sugars, amino acids or bile salts.

Spores also have an important role in the epidemiology of certain human diseases, such as anthrax, tetanus, gas gangrene and infection caused by *Clostridium difficile*.

The eradication of spores is of particular importance in some processes, e.g. the production of sterile products including pharmaceuticals and surgical instruments, in routine hospital ward and care centre cleaning, and in food preservation.

Bacterial growth

Most bacteria will grow on artificial culture media prepared from extracts from animal or plant tissues, which supply pre-formed nutrients and vitamins. However, some bacteria, e.g. *Mycobacterium leprae* (leprosy) and *Treponema pallidum*

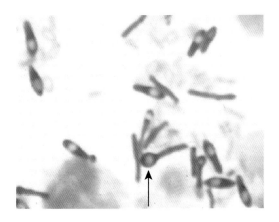

Figure 1.9 Gram-stain of *Clostridium sporogenes* (showing oval subterminal spores) and a *Clostridium tetani* with a terminal spore (arrowed).

(syphilis), cannot yet be grown *in vitro*; other bacteria, e.g. *Chlamydia* spp. and *Rickettsia* spp., only replicate intracellularly within host cells and are therefore grown in tissue culture.

Under suitable conditions (nutrients, temperature and atmosphere) a bacterial cell will increase in size and then divide by binary fission into two identical cells. These two cells are able to grow and divide at the same rate as the parent cell, provided that conditions including nutrient supply remain stable. This results in an exponential or logarithmic growth rate. The time required for the number of bacteria in a culture to double is called the generation time, e.g. *Escherichia coli* has a generation time of about 20 minutes under optimal conditions. By contrast, *Mycobacterium tuberculosis* has a generation time of 24 hours.

Requirements for bacterial growth

Most bacteria of medical importance require carbon, nitrogen, water, inorganic salts and a source of energy for growth. They have various gaseous, temperature and pH requirements, and can utilise a range of carbon, nitrogen and energy sources. Some bacteria also require special growth factors, including amino acids and vitamins.

Growth requirements are important in selecting the various culture media required in diagnostic microbiology and in understanding the tests for identifying bacteria.

Carbon and nitrogen sources

Bacteria are classified into two main groups according to the type of compounds that they can utilise as a carbon source:

1 *Autotrophs* utilise inorganic carbon from carbon dioxide and nitrogen from ammonia, nitrites and nitrates; they are of minor medical importance.
2 *Heterotrophs* require organic compounds as their major source of carbon and energy; they include most bacteria of medical importance.

Atmospheric conditions

Carbon dioxide

Bacteria require CO_2 for growth; adequate amounts are present in the air or are produced during metabolism by the microorganisms themselves. A few bacteria, however, require additional CO_2 for growth, e.g. *Neisseria meningitidis*, *Campylobacter jejuni*.

Oxygen

Bacteria may be classified into four groups according to their O_2 requirements:

1 *Obligate (strict) aerobes*: grow only in the presence of oxygen, e.g. *Pseudomonas aeruginosa*.
2 *Microaerophilic bacteria*: grow best in low oxygen concentrations, e.g. *Campylobacter jejuni*.
3 *Obligate (strict) anaerobes*: grow only in the absence of free oxygen, e.g. *Clostridium tetani*.
4 *Facultative anaerobes*: grow in the presence or absence of oxygen, e.g. *Escherichia coli*.

Temperature

Most pathogenic bacteria grow best at 37 °C. However, the optimum temperature for growth is occasionally higher, e.g. for *C. jejuni*, it is 42 °C. The ability of some bacteria to grow at low temperatures (0–4 °C) is important in food microbiology; *Listeria monocytogenes*, a cause of food poisoning, will grow slowly at 4 °C and has resulted in outbreaks of food poisoning associated with cook-chill products.

pH

Most pathogenic bacteria grow best at a slightly alkaline pH (pH 7.2–7.6). There are a few exceptions: *Lactobacillus acidophilus*, present in the vagina of post-pubescent females, prefers an acid medium (pH 4.0). It produces lactic acid, which keeps the vaginal secretions acid, thus preventing many pathogenic bacteria from establishing infection. *Vibrio cholerae*, the cause of cholera, prefers an alkaline environment (pH 8.5).

Growth in liquid media

When bacteria are added (inoculated) into a liquid growth medium, subsequent multiplication can be followed by determining the total number of live microorganisms (viable counts) at various time intervals. The growth curve produced normally has four distinct phases (Figure 1.10):

1 *Lag phase* (A): the interval between inoculation of a fresh growth medium with bacteria and the commencement of growth;
2 *Log phase* (B): the phase of exponential growth; the growth medium becomes visibly turbid at approximately 1×10^6 cells/ml;
3 *Stationary phase* (C): the growth rate slows as nutrients become exhausted, waste products accumulate, and the rate of cell division equals the rate of death; the total viable count remains relatively constant;
4 *Decline phase* (D): the rate of bacterial division is slower than the rate of death, resulting in a decline in the total viable count.

Note that the production of waste products by bacteria, particularly CO_2, and the uptake of O_2 have been utilised in the development of semi-automated instruments to detect bacterial growth in blood samples obtained from patients with suspected bloodstream infection.

Growth on solid media

Liquid growth media containing the nutrients needed for bacterial growth can be solidified with agar, a polysaccharide extracted from seaweed. Heating during sterilisation of the medium melts the agar, which then remains liquid until the temperature falls to approximately 40 °C, when it produces a transparent solid gel. Solid media are normally set in Petri dishes ('agar plates'). When spread across the surface of an agar plate, most bacteria grow as visible colonies. Each colony comprises millions of bacterial cells that emanated from either a single cell or a cluster of cells. The appearance of the bacterial colony (colonial morphology) assists in identification.

Growth on laboratory media

To grow bacteria *in vitro*, the microbiologist has to take into account the physiological requirements. Various types of liquid and solid media have been

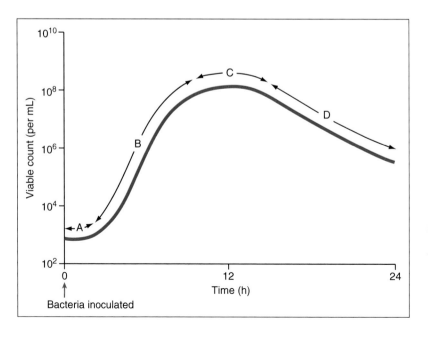

Figure 1.10 Bacterial growth curve showing the four phases: (A) lag; (B) log or exponential; (C) stationary; and (D) decline (death).

developed for the diagnostic microbiology laboratory.

Simple media

Many bacteria will grow in or on simple media, e.g. nutrient broth/nutrient agar that contains 'peptone' (polypeptides and amino acids from the enzymatic digestion of meat) and 'meat extract' (water-soluble components of meat containing mineral salts and vitamins).

Enriched media

These contain additional nutrients for the isolation of more fastidious bacteria that require special conditions for growth, e.g. agar containing whole blood (blood agar) or agar containing lysed blood (chocolate agar).

Selective media

These are designed to facilitate growth of some bacteria, while suppressing the growth of others, and include:

- *mannitol salt agar* which contains increased NaCl (salt) concentration for the recovery of staphylococci;

- *MacConkey agar*, which contains bile salts and allows the growth of bile-tolerant bacteria only; and
- *antibiotics*, which are frequently added to media to allow only certain bacteria to grow while suppressing or killing others.

Indicator media

These are designed to aid the detection and recognition of particular pathogens. They are often based on sugar fermentation reactions that result in production of acid and the subsequent colour change of a pH indicator, e.g. MacConkey agar contains lactose and a pH indicator (neutral red); lactose-fermenting bacteria (e.g. *Escherichia coli*) produce acid and form pink colonies, whereas non-lactose fermenting bacteria (e.g. *Salmonella* spp.) do not produce acid and form pale yellow colonies. This property facilitates the recognition of possible *Salmonella* colonies among normal bowel flora. Note that indicator media may also contain selective agents including antibiotics or substances such as bile salts and crystal violet to suppress growth of most Gram-positive microorganisms. MacConkey agar is therefore both a selective medium and an indicator medium.

2

Classification of bacteria

Peter Lambert
Aston University, Birmingham, UK

Bacterial taxonomy and nomenclature

The classification of microorganisms is essential for the understanding of clinical microbiology. Bacteria are designated by a binomial system, with the genus name (capital letter) followed by the species name (without capital letter), e.g. *Escherichia coli* or *Staphylococcus aureus*. Names are often abbreviated, e.g. *E. coli* and *S. aureus*.

Many nomenclature problems exist with this system that can lead to confusion, e.g. 'bacillus' refers to any rod-shaped bacteria, whereas the genus *Bacillus* includes only the aerobic spore-bearing rods. Other complications include the use of alternative terminology. *Streptococcus pneumoniae* is referred to as the pneumococcus, *Neisseria meningitidis* as the meningococcus and *Neisseria gonnorhoeae* as the gonococcus. Occasionally, collective terms are used, e.g. the term 'coliform' may indicate *E. coli* or a closely related Gram-negative bacillus found within the gut, and the term 'coagulase-negative staphylococci'

means staphylococci other than *S. aureus*. In this text, conventional terminology is used and, where appropriate, common alternatives are indicated.

Bacterial classification

Medically important bacteria can be subdivided into five main groups according to their cell shape (morphology) and staining reactions. The basic shapes of bacteria include cocci, bacilli, and spiral and variable shaped (pleomorphic) forms. Each of these morphological forms is further subdivided by their staining reactions, predominantly the Gram and acid-fast stains (Table 2.1). Bacteria are divided primarily into Gram-positive or Gram-negative microorganisms. Other characteristics, including the ability to grow in the presence (aerobic) or absence (anaerobic) of oxygen, spore formation and motility, are used to divide the groups further. Subdivision of these groups into genera is made on the basis of various factors, including culture properties (e.g. conditions required for growth and

---

Medical Microbiology and Infection Lecture Notes, Fifth Edition. Edited by Tom Elliott, Anna Casey, Peter Lambert and Jonathan Sandoe.
© 2011 Blackwell Publishing Ltd. Published 2011 by Blackwell Publishing Ltd.

colonial morphology), antigenic properties and biochemical reactions. The medically important genera based on this classification are shown in Table 2.2 (Gram-positives) and Table 2.3 (Gram-negatives).

Table 2.1 Main groups of bacteria

I	Gram-positive cocci, bacilli and branching bacteria
II	Gram-negative cocci, bacilli and comma-shaped bacteria
III	Spiral-shaped bacteria
IV	Acid-fast bacteria
V	Cell-wall-deficient bacteria

Other bacterial groups

Spiral bacteria

These are relatively slender spiral-shaped filaments, which are classified into three clinically important genera:

1 *Borrelia*: these are relatively large, motile spirochaetes and include *Borrelia vincenti* and *Leptotrichia buccalis*, which cause Vincent's angina, *Borrelia recurrentis*, which causes relapsing fever and *Borrelia burgdorferi*, which causes Lyme disease.
2 *Treponema*: these are thinner and more tightly spiralled than *Borrelia*. Examples include *Treponema pallidum* (causes syphilis) and *Treponema pertenue* (causes yaws).
3 *Leptospira*: these are finer and even more tightly coiled than the *Treponema* spp. (species plural). They are classified within the single species of

Table 2.2 Classification of Gram-positive bacterial pathogens

GRAM-POSITIVE BACTERIA

Grouping	Aerobic/anaerobic growth	Genus	Examples of clinically important species
Gram-positive cocci			
Clusters	Both	*Staphylococcus*	S. aureus, S. epidermidis, S. saprophyticus
Chains/pairs	Both	*Streptococcus* and *Enterococcus*	S. pneumoniae, S. pyogenes, E. faecalis
Chains	Anaerobic	*Peptostreptococcus*	P. magnus, P. asaccharolyticus
Gram-positive bacilli			
Sporing	Aerobic	*Bacillus*	B. anthracis, B. cereus
Non-sporing	Both	*Corynebacterium*	C. diphtheriae
	Aerobic or microaerophilic	*Listeria*	L. monocytogenes
	Anaerobic or microaerophilic	*Lactobacillus*	L. acidophilus
Sporing	Anaerobic	*Clostridium*	C. difficile, C. botulinum, C. perfringens, C. tetani
Non-sporing	Anaerobic	*Propionibacterium*	P. acnes
Branching	Anaerobic	*Actinomyces*	A. israeli
	Aerobic	*Nocardia*	N. asteroides

Table 2.3 Classification of Gram-negative bacterial pathogens

GRAM-NEGATIVE BACTERIA

Shape	Aerobic/anaerobic growth	Major grouping	Genus	Examples of clinically important species
Cocci	Aerobic		Neisseria	N. gonorrhoeae
				N. meningitidis
Cocci	Anaerobic		Veillonella	V. parvula
Bacilli		Enterobacteriaceae ('Coliforms')	Enterobacter	E. cloacae
			Escherichia	E. coli
			Klebsiella	K. pneumoniae
			Proteus	P. mirabilis
			Salmonella	S. typhimurium
			Serratia	S. marcescens
			Shigella	S. sonnei
			Yersinia	Y. enterocolitica
Bacilli	Aerobic		Pseudomonas	P. aeruginosa
Comma shaped	Both	Vibrios	Vibrio	V. parahaemolyticus
				V. cholerae
			Campylobacter	C. jejuni
			Helicobacter	H. pylori
Bacilli	Varies with genus		Bordetella	B. pertussis
			Brucella	B. abortus
			Haemophilus	H. influenzae,
				H. parainfluenzae
			Eikenella	E. corrodens
			Pasteurella	P. multocida
Bacilli	Aerobic		Legionella	L. pneumophila
Bacilli	Anaerobic		Bacteroides	B. fragilis
			Fusobacterium	F. nucleatum

Leptospira interrogans, which is divided serologically into two complexes. There are over 130 serotypes in the interrogans complex, many of which are pathogenic, including *L. icterohaemorrhagiae* (causes Weil's disease) and *L. canicola* (causes lymphocytic meningitis).

Acid-Fast Bacilli

These include the genus *Mycobacterium*. They are identified by their acid-fast staining reaction, which reflects their ability to resist decolorisation with acid, after being stained with hot carbol fuchsin, e.g. Ziehl-Neelsen stain. Mycobacteria are generally difficult to stain by Gram's method. They can be simply divided into the following main groups:

1 Tubercle bacilli: *Mycobacterium tuberculosis* and *Mycobacterium bovis* (Chapter 27)
2 Leprosy bacillus: *Mycobacterium leprae*
3 Atypical mycobacteria: some tuberculosis-like illnesses in humans are caused by other species of mycobacteria. They are sometimes also referred to as mycobacteria other than tuberculosis (MOTT). They can grow at 27°C,

42°C or 45°C; some produce pigment when growing in light and are called photochromogens, whereas others produce pigment in light or darkness and are referred to as scotochromogens. Unlike *M. tuberculosis*, other mycobacteria can be rapid growers. All these species of mycobacteria are commonly referred to as the atypical mycobacteria; examples include *Mycobacterium kansasii* (photochromogenic), *Mycobacterium avium-intracellulare* (non-pigmented) and *Mycobacterium chelonei* (fast growing).

Cell-wall-deficient bacteria

Some bacteria do not form cell walls and are called mycoplasmas. Pathogenic species include *Mycoplasma pneumoniae* and *Ureaplasma urealyticum*. It is important to distinguish mycoplasmas from other cell-wall-deficient forms of bacteria, which can be defined as either L-forms or protoplasts:

- *L-forms* are cell-wall-deficient forms of bacteria, which are produced by removal of a bacterium's cell wall, e.g. with cell-wall-acting antibiotics such as the β-lactams. L-Forms are able to multiply and their colonial morphology is similar to the 'fried egg' appearance of the mycoplasmas.
- *Protoplasts* are bacteria that have also had their cell walls removed. They are metabolically active and can grow, but are unable to multiply. They survive only in an osmotically stabilised medium.

3

Staphylococci

Tom Elliott[1] and Peter Lambert[2]
[1]University Hospitals Birmingham NHS Foundation Trust, Birmingham, UK
[2]Aston University, Birmingham, UK

Of the many species of staphylococci that are associated with humans, only a limited number are clinically important; these include *Staphylococcus aureus*, *S. epidermidis* and *S. saprophyticus*. Their principal characteristics are shown in Table 3.1.

Definition

Gram-positive cocci; usually arranged in clusters; non-motile; catalase positive; non-sporing; grow over a wide temperature range (10–42 °C), with an optimum of 37 °C; aerobic and facultatively anaerobic; grow on simple media.

Classification

1 *Colonial morphology*: *S. aureus* colonies are grey to golden yellow (Figure 3.1); *S. epidermidis* and *S. saprophyticus* colonies are white. Staphylococci may produce haemolysins, resulting in haemolysis on blood agar.
2 *Coagulase test*: *S. aureus* possesses the enzyme coagulase, which acts on plasma to form a clot. Other staphylococci (e.g. *S. epidermidis* and *S. saprophyticus*) do not possess this enzyme and are often termed, collectively, 'coagulase-negative staphylococci' (CoNS). There are three methods to demonstrate the presence of coagulase:
   (a) *tube coagulase test*: diluted plasma is mixed with a suspension of the bacteria; after incubation, clot formation indicates *S. aureus*
   (b) *slide coagulase test*: a more rapid and simple method in which a drop of plasma is added to a suspension of staphylococci on a glass slide; visible clumping indicates the presence of coagulase.
   (c) *latex agglutination test*: cells are mixed with coated latex particles; visible agglutination provides simultaneous detection of staphylococci containing coagulase and/or protein A.
3 *Deoxyribonuclease (DNAase) production*: *S. aureus* possesses an enzyme, DNAase, which depolymerises and hydrolyses DNA; other staphylococci rarely possess this enzyme.
4 *Protein A detection*: *S. aureus* possesses a cell-wall antigen, protein A; antibodies to protein A agglutinate *S. aureus* but not other staphylococci.
5 *Novobiocin sensitivity*: useful for differentiating between species of coagulase-negative staphylococci; *S. saprophyticus* is novobiocin resistant and *S. epidermidis* is sensitive.

Medical Microbiology and Infection Lecture Notes, Fifth Edition. Edited by Tom Elliott, Anna Casey, Peter Lambert and Jonathan Sandoe.
© 2011 Blackwell Publishing Ltd. Published 2011 by Blackwell Publishing Ltd.

Table 3.1 Main characteristics of staphylococci

Characteristic	S. aureus	S. epidermidis	S. saprophyticus
Coagulase	+	−	−
Deoxyribonuclease	+	−	−
Novobiocin	S	S	R
Colonial appearance	Golden-yellow	White	White
Body sites which may be colonised	Nose	Skin	Periurethra
	Mucosal surfaces	Mucosal surfaces	Faeces
	Faeces		
	Skin		
Common infections	Skin (boils, impetigo, furuncles, wound infections)	Prosthetic device-related infections e.g. artificial valves, heart, intravenous catheters, CSF shunts	Urinary tract infections in sexually active young women
	Abscesses		
	Osteomyelitis		
	Septic arthritis		
	Sepsis		
	Infective endocarditis		
	Prosthetic device-related infections		

+, present; −, absent; CSF, cerebrospinal fluid, S, sensitive R, resistant.

S. aureus

Epidemiology

S. aureus is a relatively common human commensal: nasal carriage occurs in 30–50% of healthy adults, faecal carriage in about 20% and skin carriage in 5–10%, particularly the axilla and perineum. *S. aureus* is spread via droplets and skin scales, which contaminate clothing, bed linen and other environmental sources.

Morphology and identification

On microscopy, *S. aureus* is seen as typical Gram-positive cocci in 'grape-like' clusters. It is both coagulase and DNAase positive (Figure 3.2). Other biochemical tests can be performed for full identification.

Pathogenicity

S. aureus causes disease because of its ability to adhere to cells, spread in tissues and form abscesses, produce extracellular enzymes and exotoxins (Table 3.2), combat host defences and resist treatment with many antibiotics.

Adhesins

S. aureus has a wide repertoire of adhesins known as MSCRAMMs (microbial surface components

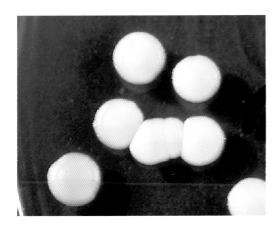

Figure 3.1 *S. aureus* colonies on a blood agar plate (2–3 mm diameter).

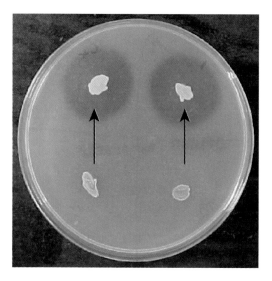

Figure 3.2 Plate containing DNA showing clear zones around DNAase-producing staphylococci (arrowed). DNAase-negative staphylococci shown below.

recognizing adhesive matrix molecules), which mediate adherence to host cells; these include protein A, fibrinogen and fibronectin-binding and collagen-binding protein.

Exotoxins and enzymes

- *Coagulase*: S. *aureus* produces coagulase, an enzyme that coagulates plasma. Coagulase results in fibrin deposition, which interferes with phagocytosis and increases the ability of the microorganism to invade tissues.
- *Other enzymes*: S. *aureus* may also produce staphylokinase (results in fibrinolysis), hyaluronidase (dissolves hyaluronic acid), proteases (degrades proteins) and lipases (solubilises lipids).
- *Haemolysin, leukotoxin and leukocidin*: several exotoxins are produced by S. *aureus*; α-toxin (haemolysin) lyses erythrocytes and damages platelets; β-toxin degrades sphingomyelin and is toxic for many types of cell, including erythrocytes; leukocidin (Panton Valentine leukocidin, PVL) lyses white blood cells and damages membranes and susceptible cells.
- *Enterotoxins*: there are six soluble enterotoxins that are produced by almost half of all S. *aureus* strains. They are heat stable (resistant at $100\,°C$ for 30 min), unaffected by gastrointestinal enzymes and are a cause of food poisoning, principally associated with vomiting.
- *Exfoliative/epidermolytic toxin*: some strains produce a toxin that can result in generalised

Table 3.2 Pathogenicity factors produced by S. aureus

Factor	Effect
MSCRAMMs	Mediate adherence to host cells
Protein A	Evade host defence/inhibits phacocytosis
Fibronectin-binding protein	Mediates binding to fibronectin
Fibrinogen-binding protein	Clumping factors
Capsule	Evade host defences
Coagulase	Generates protective fibrin layer around S. *aureus*
Staphylokinase	Fibrinolysis
Proteases	Degrade antibacterial proteins and matrix proteins
Lipases	Promote interstitial spreading of microorganism
Hyaluronidase	Degrades hyaluronic acid
α-Haemolysin	Lyses erythrocytes, damages platelets
β-Haemolysin	Degrades sphingomyelin/toxic for cells
Leukocidin/leucotoxin	Lyse white blood cells
Exotoxins, e.g. enterotoxins	Food poisoning with profuse vomiting
Superantigens, e.g. TSST, exfoliative toxin	Toxic shock syndrome, scalded skin syndrome

NB: Toxin production varies between strains of S. *aureus*.

desquamation of the skin (staphylococcal scalded skin syndrome).
- *Toxic shock syndrome toxin* (*TSST*): this is associated with shock and desquamation of skin, and is usually related to an underlying *S. aureus* infection.
- Staphylococcal enterotoxins, TSSTs and exfoliative toxin are 'superantigens', all of which bind non-specifically to specific white cells, resulting in over production of cytokines, giving rise to a toxic shock-like presentation.

Cell envelope

Over 90% of all clinical isolates of *S. aureus* strains possess a polysaccharide capsule that interferes with opsonisation and phagocytosis. *S. aureus* also possesses a cell-wall protein (protein A) that binds the Fc component of the antibody, preventing complement activation.

Antibiotic resistance

Many strains of *S. aureus* are resistant to the antibiotic meticillin and are termed 'meticillin-resistant *S. aureus*' (MRSA). Most resistance depends on the production of an additional penicillin-binding protein, which is encoded by an acquired *mecA* gene. Many strains of MRSA are now resistant to multiple antibiotics.

Laboratory diagnosis

Laboratory diagnosis is by microscopic detection of the microorganism in clinical samples, direct isolation from the infected site or blood cultures, and detection of serum antibodies to staphylococcal haemolysin and DNAase. *S. aureus* strains can be typed ('fingerprinted') by conventional methods, including biotype and antibiogram. *S. aureus* can also be genotyped by molecular methods, including pulsed field gel electrophoresis (PFGE). Typing of *S. aureus* is useful in epidemiological studies.

Treatment and prevention

Antimicrobial agents, such as flucloxacillin, remain the first-line treatment for sensitive strains of *S. aureus*; however, the increase in infections caused by MRSA has required the use of glycopeptide antibiotics such as vancomycin. Resistance to vancomycin has been reported but is still rare. MRSA can cause sepsis, ranging from wound infections to urinary tract infections and severe sepsis and septic shock. Epidemic strains of MRSA (EMRSA) have also

been recognised. Prevention of spread through effective infection control procedures, including MRSA decolonisation, is therefore important.

Associated infections

- *Skin*: boils, impetigo, furuncles, wound infections, staphylococcal scalded skin syndrome;
- *Respiratory*: pneumonia, lung abscesses, exacerbations of chronic lung disease;
- *Skeletal*: most common cause of osteomyelitis and septic arthritis;
- *Invasive*: bloodstream infection, infective endocarditis, deep abscesses (brain, liver, spleen), toxic shock syndrome;
- *Gastrointestinal*: toxin-mediated food poisoning;
- *Device related*: indwelling catheters, prosthetic joints and heart valves.

S. epidermidis

- *S. epidermidis* is both coagulase and DNAase negative and is present in large numbers on the human skin and mucous membranes.
- *S. epidermidis* is a cause of bacterial endocarditis, particularly in patients with prosthetic heart valves and in drug addicts. It is also a major cause of infections of implanted devices such as cerebrospinal shunts, hip prostheses, central venous and peritoneal dialysis catheters.
- The microorganism colonises implanted devices by attaching firmly onto artificial surfaces. Some strains also produce a slime layer (glycocalyx), which appears to facilitate adhesion and protect the microorganism from antibiotics and host defences. The increased use of implanted devices, particularly central venous catheters, has resulted in *S. epidermidis* becoming one of the most frequently isolated microorganisms from blood cultures. *S. epidermidis* occasionally causes urinary tract infections, particularly in catheterised patients. When isolated from hospitalised patients, *S. epidermidis* is often resistant to antibiotics such as flucloxacillin and erythromycin, necessitating the use of glycopeptide antibiotics (e.g. vancomycin).

S. saprophyticus

S. saprophyticus is both coagulase and DNAase negative and is frequently associated with urinary tract infections in sexually active young women, occasionally resulting in severe cystitis with haematuria.

4

Streptococci and enterococci

Anna Casey
University Hospitals Birmingham NHS Foundation Trust, Birmingham, UK

Streptococci

Definition

Gram-positive cocci arranged in pairs or chains (Figure 4.1); facultatively anaerobic; non-sporing; non-motile; catalase-negative; most are capsulate; optimum growth at 37 °C; sometimes require enriched media; many species exhibit characteristic haemolysis on blood agar. Many streptococci are human commensals (most notably of the upper respiratory tract).

Classification

Streptococci are classified by:

1 *The type of haemolysis observed on blood agar:*
   (a) α-*haemolysis*: a greenish zone forms around colonies due to partial haemolysis of erythrocytes (Figure 4.2). An example of an α-haemolytic species is *Streptococcus pneumoniae.*
   (b) β-*haemolysis*: a clear zone forms around colonies due to complete haemolysis of erythrocytes (Figure 4.2).

(c) γ-*haemolysis*: no zone is formed, as erythrocytes are not lysed. These streptococci are more commonly referred to as non-haemolytic streptococci.
2 *Serological detection of cell wall antigens*: streptococci can be classified alphabetically according to the possession of specific cell wall antigens (Lancefield groups A–H and K–V). Antibodies that react with these antigens are used to group streptococci and are particularly useful in the identification of β-haemolytic species. These groups are important to distinguish, as they can cause specific infections.
3 *Biochemical reactions*: some streptococci are difficult to classify by the above characteristics, therefore biochemical tests can be useful in their identification.

α-Haemolytic streptococci

Streptococcus pneumoniae (pneumococcus)

Epidemiology

S. pneumoniae is a commensal of the upper respiratory tract.

Medical Microbiology and Infection Lecture Notes, Fifth Edition. Edited by Tom Elliott, Anna Casey, Peter Lambert and Jonathan Sandoe.

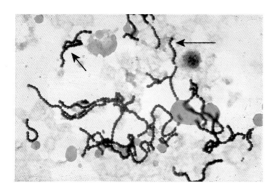

Figure 4.1 Gram stain of streptococci showing long chains.

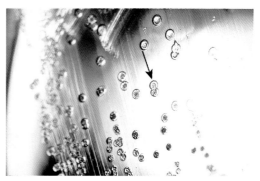

Figure 4.3 *Streptococcus pneumoniae* colonies (arrowed) with a characteristic 'draughtsman'-like appearance (1 mm diameter).

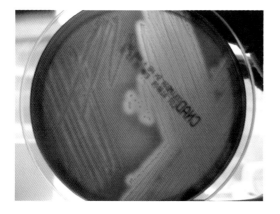

Figure 4.2 Colonies (each 0.5 mm diameter) of α- (left) and β-haemolytic (right) streptococci on a blood agar plate.

Morphology and identification

Cocci are most commonly observed in pairs or chains and often have a polysaccharide capsule. Their growth is enhanced in the presence of additional carbon dioxide (CO_2) and colonies are typically disc shaped with central depressions (giving a 'draughtsmen' appearance) (Figure 4.3). *S. pneumoniae* may be differentiated from the 'viridans' streptococci by its sensitivity to optochin and its solubility in bile salts.

Pathogenicity

There are in excess of 80 antigenic types of pneumococcal polysaccharide capsules. A limited number of serotypes account for the majority of cases of infection. The capsule inhibits phagocytosis, unless antigen-specific opsonic antibody is present. Pneumococci also produce pneumolysin, a membrane-damaging exotoxin.

Associated infections

- *Respiratory tract*: otitis media, sinusitis, lower respiratory tract infection (particularly community-acquired pneumonia);
- *Musculoskeletal*: septic arthritis;
- *Gastrointestinal*: spontaneous bacterial peritonitis;
- *Central nervous system*: meningitis.

Laboratory diagnosis

This is by microscopy and microbiological culture of specimens from the infected site, e.g. sputum, blood, peritoneal fluid or CSF. Direct detection of pneumococcal antigen in specimens can be undertaken by various techniques. Pneumococcal DNA can be detected in blood, CSF and other samples by PCR.

Treatment and prophylaxis

S. pneumoniae is sensitive to a wide range of antibiotics. However, penicillin-resistant strains have now emerged worldwide (Chapter 39).

A pneumococcal conjugate vaccination (PCV) schedule is currently recommended in infants. In addition, a pneumococcal polysaccharide vaccine (PPV) is recommended for adults 65 years of age or older, and for patients at particular risk of infection. Such patients include those with chronic illness such as renal, heart, liver or lung disease, diabetes mellitus, splenic dysfunction or another form of immunodeficiency. Penicillin prophylaxis may also be given either instead of, or in addition to, immunisation, particularly in patients who have undergone splenectomy.

'Viridans' or 'oral' streptococci

The 'viridans' streptococci are a group of α- or non-haemolytic streptococci, which are predominantly found in the oral cavity and so are commonly referred to as the 'oral' streptococci. Examples include the *Streptococcus mitis, Streptococcus mutans, Streptococcus salivarius* and *Streptococcus sanguinis* groups.

Epidemiology

The 'viridans' streptococci are commensals of the upper respiratory tract.

Morphology and identification

They are mostly resistant to optochin and insoluble in bile salts. Biochemical tests are often used for their identification.

Pathogenicity

Various carbohydrates facilitate the attachment of these streptococci to teeth adjacent to the gingivae. Some species, particularly *S. mutans*, produce acid involved in the development of dental caries.

Associated infections

- *Cardiovascular*: they are a common cause of infective endocarditis;
- *Dental*: these streptococci, particularly *S. mutans*. are the most common cause of dental caries and periodontal disease.

Laboratory diagnosis

Diagnosis is by isolation of the microorganism from infected sites.

Treatment and prophylaxis

The 'viridans' streptococci are usually sensitive to a wide range of antibiotics. Infections are often treated with penicillin. In the UK, antimicrobial prophylaxis is no longer recommended to prevent endocarditis

in patients with valve disease who are undergoing dental procedures. In European and North America guidelines, prophylaxis is still recommended for selected dental procedures in high risk patients.

β-Haemolytic streptococci

Group A (*Streptococcus pyogenes*)

Epidemiology

S. pyogenes is an upper respiratory tract commensal.

Morphology and identification

Group A streptococci will not grow on media containing bile. The identity of *S. pyogenes* is normally confirmed by Lancefield grouping and biochemical testing. Strains of *S. pyogenes* can be further differentiated according to the presence of surface proteins M, R and T (Griffith types). Epidemiological typing can be carried out, based on the possession of different M-proteins.

Pathogenicity

S. pyogenes produces a wide range of virulence factors including:

- *A capsule composed of hyaluronic acid*: provides protection against phagocytosis.
- *Fimbriae/pili*: facilitate adherence to host cells. They consist of lipoteichoic acid (an adherence factor) and M-protein.
- *M-proteins*: surface proteins which are anti-phagocytic and also bind host proteases.
- *F-proteins*: surface proteins that bind to fibronectin.
- *Streptolysins (haemolysins)*: streptolysins O and S lyse erythrocytes and are cytotoxic to leukocytes and other cell types.
- *Other enzymes*: include streptokinase (prevents the formation of a fibrin mesh), hyaluronidase (breaks down hyaluronic acid in connective tissue), deoxyribonucleases (DNAases), nicotinamide adenine dinucleotidase (NADase) and C5a peptidase (inactivates the C5a component of the complement system).
- *Streptococcal pyrogenic exotoxins (erythrogenic toxins)*: responsible for the rash of scarlet fever.

These are 'superantigens', which facilitate release of cytokines, potentially leading to shock.

Associated infections

- *Respiratory tract*: pharyngitis, sinusitis, tonsillitis, otitis media, pneumonia;
- *Musculoskeletal*: septic arthritis;
- *Gastrointestinal*: spontaneous bacterial peritonitis;
- *Skin and soft tissue*: cellulitis, impetigo, erysipelas, scarlet fever, wound infection, necrotising fasciitis;
- *Genitourinary*: puerperal sepsis;
- *Cardiovascular*: infective endocarditis.

Post-infection complications

Antibodies produced as a result of infection with *S. pyogenes* may cause non-pyogenic complications at other anatomical sites post-infection. Indeed, rheumatic fever and acute glomerulonephritis may develop up to 3 weeks after the streptococcal infection. Inflammation of the cardiac muscle occurs in rheumatic fever, whilst acute glomerulonephritis is characterised by inflammation of the renal glomerulus.

Laboratory diagnosis

Diagnosis is by isolation of the microorganism from infected sites (e.g. throat, skin, blood). The detection of serum antibodies to streptolysin O (ASOT: anti-streptolysin O titre) is particularly useful for the diagnosis of post-infection complications, such as rheumatic fever or acute glomerulonephritis. This is because the microorganism is often no longer present at the time of clinical presentation.

Treatment

S. pyogenes is sensitive to many antibiotics. Penicillin remains the drug of choice for treatment of infection with this microorganism.

Group B (*Streptococcus agalactiae*)

Epidemiology

S. agalactiae forms part of the normal faecal, perineal and vaginal flora in females.

Morphology and identification

These microorganisms grow readily on blood agar and are identified by Lancefield grouping. Group B streptococci will grow on media containing bile.

Pathogenicity

The virulence factors for group B streptococci are less well defined than for group A. However, more type-specific antigens and lipoteichoic acid are present in strains isolated from serious infection, thus these factors appear to be important in its virulence.

Associated infections

- *Respiratory tract*: pneumonia in neonates and the elderly;
- *Musculoskeletal*: septic arthritis, osteomyelitis;
- *Skin and soft tissue*: cellulitis;
- *Genitourinary*: (in the post-partum period) septic abortion, endometritis, urinary tract infections;
- *Cardiovascular*: infective endocarditis;
- *Central nervous system*: neonatal meningitis (neonatal acquisition of *S. agalactiae* is most frequently via transmission from the colonised mother *in utero* or at the time of birth.

Laboratory diagnosis

This is by isolation from the infected site. Direct detection of antigen in body fluids can be undertaken by various techniques.

Treatment

Penicillin is the drug of choice for treatment of infection with *S. agalactiae*.

Group C and G β-haemolytic streptococci

- Group C and G streptococci contain multiple species.
- They will not grow on media containing bile and are identified by Lancefield grouping and other commercial identification kits.
- Whilst infection with these microorganisms is less common, it can be severe. Examples of infections caused by these microorganisms include respiratory tract, puerperal and skin

infection, endocarditis, meningitis, bacteraemia and the post-streptococcal infection complication, acute glomerulonephritis.
- Infections are often treated with penicillin.

Streptococcus anginosus group (formerly known as the Streptococcus milleri group)

- This group includes *Streptococcus anginosus*, *Streptococcus constellatus* subspecies *constellatus*, *S. constellatus* subspecies *pharynges* and *Streptococcus intermedius*.

- The *S. anginosus* group does not fall neatly into the normal classification of streptococci. They are often α-haemolytic, but may be β- or non-haemolytic.
- Growth of these microorganisms is enhanced by low O_2 tension and supplemented CO_2. Members of this group will grow on media containing bile.
- Strains most often possess Lancefield group F antigens, but can possess A, C or G antigens or none.
- Members of the *S. anginosus* group are commensals of the gastrointestinal and female genital tract, and are a common cause of brain, chest and liver abscesses.
- These microorganisms are sensitive to penicillin; however, antibiotic combinations such as penicillin and metronidazole are often required for the treatment of deep-seated abscesses due

Table 4.1 Examples of infections caused by streptococci and enterococci

Microorganism	Examples of clinical infections
α-*haemolytic streptococci*	
S. pneumoniae	Otitis media/sinusitis
	Pneumonia
	Meningitis
'Viridans' streptococci	Dental caries
	Endocarditis
β-*haemolytic streptococci*	
Group A (S. pyogenes)	Pharyngitis, otitis media/sinusitis
	Cellulitis, erysipelas, necrotising fasciitis, scarlet fever (toxin-mediated), septic arthritis
	Streptococcal toxic shock syndrome, puerperal sepsis
	Rheumatic fever, acute glomerulonephritis (post-infectious complications)
Group B (S. agalactiae)	Neonatal: pneumonia, meningitis, bloodstream infection
	Puerperal sepsis
	Pneumonia
Group C and G	Pharyngitis
	Cellulitis,
	Puerperal sepsis
	Endocarditis
S. anginosus group	Deep abscesses
Enterococci	Urinary tract infection
(e.g. E. faecalis)	Biliary tract infection
	Peritonitis
	Endocarditis

to the presence of other bacteria such as anaerobes.

Enterococci (previously classified as streptococci)

Enterococcus faecalis and *Enterococcus faecium* are most commonly associated with human infection; however, infection with other enterococcal species also occurs.

Definition

Gram-positive cocci arranged in pairs or chains; facultatively anaerobic; non-sporing; non-motile (except *Enterococcus casseliflavus* and *Enterococcus gallinarum*); mostly catalase-negative (some strains produce a pseudocatalase); some strains are encapsulated; can grow over wide temperature range.

Epidemiology

Enterococci are commensals, most notably of the gastrointestinal and vaginal tract.

Morphology and identification

On blood agar they appear α-, β- or sometimes non-haemolytic. Enterococci belong to Lancefield group D. Speciation can be performed using biochemical tests. They will grow on media containing bile and hydrolyse aesculin in the presence of 40% bile. Since group D streptococci (i.e. the *Streptococcus bovis* group) also share these properties,

differentiation is achieved by the fact that group D streptococci, unlike enterococci, are unable to hydrolyse pyrrolidonyl-β-naphthylamide (PYR) and arginine and are not heat resistant.

Pathogenicity

Enterococcal strains can produce cytolysin, which causes lysis of a variety of cells, including erythrocytes and other mammalian cells. Other virulence factors include gelatinase, hyaluronidase, aggregation substance, Enterococcal Surface Protein (a surface adhesin) and extracellular superoxide production.

Associated infections

They cause a number of (mainly healthcare-associated) infections. These include:

- *Gastrointestinal*: peritonitis;
- *Genitourinary*: urinary tract infection;
- *Cardiovascular*: infections associated with indwelling catheters, infective endocarditis.

Laboratory diagnosis

Diagnosis is by isolation of the microorganism from infected sites.

Treatment

Enterococcal infections are often treated with ampicillin. Enterococci, (particularly *E. faecium*), have developed resistance to penicillin. In addition, the emergence of resistance to glycopeptide, antibiotics such as vancomycin is of concern. These bacteria are referred to as 'vancomycin-resistant enterococci' (VRE) (Chapter 39).

Table 4.1 lists the infections most commonly caused by streptococci and enterococci.

5

Clostridia

Tony Worthington
Aston University, Birmingham, UK

Definition

Large Gram-positive bacilli (Figure 5.1); strictly an-aerobic; spore-forming; fermentative. Whilst many *Clostridium* species exist, only some are of medical importance, including *C. perfingens, C. difficile, C. tetani, C. botulinum, C. septicum and C. tertium.*

Epidemiology

Clostridia are widely distributed in the environment and in the gastrointestinal tract of mammals. They produce highly resistant, transmissible spores, which can survive desiccation, ultraviolet and gamma radiation, extreme temperatures, starvation and disinfection. Spores of clostridia are the vector of infection.

Classification

Based on morphology, biochemical activity, fatty acid production and gene sequencing techniques.

C. perfringens

Morphology and identification

Non-motile, sub-terminal spores. Forms irregular, spreading colonies on blood agar surrounded by a double zone of β-haemolysis (inner zone of complete lysis due to θ-toxin and wider outer zone of partial haemolysis due to α-toxin). Five types (A to E) of *C. perfringens* are recognised based on surface antigens and the types of toxin produced:

1 *Type A strains*: commonly found in human infections; produce only α-toxin
2 *Type B to E strains*: commonly found in animals (lambs, goat, cattle); produce α- and other toxins.

Pathogenicity

Toxin and enzyme production: α-toxin (phospholipase C) is associated with toxaemia seen in gas gangrene; hyaluronidase breaks down cellular cement facilitating spread; collagenase/proteinase – liquefaction of muscle; lipase-lipid breakdown.

Medical Microbiology and Infection Lecture Notes, Fifth Edition. Edited by Tom Elliott, Anna Casey,
Peter Lambert and Jonathan Sandoe.
© 2011 Blackwell Publishing Ltd. Published 2011 by Blackwell Publishing Ltd.

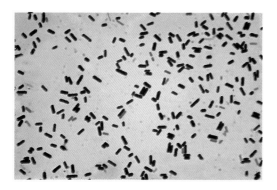

Figure 5.1 Gram stain of C. *perfringens* showing Gram-positive bacilli with square ends (5 μm × 1 μm).

Associated infections

- *Skin and Soft tissue*: gas gangrene, cellulitis;
- *Gastrointestinal*: necrotising enteritis, food poisoning;
- *Gynaecological*: septic abortion.

Laboratory diagnosis

Gram stained smears and culture of clinical samples, e.g. blood, pus and tissue may provide evidence of clostridial infection. Recovery of *C. perfringens* on simple or selective agar provides a definitive diagnosis. Identification of *C. perfringens* is determined through biochemical tests (e.g. API 20A, Rapid ID 32A kits). Confirmation of α-toxin and lipase production is established on egg-yolk agar (Nagler plate); toxin-producing strains generate a zone of opalescence around the colonies, which can be inhibited by specific antitoxin to α-toxin.

Treatment and prevention

Gas gangrene: surgical debridement, immediate antibiotic therapy with high dose benzylpenicillin and/or metronidazole and supportive measures. Co-infecting microorganisms may be present, therefore additional antibiotics may be required. Prophylactic benzylpenicillin may be given for dirty wounds and lower limb amputation.

Food poisoning: self limiting; no antimicrobial therapy warranted.

C. difficile

Morphology and identification

Motile; sub-terminal spores. Forms colonies with irregular edges and a ground glass appearance on blood agar (Figure 5.2). Colonies have a typical 'horse manure' odour.

Epidemiology

Ubiquitous in the environment and colonises the intestine of 50% of healthy neonates and 4% of healthy adults. A major cause of healthcare-associated infection in the 21st century; patients taking antibiotics, e.g. cephalosporins, clindamycin are at increased risk of developing *C. difficile* antibiotic associated diarrhoea. This is due to suppression of the normal bowel flora and subsequent overgrowth of *C. difficile*. Infection may be endogenous or exogenous (through ingestion of environmental spores).

Pathogenicity

Produces two major toxins: Toxin A (enterotoxin) and Toxin B (cytotoxin). A further binary toxin is present in some strains. Toxin A induces cytokine production with hypersecretion of fluid. Toxin B induces depolymerisation of actin with loss of cytoskeleton. Adhesin factor and hyaluronidase production are also associated virulence factors. Hypervirulent, hypertoxin producing strains now recognised (e.g. ribotype 027, 078).

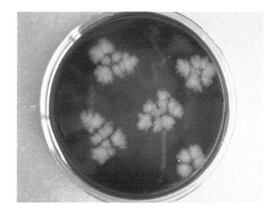

Figure 5.2 Colonies (∼5–8 mm diameter) of *C. difficile* on blood agar. They appear grey in colour, with irregular edges.

Associated infections

- *Gastrointestinal*: antibiotic associated diarrhoea, pseudomembranous colitis, fulminant colitis.

Laboratory diagnosis

Direct detection of toxin in faeces by various methods: cell toxicity neutralisation assay, commercial assays (e.g. ELISA, latex agglutination) and polymerase chain reaction (PCR). Culture of *C. difficile* on selective agar (e.g. Cycloserine Cefoxatime Fructose Agar); genotyping of isolates by ribotyping where necessary. Assay for glutamate dehydrogenase (GDH) and lactoferrin in faecal samples.

Treatment and prevention

Treatment: Oral Vancomycin or Metronidazole. Prevention of *C. difficile* is multifactoral and includes: clinical awareness, judicious use of antibiotics, infection control strategies, e.g. hand hygiene, environmental decontamination and cleanliness.

C. tetani

Morphology and identification

Motile; terminal spore ('drumstick' appearance); produces a thin spreading film of growth without discrete colonies on blood agar; motile via numerous peritrichous flagella.

Epidemiology

C. tetani is present in mammalian intestines and the environment (particularly manured soil). Spores are ubiquitous in nature. Incidence of tetanus varies worldwide; more common in developing tropical and subtropical countries; infection is inversely related to living standards, preventative medicine and wound management.

Pathogenicity

Many strains are highly toxigenic, producing oxygen-labile haemolysin (tetanolysin) and a potent neurotoxin (tetanospasmin). Tetanospasmin blocks neurotransmitter release, resulting in the characteristic motor spasms associated with tetanus (e.g. lockjaw, arching of the back).

Associated infections

- *Neurological*: tetanus.

Laboratory diagnosis

Demonstration of characteristic 'drumstick' bacilli in clinical samples, followed by anaerobic culture on selective or blood agar; serological detection of circulating neurotoxin by enzyme immunoassay.

Treatment and prevention

Treatment includes administration of human tetanus immunoglobulin and benzylpenicillin or metronidazole. Surgical debridement and cleansing of wounds is important in successful treatment. Prevention includes administration of the tetanus toxoid vaccine.

C. botulinum

Morphology and identification

Toxin producing; subterminal spores; motile with peritrichous flagella. Seven main types of *C. botulinum* are recognised (A–G), based on antigenically distinct toxins with identical actions.

Epidemiology

Ubiquitous saprophyte occurring in soil, vegetation, fruit and manure. Infection arises through consumption of contaminated food or wound contamination. Human infection is commonly caused by types A, B and D. Infection in the UK is rare.

Pathogenicity

Production of potent neurotoxin which blocks the release of acetylcholine at neuromuscular junctions, resulting in flaccid paralysis.

Associated infections

- *Neurological*: botulism, wound botulism, infant botulism.

Laboratory diagnosis

Detection of the microorganism or its toxin in food; toxin may be demonstrated in patient's blood by toxin-antitoxin neutralisation assay.

Treatment and prevention

Treatment includes administration of human tetanus immunoglobulin and benzylpenicillin or metronidazole. Surgical debridement and cleansing of wounds is important. Prevention includes administration of the tetanus toxoid vaccine.

Other clostridial infections

C. septicum is associated with non-traumatic myonecrosis more often in immunocompromised patients. *C. tertium* is associated with traumatic wound infection.

6

Other Gram-positive bacteria

Anna Casey
University Hospitals Birmingham NHS Foundation Trust, Birmingham, UK

In addition to the microorganisms presented in Chapters 3, 4 and 5, various other Gram-positive bacteria may cause human infection. Some of the important pathogens are outlined in alphabetical order in this chapter.

Actinomyces

The *Actinomyces* genus contains a large number of species. *A. israelii* is the most common (but not the only) cause of human actinomycosis.

Definition

Gram-positive bacilli: varying from short pleomorphic bacilli to branching filaments; anaerobic and micro-aerophilic; non-sporing; non-motile; most species are catalase-negative; growth is optimal on enriched media, such as blood agar at 37 °C.

Epidemiology

Pathogenic species do not exist widely in the environment. They are commensals of the oral cavity, large intestine and female genital tract.

Morphology and identification

Filaments may aggregate to form visible granules (sulphur granules) in pus. Specimens from infected tissues can be placed into sterile water to separate out these granules. They are then crushed and subjected to Gram and modified Ziehl-Neelsen staining and microbiological culture. Colonies may take 10 days to appear. *Actinomyces* are normally non-acid fast and identification can be confirmed using commercial identification kits, gas-liquid chromatography and 16S ribosomal RNA gene sequencing and analysis.

Pathogenesis

Mycelial masses penetrate human tissue.

Associated infections

- *Maxillofacial*: mandibular abscesses, often associated with dental extraction or trauma may manifest as discharging skin lesions;
- *Respiratory*: possible role in chronic tonsillitis;
- *Gastrointestinal*: intra-abdominal infection (may follow appendectomy or spread from uterine infection);
- *Thoracic* infection;
- *Genitourinary*: uterine infection is associated with the use of intrauterine contraceptive devices (*A. israelii*).

Laboratory diagnosis

Direct isolation of the microorganism from clinical specimens.

Treatment

Antibiotic therapy such as penicillin (for up to 12 months) may need to be combined with surgical intervention.

Bacillus

The *Bacillus* genus contains numerous species, many of which are not of clinical importance. Two important human pathogens – *Bacillus anthracis* and *Bacillus cereus* cause anthrax and food poisoning, respectively.

Definition

Gram-positive bacilli often arranged in chains; aerobic (some species are obligate aerobes and some facultative anaerobes); spore-forming; most species are motile; usually catalase-positive; some species are capsulate; grow over a wide temperature range on simple media.

B. anthracis

Epidemiology

Anthrax is principally a zoonotic disease and is common in some parts of the developing world. Human infections can be classified as: non-industrial (direct human contact with infected animals) or industrial (processing of animal products by humans). Spores can survive in the soil for long periods of time and are relatively resistant to chemical disinfectants and heat.

Infection with *B. anthracis* in the UK is rare but is normally associated with handling imported animal products. Recent UK cases have occurred in intravenous drug users, probably as a result of contaminated heroin. Anthrax has been used as a biological weapon.

Morphology and identification

Can grow under anaerobic conditions; its non-motility allows it to be distinguished from other *Bacillus* species; virulent strains are capsulate; do not produce a zone of haemolysis on blood nor a zone of precipitation on egg yolk agar (i.e. does not produce lecithinase). Identification is normally confirmed by morphological and biochemical tests.

Pathogenicity

Virulent strains of *B. anthracis* possess a protein capsule, which prevents phagocytosis. This microorganism also produces a plasmid-encoded exotoxin, which is composed of three proteins: protective antigen, oedema factor and lethal factor. Protective antigen is concerned with receptor binding and therefore the attachment and translocation of oedema factor and lethal factor into the cell. Oedema factor causes impairment of macrophage function and lethal factor lysis of macrophages.

Associated infections

Types of anthrax infection include:

- *Skin and soft tissues*: cutaneous anthrax is the predominant clinical manifestation. Development of a necrotic skin lesion (malignant pustule) occurs.
- *Respiratory*: ('wool-sorter's disease'): spores are inhaled (often from wool fibres) causing pulmonary oedema, haemorrhage and commonly, death.
- *Gastrointestinal*: consumption of contaminated meat results in haemorrhagic diarrhorea. This type of anthrax can also result in death.

Laboratory diagnosis

Normally by direct isolation of the microorganism from infected sites, i.e. sputum or specimens from skin lesions. A safety cabinet should be used to handle such specimens.

Treatment and prevention

B. anthracis is sensitive to many antibiotics. Common therapeutic agents used are penicillin, erythromycin, ciprofloxacin or doxycycline. Ciprofloxacin or doxycycline may be given for post-exposure prophylaxis. Anthrax vaccinations are available for individuals at high risk, e.g. military personnel, veterinary practitioners and farm workers. Livestock in endemic areas may also be vaccinated.

B. cereus

B. cereus can grow under anaerobic conditions, is motile and it does not produce lecithinase; however, unlike *B. anthracis*, it produces a zone of haemolysis on blood agar. This microorganism is an important cause of food poisoning, particularly associated with rice dishes and cereals. Pathogenicity is related to the production of enterotoxins. Food poisoning can present as the emetic form, which has a short incubation period (typically 1–6 hours) and is characterised by nausea and vomiting, or as the diarrhoeal form, for which the incubation period is longer (typically 8–16 hours). Food-poisoning is self-limiting, therefore antimicrobial therapy is not normally required. *B. cereus* is an infrequent cause of non-gastrointestinal infections, including ocular infections, pneumonia and endocarditis.

Corynebacteria

The *Corynebacterium* genus consists of several species, most of which are human commensals. Some species cause human infection. These include *Corynebacterium diphtheriae, Corynebacterium pseudotuberculosis, Corynebacterium ulcerans, Corynebacterium jeikeium* and *Corynebacterium urealyticum*.

Definition

Pleomorphic Gram-positive bacilli arranged singly or in clusters (giving the appearance of Chinese letters); facultatively anaerobic; non-sporing; non-motile; catalase-positive; non-capsulate; growth at optimum of 37 °C; growth improved by addition of serum or blood.

C. diphtheriae

C. diphtheriae is the cause of diphtheria, an upper respiratory tract infection with cardiac and neurological complications.

Epidemiology

Infection is normally spread via nasopharyngeal secretions from people who are infected or who are carriers of the microorganism. Diphtheria is rare in developed countries.

Morphology and identification

- Microbiological medium containing tellurite, e.g. Hoyle's tellurite, is often used for culture of throat swabs from patients with suspected diphtheria. This selective medium allows the growth of *Corynebacterium* spp. whilst suppressing commensals of the upper respiratory tract. Colonies of *C. diphtheriae* are grey-black in colour.
- *C. diphtheriae* can be differentiated into four subspecies: *var. gravis, var. mitis, var. intermedius* and *var. belfanti*. This and differentiation from other species can be achieved by colonial morphology, biochemical tests and haemolytic activity.
- Toxigenic strains can be confirmed by the Elek test (a precipitation reaction in agar), enzyme immunoassay (EIA) or polymerase chain reaction (PCR)-based techniques.

Pathogenicity

- All subspecies, except *var. belfanti*, may produce the diphtheria exotoxin. It is a heat-stable polypeptide comprised of fragment A and fragment B. Fragment A is involved with the translocation of fragment B into the cell, the latter fragment then causes cell death by inhibiting protein synthesis. The gene which codes for production of this toxin is carried on a bacteriophage and is then integrated into the bacterial chromosome.
- Toxin-producing strains of *C. diphtheriae* multiply in the pharynx and the exotoxin produced causes necrosis of the epithelial cells.

Associated infections

- *Respiratory*: Diphtheria: the main clinical symptoms are a sore throat, thick pharyngeal pseudomembrane, bullneck (oedema of the neck), fever, fatigue and headache.
- *Bloodstream infection*: The toxin may then cause damage to myocardial, neural and renal cells.
- *Skin and soft tissue*: Diphtheria toxin can also cause cutaneous ulceration.

Laboratory diagnosis

Direct isolation of the microorganism from throat swabs; however, laboratories in the developed world do not routinely culture throat swabs for *C. diphtheriae*, as cases are increasingly rare.

Treatment and prevention

Penicillin or erythromycin can be used to eradicate the microorganisms. Diphtheria antitoxin is used for passive immunisation of suspected cases of diphtheria only. In developed countries, children are routinely immunised with a toxoid vaccine. Contacts should be given antibiotic prophylaxis and a reinforcing dose of vaccine if previously vaccinated (a full immunisation course is required if not vaccinated). Travellers to areas of the world affected by diphtheria should also receive a reinforcing dose of vaccine (again, a full immunisation course is required if not previously vaccinated).

Other *corynebacteria*

Other *Corynebacterium* species occasionally cause infections. *C. ulcerans* and *C. pseudotuberculosis* can also be toxigenic, causing diphtheria-like infection. *Corynebacterium* spp. are skin commensals and can cause infections when the integrity of the skin is compromised. For example, *C. jeikeium* is a cause of cutaneous infections, infection associated with the use of indwelling medical devices and infective endocarditis. *C. urealyticum* is a cause of urinary tract infection.

Erysipelothrix

In the *Erysipelothrix* genus, only *E. rhusiopathiae* causes infection in humans. It is a facultatively anaerobic, non-sporing, non-motile, catalase-negative, non-capsulate Gram-positive bacillus, which may form long filaments. It produces a zone of α-haemolysis on blood agar. This microorganism can be distinguished from other Gram-positive bacilli based on biochemical characteristics. *E. rhusiopathiae* can cause a type of cellulitis in humans ('erysipeloid'), particularly in people who work with animal products. *E. rhusiopathiae* is also an infrequent cause of endocarditis. Penicillin is often used for treatment.

Listeria

There are several species of *Listeria*; however, most cases of human listeriosis are caused by *Listeria monocytogenes*.

Definition

Gram-positive bacilli occurring singly or in short chains; facultatively anaerobic; non-sporing; motile (at $<30\,^{\circ}$C); catalase-positive; non-capsulate; optimum growth at $37\,^{\circ}$C; strains are commonly β–haemolytic on blood agar.

Epidemiology

L. monocytogenes is widely distributed in the environment and the intestinal tract of some animals and humans. It can contaminate a variety of foods, including raw poultry and meat and can cause outbreaks of food poisoning. It also causes infection, predominantly in neonates, pregnant women, the immunocompromised and the elderly.

Morphology and identification

Listeria spp. can be distinguished from other Gram-positive bacilli by biochemical tests and by their characteristic 'tumbling' motility at less than $30\,^{\circ}$C in broth cultures.

Pathogenicity

L. monocytogenes is an intracellular pathogen that can survive within phagocytic cells. Pathogenic strains produce a haemolysin, listeriolysin O, which is responsible for survival of the bacteria intracellularly.

Associated infections

- *Maternal infection*: this is rare, prior to 20 weeks gestation and is characterised by back pain, pyrexia, sore throat and headache. The foetus may or may not become infected. If the latter occurs, this may result in abortion or stillbirth;
- *Neonatal infection*: early-onset infection (up to 2 days following birth) is contracted *in utero*, normally takes the form of disseminated infection and is associated with a high mortality rate. Late-onset infection (5 or more days following birth) can be contracted as a result of cross-infection, normally results in meningitis and is associated with a lower rate of mortality;
- *Central nervous system*: meningitis (mostly in the elderly and immunocompromised);
- *Cardiovascular*: endocarditis (rare).

Laboratory diagnosis

By direct isolation of the microorganism from clinical specimens, such as blood cultures or CSF; identification is based on the characteristics outlined above. Pregnant staff should not work with suspected cultures of *Listeria* spp.

Treatment

L. monocytogenes is sensitive to several antibiotics; penicillin or ampicillin are often prescribed (note: not sensitive to cephalosporins).

Nocardia

Nocardia spp. are similar to *Actinomyces*. They are non-sporing, non-motile Gram-positive bacilli, which form branching hyphae; however, they only grow aerobically, are catalase-positive and are usually acid-fast. *Nocardia* species are found widely in the environment and some are human oral commensals. Human infection is, however, rare. Many species exist, several of which cause nocardiosis. Examples of human pathogens include *N. asteroides* and *N. brasiliensis*. *Nocardia* spp. predominantly cause respiratory infection acquired via inhalation of the bacilli, and also cutaneous infection arising from inoculation of the microorganism into the skin. Complications, such as secondary abscesses in other anatomical sites, may occur. The microorganism can be grown from various clinical samples but may require extended incubation. Treatment requires the use of antibiotics, such as co-trimoxazole or minocycline, for up to 12 months.

Peptostreptococcus

Strictly anaerobic Gram-positive cocci from several genera may be isolated from clinical specimens. Most clinically significant species belong to the genus *Peptostreptococcus*. They are commensals of many areas of the human body, including the intestinal and genitourinary tracts. *Peptostreptococcus* spp. can cause abscesses at many anatomical sites, normally in association with other bacteria. They are mostly sensitive to penicillin and metronidazole.

Propionibacteria

Propionibacteria are facultatively anaerobic, non-sporing, non-motile, catalase-positive (with the exception of *Propionibacterium propionicum*) Gram-positive pleomorphic bacilli that may bifurcate or branch. They grow better anaerobically, are non-acid fast and can be identified further using commercial identification kits. Propionibacteria constitute part of the normal flora of skin, conjunctiva, oral cavity and intestinal tract. They are normally non-pathogenic; however, they are an infrequent cause of a variety of infections in the immunocompromised and patients with prosthetic devices.

The most common pathogenic species is *Propionibacterium acnes*. Its association with acne vulgaris is widely accepted and it is also associated with cases of endophthalmitis, endocarditis, sarcoidosis and prosthetic joint infection. This microorganism is susceptible to most antibiotics (however, not metronidazole).

Rhodococcus

This genus contains several species, some of which cause human disease. They are aerobic, non-sporing, non-motile, catalase-positive Gram-positive bacilli. They vary from short bacilli to branched filaments, which then fragment into cocci. These cocci then produce bacilli when sub-cultured. They are normally partially acid-fast.

R. equi is the major species of clinical importance. It is widely distributed in the environment and is an opportunistic pathogen affecting severely immunocompromised patients, such as those infected with AIDS or those who have undergone organ transplantation. Most infections are respiratory; however, other infection types occur, including bacteraemia and abscesses at various anatomical sites. The diagnosis of infection is normally made via direct isolation of the microorganisms from clinical specimens such as blood or those from bronchoscopy. Several antibiotics are used for treatment, including vancomycin or ciprofloxacin (for ~4 weeks).

Tropheryma whipplei

T. whipplei, a Gram-positive bacillus is the aetiological agent of Whipple's disease. This is a rare multi-system chronic infection involving, most notably, the gastrointestinal tract but also other anatomical sites. This disease is more prevalent in middle-aged Caucasian males and common symptoms include diarrhoea, malabsorption, weight loss and arthralgia. Culture of this intracellular pathogen is difficult; however, novel immunohistochemistry and serological tests have been developed and can assist in establishing the diagnosis. Antimicrobial therapy for one to two years with co-trimoxazole is often used to prevent recurrence.

7

Gram-negative cocci

Jonathan Sandoe
Leeds Teaching Hospitals NHS Trust and University of Leeds, Leeds, UK

Neisseria

The genus *Neisseria* consists of Gram-negative cocci and includes two important human pathogens: *N. gonorrhoeae* (gonococcus) and *N. meningitidis* (meningococcus) (Table 7.1). Some *Neisseria* species are normal commensals of the human upper respiratory tract.

N. gonorrhoeae

Definition

Gram-negative kidney-shaped cocci, usually in pairs (diplococci) (Figure 7.1), aerobic.

Epidemiology

- Obligate human parasite;
- Many women are asymptomatic and may act as a reservoir of infection;
- Highly transmissible by sexual contact;
- Vertical transmission to neonates may occur during passage through an infected birth canal;
- Occurs worldwide;
- Infections are most common among sexually active young adults;
- Genotypic (PFGE, AFLP) typing may be undertaken to differentiate between strains of gonococci, e.g. in child abuse cases.

Laboratory identification

Provisional identification can be made by microscopy if kidney-shaped Gram-negative diplococci are seen in pus cells. Confirmation is based on cultures: growth on gonococcal selective media, colonial morphology, Gram-stain appearance, positive oxidase reaction, catalase production, biochemical reactions (including carbohydrate fermentation) and immunological tests (for detection of specific gonococcal antigens). Gonococcal DNA can also be detected directly from clinical samples, using various molecular methods.

Pathogenicity

Gonococci have cell-surface pili, which aid adherence to mucosal surfaces of the cervix, urethra, rectum and upper respiratory tract, thus initiating infection. Other virulence factors include IgA proteases. Gonococci can survive intracellularly within polymorphonucleocytes (PMNs) and some strains are also able to resist serum lysis. Re-infections occur, because protective immunity does not develop.

Associated infections

- *Genitourinary*: urethritis (Figure 7.2), cervicitis; complications include epididymitis, prostatitis,

Table 7.1 Gram-negative cocci and associated infections

GRAM-NEGATIVE COCCI	
N. meningitidis	Meningitis
	Bloodstream infection
N. gonorrhoeae	Urethritis, cervicitis
	Epididymitis
	Pelvic inflammatory disease
	Neonatal ophthalmia
	Bloodstream infection
	Arthritis
Moraxella catarrhalis	Upper and lower respiratory tract infections

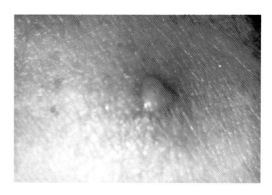

Figure 7.3 Gonococcal skin lesion.

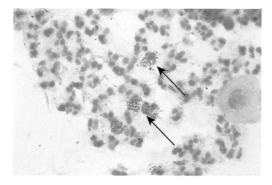

Figure 7.1 Intracellular Gram-negative diplococci (arrowed) of *Neisseria gonorrhoeae* (0.8 μm diameter) in neutrophils.

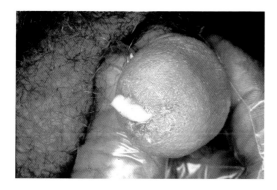

Figure 7.2 Gonococcal urethral discharge.

urethral stricture, pelvic inflammatory disease and sterility;
- *Gastrointestinal*: proctitis (asymptomatic in many);
- *Occular*: hyper-acute conjunctivitis, periorbital cellulitis;
- *Blood*: bloodstream infection (disseminated gonococcal infection, Figure 7.3), endocarditis (rare);
- *Musculoskeletal*: septic arthritis (uncommon).

Microbiological diagnosis

- A diagnosis can be confirmed by microscopy, culture and/or molecular analysis of pus and secretions from various sites (depending upon the infection): cervix, urethra, rectum, conjunctiva, throat and synovial fluid.
- Clinical samples are cultured on enriched selective media and identified as above.
- Specimens should be rapidly transported to the laboratory, because gonococci die readily on drying.
- Blood cultures should be sent before antimicrobial therapy is commenced when disseminated infection is suspected, e.g. in sexually active patients with septic arthritis.
- Serology is not helpful in the diagnosis of gonococcal infection.

Treatment and prevention

Resistance to penicillins is common and resistance to quinolones (e.g. ciprofloxacin) is increasing. Most strains remain susceptible to cephalosporins (e.g. ceftriaxone). Single-dose therapies are recommended to increase patient compliance. No vaccine is available. Prevention of gonorrhoea includes sex education, promotion of public awareness and the use of condoms. Contact tracing is essential in preventing further spread of disease.

N. meningitidis

Definition

Gram-negative kidney-shaped cocci, usually in pairs (diplococci); aerobic.

Epidemiology

- Humans are the only natural host.
- Ten percent of the population are asymptomatic carriers in the upper respiratory tract.
- Spread from human to human is via droplets or direct contact.
- Sporadic cases, clusters and epidemics occur worldwide.
- Serotyping (performed by reference laboratories) can be used to identify outbreaks. At least 13 serogroups of meningococci have been identified. Typing is based on capsular polysaccharides; the most important groups are A, B, C, D, X, Y and W-135. In the UK, the majority of cases are caused by group B and group C is now uncommon.
- Patients with genetic or drug induced defects of the later components of the complement system are predisposed to meningococcal infections.
- In temperate climates most infections occur in patients aged less than 5 years or 15–19 years.

Laboratory identification

Provisional identification is by microscopy when kidney-shaped, Gram-negative cocci are seen within polymorphonucleocytes. Confirmation of identification is based on cultures: colonial morphology, Gram-stain appearance, positive oxidase test and biochemical reactions (including carbohydrate fermentation).

Pathogenicity

A polysaccharide capsule protects against phagocytosis and promotes intracellular survival. Cell-wall endotoxins (lipopolysaccharide) are important in the pathogenesis of severe meningococcal disease. Colonisation of nasopharynx occurs; local invasion may follow with bacteraemia and meningeal involvement.

Associated infections

- *Central nervous system*: meningitis;
- *Blood*: bloodstream infection ('septicaemia') without meningitis (less common);
- *Musculoskeletal*: osteomyelitis, septic arthritis;
- *Occular*: conjunctivitis;
- *Genitourinary*: urethritis;
- *Respiratory*: pneumonia (rare);
- *Cardiovascular*: pericarditis (rare).

Microbiological diagnosis

- *Specimens*: cerebrospinal fluid (CSF) or pus for microscopy, culture, antibiotic susceptibility testing and PCR;
- *Blood cultures*: should also be sent, in addition to a blood sample for PCR;
- *Nasopharyngeal swabs*: can determine carriage of meningococci.

Treatment

Penicillin or cefotaxime are first-line treatments, chloramphenicol is still used for patients with a true penicillin allergy; rifampicin or ciprofloxacin should also be given to eradicate nasopharyngeal carriage, except in patients treated with certain cephalosporins.

Prevention includes antibiotic prophylaxis for close contacts. Meningococcal group C vaccine (group B vaccine being developed) and tetravalent (A, C, Y, W135) polysaccharide vaccine are available for travellers to high incidence areas.

Moraxella catarrhalis

Definition

Gram-negative diplococci and tetrads; aerobic.

Epidemiology

- Part of the normal flora of the upper respiratory tract;
- Opportunistic pathogen;
- Transmission results from direct contact with contaminated secretions or droplets;
- Most infections occur in the young or patients with underlying respiratory disease.

Laboratory identification

- *Microscopy*: Gram-negative diplococci;
- Colonies may be characteristically nudged across the surface of the agar plates with a bacteriological loop much like a 'hockey puck';
- Reduces nitrates and oxidase, catalase and DNAse positive;
- Distinguished from *Neisseria* species by butyrate esterase detection (Tributyrin test).

Pathogenicity

Some strains of *M. catarrhalis* possess fimbriae that aid adherence to respiratory epithelium. Cell-wall endotoxin (lipopolysaccharide) may play a role in the disease process.

Associated infections

Respiratory: otitis media, sinusitis, bronchitis, pneumonia.

Laboratory diagnosis

- Specimens of sputum, bronchoalveolar lavage fluid, tympanocentesis fluid and sinus aspirates for culture and microscopy;
- Serological tests are not used.

Treatment

Most clinical isolates produce β-lactamase and are resistant to amoxicillin. Infection may be treated with co-amoxiclav (amoxicillin plus clavulanate – a β-lactamase inhibitor), tetracyclines (not children) or cephalosporins.

Other Gram-negative cocci

Other Gram-negative cocci, such as *Neisseria subflava*, *Neisseria lactamica* and *Veillonella* species, are part of the normal flora of the upper respiratory tract and rarely cause disease.

8

Enterobacteriaceae

Peter Lambert
Aston University, Birmingham, UK

The Enterobacteriaceae include the following genera: *Escherichia, Enterobacter, Klebsiella, Proteus, Serratia, Shigella, Salmonella* and *Yersinia* (Table 8.1).

They are Gram-negative bacilli, which are found as commensals in the intestinal tract of mammals. They are also referred to as coliforms or enteric bacteria.

Definition

Aerobic and facultatively anaerobic growth; optimal growth normally at 37 °C; grow readily on simple media; ferment wide range of carbohydrates; oxidase-negative; some are motile; bile-tolerant and grow readily on bile-salt-containing media, e.g. MacConkey's agar.

Morphology and identification

- Fermentation of lactose to produce pink colonies on MacConkey's agar is characteristic of *Escherichia, Enterobacter* and *Klebsiella. Salmonella, Shigella, Serratia, Proteus* and *Yersinia* do not ferment lactose and form pale colonies on MacConkey's agar.
- Various tests are used for identification:
  - (a) oxidase (negative);
  - (b) carbohydrate fermentation reactions;
  - (c) production of urease (which splits urea with release of ammonia);
  - (d) hydrogen sulphide production;
  - (e) amino acid decarboxylation;
  - (f) indole production.

  Commercial kits based on these biochemical tests are available for identification of the Enterobacteriaceae.
- Enterobacteriaceae possess a variety of antigens: these may include lipopolysaccharide ('O'), flagellar ('H') and capsular polysaccharide ('K') antigens. These are used to subdivide (serotype) some genera and species, e.g. *Escherichia, Salmonella.*

Escherichia

The genus *Escherichia* currently contains several species. However, *E. coli* (Figure 8.1) is the species most frequently isolated from humans.

Epidemiology and associated infections

Although *E. coli* is a harmless commensal of the human intestine, some strains (identified as particular O, H, and K serotypes) can cause infections of the gastrointestinal tract, urinary tract, biliary tract, lower respiratory tract, bloodstream, haemolytic-uraemic syndrome (HUS), haemorrhagic colitis and neonatal meningitis.

Medical Microbiology and Infection Lecture Notes, Fifth Edition. Edited by Tom Elliott, Anna Casey,
Peter Lambert and Jonathan Sandoe.
© 2011 Blackwell Publishing Ltd. Published 2011 by Blackwell Publishing Ltd.

Table 8.1 Enterobacteriaceae infections

Genus/species	Common infections
Escherichia coli	Urinary tract infection
	Intra-abdomal infection
	Wound infection
Klebsiella spp	Urinary tract infection
	Pneumonia
	Intravascular catheter-related infection
Enterobacter spp	Hospital-acquired pneumonia
Serratia spp	Wound infection
Proteus spp	Urinary tract infection
Salmonella serotypes Typhi and Paratyphi	Enteric fever and bloodstream infection
Other salmonellae	Enteritis
Shigella spp	Enteritis
Yersinia enterocolitica	Enteritis
Yersinia pestis	Plague
Yersinia pseudotuberculosis	Mesenteric adenitis

Pathogenicity

- Specific fimbriae facilitate adherence to mucosal surfaces and colonisation of the intestinal and urinary tracts.
- The lipopolysaccharide (endotoxin) in the cell wall is liberated when Gram-negative bacteria lyse, resulting in production of inflammatory mediators (cytokines and nitric oxide) and complement activation. This results in endotoxic shock and intravascular coagulopathy.

- The K1 capsular polysaccharide antigen is associated with neonatal meningitis.
- A number of distinct infections are mediated by the different protein toxins produced by *E. coli*.
- VTEC (verocytotoxin-producing *E. coli*, particularly the O157:H7 serotype, are an important cause of diarrhoea and HUS. These are also referred to as enterohaemorrhagic *E. coli* (EHEC).
- Most are sporadic cases and have the following key features:
  o zoonotic infections mainly from cattle, but also from vegetables washed in contaminated water;
  o low infecting dose;
  o acquired by eating undercooked contaminated meat and vegetables;
  o damage gut endothelium, resulting in haemorrhagic colitis;
  o HUS occurs in about 5% of patients, which results in renal failure, oliguria, thrombocytopenia.

Diarrhoea caused by other *E. coli*:

- *Enteropathogenic* (*EPEC*): cause of infantile diarrhoea;
- *Enterotoxigenic* (*ETEC*): travellers' diarrhoea, non-invasive;

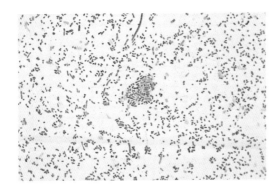

Figure 8.1 Gram stain of *Escherichia coli* showing Gram-negative bacilli ($2\,\mu m \times 0.5\,\mu m$).

- *Enteroinvasive* (*EIEC*): causes dysentery-like illness;
- *Enteroaggregative* (*EAEC*): watery diarrhoea without fever.

Laboratory diagnosis

- Diagnosis is by direct isolation of the microorganism from clinical samples, e.g. faeces, urine and blood.
- Identification of some pathogenic strains, e.g. VTEC, EPEC, may be achieved by serotyping.

Antibacterial therapy

E. coli is commonly resistant to penicillin and ampicillin by production of β-lactamase enzymes. Production of extended spectrum β-lactamases (ESBLs), which inactivate many penicillins and cephalosporins, is an increasing problem. Antibiotics often used to treat *E. coli* infections include the cephalosporins, trimethoprim, ciprofloxacin and aminoglycosides; strains isolated from hospitalised patients are often more resistant to antibiotics and therefore local antibiotic sensitivity patterns need to be considered.

Klebsiella

The genus *Klebsiella* contains a number of species, including *K. pneumoniae* and *K. oxytoca*; these can be distinguished on the basis of biochemical tests. Pathogenicity is associated with capsular polysaccharide and lipopolysaccharide (endotoxin) production. There are many capsular serotypes. Klebsiellae are widespread in the environment and in the intestinal flora of humans and other mammals. Infections are often opportunistic and associated with hospitalisation, particularly in high-dependency units. They include pneumonia, urinary tract and wound infection, and neonatal meningitis. Outbreaks of healthcare-associated infection occur.

Klebsiella spp. often produce β-lactamases and are resistant to ampicillin. Cephalosporins (e.g. cefotaxime), β-lactamase-inhibitor/penicillin combinations (e.g. co-amoxiclav) and aminoglycosides (e.g. gentamicin) can be used to treat *Klebsiella* infections, but multiply resistant strains may limit antibiotic choice. Extensive use of broad-spectrum antibiotics in hospitalised patients has led to development of multi-drug-resistant strains that produce ESBLs.

Enterobacter and Serratia

Enterobacter and *Serratia* spp. are closely related to *Klebsiella* spp. Infections occur principally in hospitalised patients and include the lower respiratory and urinary tracts. Hospital cross-infection with antibiotic-resistant strains is a particular problem. ESBL production in strains of *Enterobacter* is an increasing problem.

Salmonella

The genus *Salmonella* contains a large number of species (more correctly, serotypes). *Salmonella* serotype Typhi and *Salmonella* serotype Paratyphi cause enteric fever (typhoid or paratyphoid); other salmonellae cause enteritis.

Classification

- Over 2,000 serotypes are distinguished, most of which belong to the species *S. enterica*. However, many of these have been given binomial names (e.g. *Salmonella typhimurium* and *Salmonella enteritidis*), although they are not separate species. In clinical practice, laboratories identify microorganisms according to their binomial name.
- *Salmonella* spp. have both H and O antigens. There are over 60 different O antigens, and individual strains may possess several O and H antigens; the latter can exist in variant forms, termed 'phases'. *Salmonella* serotype Typhi also has a capsular polysaccharide antigen referred to as 'Vi' (for virulence), which is related to invasiveness.
- Agglutination tests with antisera for different O and H antigens form the basis for the serological classification of *Salmonella* spp. Further strain differentiation of *Salmonella* spp. for epidemiological purposes can be achieved by phage typing.

Epidemiology

Salmonella spp. are commensals of many animals, including poultry, domestic pets, birds and humans. Transmission is via the faecal-oral route. The infective dose is relatively high ($\sim10^6$ microorganisms) and multiplication in food is important for effective transmission. A chronic carrier state can occur.

Morphology and identification

- *Salmonella* spp. are motile and produce acid, and occasionally gas, from glucose and mannose.
- They are resistant to sodium deoxycholate, which inhibits many other Enterobacteriaceae. Deoxycholate agar is used as a selective media to isolate *Salmonella* spp. from stool specimens.
- *Salmonella* spp. do not ferment lactose and form pale colonies on MacConkey's medium; on xylose lysine deoxycholate (XLD) agar, many *Salmonella* spp. form pale colonies with black centres as a result of H_2S production. This aids recognition of *Salmonella* colonies in mixed cultures.
- Further biochemical tests are required for definitive identification. Serotyping of O and H antigens by slide agglutination is used for speciation.

Pathogenicity

Salmonella spp. can survive the acidic pH of the stomach and invade the gut, resulting in an inflammatory response and subsequent diarrhoea.

Associated infections

- *Salmonella infections*: (caused by non-typhoid salmonellae;
- *Enterocolitis/gastroenteritis*: rarely associated with bloodstream infection, osteomyelitis, septic arthritis or abscesses;
- *Enteric fever*: caused by *Salmonella* serotype Typhi and *Salmonella* serotype Paratyphi. Enteric fever is prevalent in Asia, South America and Africa; approximately 300 cases per year in the UK. *Salmonella* spp. may persist in biliary and urinary tracts after recovery.

Laboratory diagnosis

- *Enterocolitis*: culture of stool samples on selective media, e.g. XLD, DCA (deoxycholate citrate agar), and enrichment media, e.g. selenite broth; identification of *Salmonella* spp. by biochemical and agglutination tests. Phage typing can be used for typing individual strains.

- *Enteric fever*: isolation of *Salmonella* serotypes Typhi or Paratyphi from blood cultures (first week of infection), urine (second week) or faeces (first week onwards). Serology (Widal's test) is now rarely performed, because of unreliable results.

Treatment and prevention

- *Enteric fever*: ciprofloxacin (though resistance is increasing);
- *Enterocolitis*: self-limiting; antibiotics (e.g. ciprofloxacin and cefotaxime) reserved for severe or invasive infection, particularly in the elderly, very young or 'immunocompromised' individuals;
- Typhoid immunisation; avoidance of contaminated water/food.

Shigella

Classification

The main pathogenic species are S. *sonnei*, S. *boydii*, S. *dysenteriae* and S. *flexneri*. They are distinguished by biochemical reactions and antigenic characteristics ('O' antigens).

Epidemiology

Obligate human pathogens with no animal reservoirs; transmission via faecal-oral route with low infective dose (10–200 microorganisms). Direct person-to-person spread is common; chronic carrier state is rare.

Morphology and identification

Shigella spp. are non-motile (they have no flagella). They are resistant to sodium deoxycholate and grow on deoxycholate agar (see *Salmonella*). They are non-lactose or late lactose (S. *sonnei*) fermenters. Further biochemical tests are carried out for definitive identification and serotyping by slide agglutination is used for speciation.

Pathogenicity

Shigella spp. express an intestinal adherence factor, which aids colonisation within the gut. They cause disease by invasion and destruction of the colonic mucosa, and also produce an enterotoxin (cytotoxin) known as Shiga toxin, which can cause microangiopathy, HUS and thrombocytopenic purpura.

Associated infections

Self-limiting diarrhoeal illness, dysentery (diarrhoea with blood and pus, fever, abdominal pain) (HUS and bloodstream infection are rare).

Laboratory diagnosis

Stool culture on selective media, e.g. XLD.

Treatment

Antibiotics (e.g. ciprofloxacin) reserved for severe cases (often caused by *S. dysenteriae*).

Proteus

The genus *Proteus* contains a number of species, e.g. *P. mirabilis* and *P. vulgaris*. Characteristics include:

- non-lactose fermenting, produce pale colonies on MacConkey's agar;
- motile, tendency to 'swarm' on blood agar;
- important cause of urinary tract and occasionally abdominal wound infection.

Yersinia

The genus *Yersinia* contains three human pathogens: *Y. pestis*, *Y. pseudotuberculosis* and *Y. enterocolitica*; these species are identified by biochemical tests.

Y. pestis

Y. pestis is the cause of plague (black death). Although mainly of historical interest in Europe, plague remains endemic in some areas of the world. It is primarily a pathogen of rodents and is transmitted to humans via infected fleas; lymph nodes associated with the flea bite enlarge to form a bubo (bubonic plague). Bloodstream invasion and pneumonia may follow (pneumonic plague). Person-to-person spread via droplets occurs in pneumonic plague. *Y. pestis* can be isolated from blood, bubo aspiration, sputum, throat swabs and skin scrapings. Treatment for *Y. pestis* infection is with an aminoglycoside or tetracycline. Laboratory diagnosis is by microscopy and culture of clinical material.

Y. pseudotuberculosis

This is primarily an animal pathogen, but in humans it is an occasional cause of mesenteric adenitis, rarely septicaemia. It is probably transmitted to humans via contaminated food. Laboratory diagnosis is through culture of faeces on selective agar, e.g. CIN agar and cold enrichment of faeces.

Y. enterocolitica

Y. enterocolitica causes diarrhoeal disease, terminal ileitis and mesenteric adenitis. Infection may be complicated by septicaemia or reactive polyarthritis. A zoonotic infection of domestic and wild animals, transmission is via the faecal-oral route. Laboratory diagnosis is by culture of faeces on selective agar, e.g. CIN agar, cold enrichment of faeces, culture of blood specimens or serology.

Haemophilus and other fastidious Gram-negative bacteria

Jonathan Sandoe
Leeds Teaching Hospitals NHS Trust and University of Leeds, Leeds, UK

This chapter includes an arbitrary collection of Gram-negative coccobacilli, which are described collectively because of common characteristics, rather than being part of a formal classification system. They are all Gram-negative bacteria that can be difficult to culture and usually are members of the normal microbial flora of humans or animals. Most are therefore opportunistic pathogens. Infections associated with fastidious Gram-negative bacteria are outlined in Table 9.1.

Haemophilus influenzae

Description/definition

Gram-negative bacilli; fastidious growth requirements; aerobic and anaerobic growth.

Epidemiology

- Common commensal in the upper respiratory tract;
- Capsulated (more pathogenic) strains are also carried in a small number of healthy individuals;
- Carriers are an important reservoir for invasive disease;
- Transmission is by respiratory secretions and droplets;
- Most infections occur in children and patients with underlying respiratory disease;
- Type b strains (see Pathogenicity) were a common cause of invasive infection, particularly in small children (aged 6 months to 5 years), prior to introduction of the Hib vaccine.

Laboratory identification

- Gram-negative bacilli;
- Variable oxidase reaction;
- Nutritionally demanding and grows only on enriched media containing haemin (factor X) and nicotinamide adenine dinucleotide (factor V);
- Simple nutrient agar contains no X or V factor and strains of *H. influenzae* will only grow around paper discs containing both these factors (Figure 9.1);

Medical Microbiology and Infection Lecture Notes, Fifth Edition. Edited by Tom Elliott, Anna Casey, Peter Lambert and Jonathan Sandoe.
© 2011 Blackwell Publishing Ltd. Published 2011 by Blackwell Publishing Ltd.

Table 9.1 Infections associated with fastidious Gram-negative bacteria

Genus	Species	Associated infections
Bordetella	B. pertussis	Whooping cough
	B. parapertussis	Whooping cough-like syndrome
Brucella	B. abortus	Brucellosis
	B. melitensis	
	B. suis	
	B. canis	
Haemophilus	H. influenzae (type b)	Meningitis*
		Epiglottitis*
		Bone and joint infections*
		Exacerbations of chronic lung disease
	H. parainfluenzae	Exacerbations of chronic lung disease
	H. ducreyi	Genital ulcers (chancroid)
Pasteurella	P. multocida	Cellulitis after animal bites

*Usually in non-vaccinated children.

- Grows on 'chocolate agar' but not on blood agar (blood agar contains factor X but insufficient factor V. Heat treatment of blood before incorporation in agar produces a medium known as 'chocolate agar', which contains both factors for *H. influenzae* to grow);
- Serotyping by agglutination tests can be carried out on capsulated strains, when isolated from invasive infections.

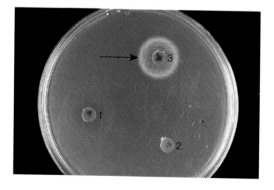

Figure 9.1 Nutrient agar plate with discs containing (1) Haemin; (2) NAD; (3) both. *Haemophilus influenzae* requires both factors for growth (arrowed).

Pathogenicity

Strains may be capsulated or non-capsulated. The polysaccharide capsule of certain strains is a major virulence factor. Capsulated strains are divided into six serotypes (designated a–f) on the basis of polysaccharide capsular antigens. *H. influenzae* type b is particularly pathogenic. Antibodies to the type b capsule protect against invasive infections.

Non-type b capsulated strains occasionally cause invasive infections. Non-capsulated strains are an important cause of respiratory tract infections.

Another component of the cell wall of *H. influenzae* that contributes to pathogenesis is lipopolysaccharide (LPS), which has similar biological activity to other Gram-negative endotoxins. *H. influenzae* also possesses pili (fimbriae) and expresses a surface protein called Hia, both of which facilitate adherence to cells of the respiratory tract.

Associated infections

- *Respiratory:* pneumonia, epiglottitis, otitis media, sinusitis, exacerbation of chronic lung disease;

- *Central nervous system*: meningitis;
- *Musculoskeletal*: osteomyelitis, septic arthritis (uncommon);
- *Skin and soft tissues*: cellulitis (including orbital cellulitis);
- *Cardiovascular*: endocarditis (rare).

Laboratory diagnosis

- *Respiratory*: send respiratory secretions for culture and sensitivity. Epiglottitic swabs for microscopy and culture should be collected under direct vision by an ENT specialist. Sinus washout fluid can be cultured.
- *Central nervous system*: send cerebrospinal fluid (CSF) for microscopy and culture.
- *Musculoskeletal*: send bone or synovial fluid for microscopy and culture.
- *Skin and soft tissues*: skin swabs are rarely helpful in cellulitis.
- *Cardiovascular*: send 3 sets of blood cultures if endocarditis suspected.

Treatment and prophylaxis

β-lactamase production and intrinsic resistance to ampicillin and many other β-lactam antibiotics is common, so treatment is directed by susceptibility testing. Third-generation cephalosporins, e.g. cefotaxime or ceftriaxone, are common empirical therapy for serious infections.

A vaccine ('Hib') to the type b polysaccharide capsule has led to a large reduction in the number of invasive *H. influenzae* type b infections. Rifampicin is used for the prophylaxis of contacts of cases of *H. influenzae* type b meningitis, and as an adjunct to therapy to reduce nasopharyngeal carriage.

H. parainfluenzae and *Aggregatibacter aphrophilus*

These species are members of the normal upper respiratory tract flora. *H. aphrophilus* and *H. paraphrophilus* have been recently renamed *Aggregatibacter aphrophilus*. They are generally not pathogenic, but occasionally cause infective endocarditis.

H. aegyptius

H. aegyptius causes an acute purulent conjunctivitis, in seasonal endemics, particularly in hot climates.

H. ducreyi

H. ducreyi causes genital ulcers (chancroid), a sexually transmitted infection seen in Africa, Asia, Latin America and many parts of Europe.

HACEK

Some species of *Haemophilus* belong to the group of Gram-negative bacilli called 'HACEK' (*Haemophilus*, *Aggregatibacter actinomycetemcomitans* (formerly *Actinobacillus actinomycetemcomitans*), *Cardiobacterium hominis*, *Eikenella corrodens* and *Kingella* species). This group of microorganisms is responsible for 5–10% of cases of infective endocarditis, involving native valves. The HACEK group is also associated with infections, including peritonitis, otitis media, bacteraemia, periodontal infection and some species, e.g. *Kingella*, cause bone and joint infections in young children (Chapter 36).

Eikenella corrodens

E. corrodens is a Gram-negative bacillus that forms typical pitting colonies on solid agar. It grows aerobically and anaerobically on complex media; colonies may take 5 days to appear on agar plates. The microorganism is found as a normal commensal of the human upper respiratory tract and may be isolated from a variety of infections, including dental abscesses, soft-tissue infections of the neck, pulmonary and abdominal abscesses and wound infections after human bites (normally in association with other microorganisms such as anaerobes, coliforms and streptococci). *E. corrodens* is a rare cause of endocarditis.

Cardiobacterium hominis

C. hominis is a Gram-negative bacillus with tapering ends. It has a tendency to form long filaments. It grows best on enriched media in a microaerophilic environment with additional CO_2. *C. hominis* is a normal commensal of the human upper respiratory tract and is a rare cause of bacterial endocarditis.

Brucella

Definition

Small, Gram-negative coccobacilli; grows slowly aerobically. The genus *Brucella* contains four species responsible for human infections: *Brucella melitensis*, *B. abortus*, *B. suis* and *B. canis*.

Epidemiology

* Worldwide distribution, but great variation in incidence of infection;
* Zoonotic infection (the main reservoir is in animals and transmission occurs from animals to humans);
* The main reservoirs for infection are goats and sheep (*B. melitensis*), cattle (*B. abortus*), pigs (*B. suis*) and dogs (*B. canis*);
* In the UK, *B. melitensis* is the most common species isolated, but is rare. (Fewer than 20 cases are reported per year in the UK);
* *B. melitensis* is found most commonly in the Mediterranean area;
* Infection is associated with close contact with farm animals, e.g. farm workers, veterinary surgeons, or occurs as a result of ingestion of unpasteurised cows' or goats' milk.

Laboratory identification

Microscopy: Gram-negative bacilli. *Brucella* species are aerobic; they require CO_2 for growth and are slow growers, requiring 2–3 weeks for colonies to be visible. Identification is based on Gram stain, colony morphology, growth characteristics and biochemical reactions.

Pathogenicity

Brucella species are intracellular pathogens that are capable of surviving and replicating within phagocytic cells. The principal virulence factor is the cell wall lipopolysaccharide (LPS). Infection with *Brucella* is typical of an intracellular pathogen, with the formation of multiple granulomatous lesions in several organs.

Associated infections

Brucellosis is an infection with non-specific symptoms including fevers, sweats, general malaise, headaches, depression and anorexia. Onset can be acute or insidious. Localised infection can occur:

* *Central nervous system*: acute or chronic meningitis, brain abscess;
* *Gastrointestinal*: liver abscesses/granulomas, hepatitis;
* *Musculoskeletal*: vertebral osteomyelitis and discitis, sacroiliitis, septic arthritis;
* *Cardiovascular*: infective endocarditis;
* *Respiratory*: pneumonia, lung abscess.

Laboratory diagnosis

* Diagnosis is made by direct isolation from blood cultures, CSF or culture of aspirated bone marrow after prolonged incubation. *Note*: routine blood cultures are normally incubated for 3–7 days, therefore it is important to inform the laboratory if brucellosis is suspected.
* Serological tests, including ELISA (enzyme-linked immunosorbent assay) to detect serum antibodies against *Brucella* are available; these aid diagnosis because many patients present late in their illness.

Treatment and prevention

Prolonged treatment is necessary with a tetracycline (6 weeks) and an aminoglycoside (2–3 weeks), or tetracycline and rifampicin (6 weeks). This reflects the intracellular location of the microorganisms.

Prevention is achieved by eradication of *Brucella* in the animal population and avoidance of raw milk and associated products.

Bordetella

The genus *Bordetella* contains eight species but *B. pertussis* (the cause of whooping cough) and *B. parapertussis* account for most human infections.

Definition

Small coccobacilli; obligate aerobes; fastidious growth requirements.

Epidemiology

B. pertussis is a human pathogen with no animal reservoir. It is readily transmissible by droplet spread from infected people. Mainly affects young children, but adults can occasionally be infected.

Pathogenicity

A variety of virulence factors has been described, including adhesins, cytotoxins and haemolysins. Lung inflammation ensues.

Associated infections

- *Respiratory*: whooping cough (pertussis), pneumonia occasionally complicated by respiratory failure and haemorrhage (e.g. subconjunctival haemorrhage or intracerebral haemorrhage secondary to coughing bouts).

Laboratory diagnosis

Culture of pernasal swabs on specialised agar, e.g. Bordet–Gengou (charcoal blood agar). Colonies may take 2–3 days to grow.

Treatment and prevention

Erythromycin may be given to reduce infectivity. If given during the incubation period, it may reduce clinical symptoms. Immunisation with DTP (diphtheria, tetanus, pertussis triple vaccine) during childhood is widely used.

Pasteurella

Pasteurella multocida is the only common human pathogen in this genus. The microorganism is found as part of the normal oral flora of cats and dogs. Human infections usually arise after animal bites and results in a local cellulitis, sometimes with bloodstream infection. Laboratory diagnosis is by culture of the microorganism, usually from blood culture samples or wound swabs. Treatment is with penicillin.

Capnocytophaga species

These Gram-negative bacilli grow slowly (often taking >5 days) on complex media and have an absolute requirement for CO_2. They are normal commensal of the oral cavity of human and animals. *Capnocytophaga canimorsus* is a normal commensal of dogs and can cause severe sepsis, notably in splenectomised patients and often with a history of dog bites. Human *Capnocytophaga* spp. can cause infection in immunocompromised patients, particularly when oral mucosal ulceration is also present, and are a rare cause of infection in immunocompetent patients (e.g. lung abscess, endocarditis).

Streptobacillus moniliformis

S. moniliformis is a short Gram-negative bacillus that grows slowly on complex media. A commensal of healthy rats, it is one cause of rat-bite fever in humans (the other aetiological microorganism being *Spirillum*), an infection characterised by fever, vomiting, headache, arthralgia and a rash. *S. moniliformis* is also the cause of 'streptobacilliary fever', sometimes called Haverhill fever, after the first recorded epidemic of the infection at Haverhill, USA. Outbreaks have occurred in the UK and may be associated with the consumption of unpasteurised milk.

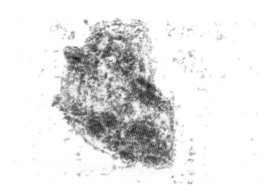

Figure 9.2 Microscopy of vaginal discharge, showing a single epithelial cell (clue cell), with numerous microorganisms attached.

Gardnerella vaginalis

G. vaginalis is a Gram-negative bacillus that occasionally appears Gram positive ('Gram variable'). It grows aerobically and anaerobically on complex media. It is a normal commensal of the vaginal flora, but is associated with bacterial vaginosis, a condition characterised by an 'ammonia smelling' vaginal discharge and the presence of clue cells (Figure 9.2).

Pseudomonas, Legionella and other environmental Gram-negative bacilli

Peter Lambert
Aston University, Birmingham, UK

This chapter includes bacteria that are found in the environment, but can colonise and infect humans.

Pseudomonas, Burkholderia and Stenotrophomonas

Species from the genera *Pseudomonas*, *Burkholderia* and *Stenotrophomonas* were all previously classified in the *Pseudomonas* genus. They are widely distributed in nature; *P. aeruginosa* is the most important pathogenic species in humans. They are sometimes collectively referred to as 'pseudomonads'.

Definition

Gram-negative bacilli; strict aerobes; grow on simple media at a wide temperature range; motile; non-capsulated; some species pigmented.

P. aeruginosa

Epidemiology

- *P. aeruginosa* is an important microorganism in healthcare-associated infection. It is a normal commensal in the human gastrointestinal tract, but may colonise other sites when host defences are compromised, including burns and leg ulcers, the respiratory tract of patients with cystic fibrosis or bronchiectasis, and the urinary tract of patients with long-term, indwelling, urethral catheters.
- *P. aeruginosa*, as with other members of the genus, has the ability to grow with minimal nutrients, e.g. in water and in the presence of some disinfectants; these properties are the key to its role as a hospital pathogen.

Morphology and identification

The microorganism grows on most media, producing a characteristic greenish pigment. It can be distinguished from the Enterobacteriaceae by

Medical Microbiology and Infection Lecture Notes, Fifth Edition. Edited by Tom Elliott, Anna Casey, Peter Lambert and Jonathan Sandoe.
© 2011 Blackwell Publishing Ltd. Published 2011 by Blackwell Publishing Ltd.

its oxidative metabolism (oxidase-positive) and the inability to grow anaerobically, except on nitrate. The different species of the genus *Pseudomonas* can be distinguished by biochemical tests.

Pathogenicity

P. aeruginosa is relatively non-pathogenic; it characteristically causes infections in hospitalised patients, particularly those who are immunocompromised. The microorganism produces several enzymes that allow spread through tissues (elastase) and a protease that breaks down IgA on mucosal surfaces. It also produces cytotoxins (exotoxin A) and other factors that inhibit host defences, including a rhamnolipid and an alginate exopolysaccharide.

Associated infections

P. aeruginosa principally causes opportunist infections including:

- *Skin and soft tissues*: infections associated with burns and cutaneous ulcers;
- *Respiratory tract*: ventilator-associated pneumonia and hospital acquired pneumonia (Chapter 26); and lower respiratory tract infections in cystic fibrosis and bronchiectasis patients;
- *Urinary tract*: associated with long-term urethral catheterisation;
- *Invasive*: bloodstream infection can follow primary infection at any site, but is more common in immunocompromised patients;
- *Eye*: contact lens-associated infections;
- *Ear nose and throat*: otitis externa.

Laboratory diagnosis

Isolation of the microorganism from relevant body sites. The isolation of *P. aeruginosa* from several patients may suggest hospital cross-infection. In such circumstances, strains of *P. aeruginosa* can be further characterised by serotyping or molecular biological techniques.

Treatment

One of the characteristics of *P. aeruginosa* is resistance to antibiotics; some newer antibiotics have been designed specifically to combat *P. aeruginosa*. Clinically important anti-pseudomonal antibiotics include:

- aminoglycosides (e.g. gentamicin);
- broad-spectrum penicillin/beta-lactamse inhibiter combinations (e.g. piperacillin/tazobactam);
- third-generation cephalosporins (e.g. ceftazidime);
- carbapenems (e.g. imipenem and meropenem);
- monobactams (e.g. aztreonam);
- quinolones (e.g. ciprofloxacin).

In hospital units where antibiotics are used frequently (e.g. special care baby units, ICUs, cystic fibrosis clinics), *P. aeruginosa* isolates may become resistant to these antibiotics. Isolation of patients colonised by multi-resistant *P. aeruginosa* strains is an important part of controlling hospital infections.

Burkholderia cenocepacia (formerly *cepacia*)

This microorganism has recently been recognised as an important cause of lower respiratory tract infection in patients with cystic fibrosis; it occurs in moist environments and hospitals. Treatment of infection is with meropenem.

Burkholderia pseudomallei

This microorganism has a characteristic safety pin appearance on Gram-staining (bi-polar staining). It causes melioidosis, is resistant to aminoglycosides, but sensitive to ceftazidime.

Stenotrophomonas maltophilia (formerly *Pseudomonas* or *Xanthomonas*)

This microorganism is a cause of hospital-acquired infections and is often multiply antibiotic resistant; it causes pneumonia, particularly in compromised patients, e.g. ventilated or cancer patients; also related to intravascular device infections. Treatment with trimethoprim-sulfamethaxole

---

Legionella

Legionella pneumophila was first recognised after investigations into an outbreak of respiratory illness in delegates at an American Legion Convention in Philadelphia, USA, in 1976. Other *Legionella* species can also cause human infection.

Definition

Gram-negative bacilli; obligately aerobic, slow-growing bacteria with fastidious growth requirements.

Epidemiology

- Environmental microorganisms, found in soil and water;
- Water systems, particularly heating systems and water-cooled air-conditioning plants can be a reservoir for infection and source of outbreaks;
- Although relatively fastidious in its growth requirements, the microorganism grows in water at temperatures between 20 and 45 °C; this may be related to growth within amoebae, which are found naturally in the same environment or to its ability to survive in biofilms;
- *Legionella* species are also relatively chlorine tolerant;
- Transmission occurs through aerosolisation of water contaminated with legionellae;
- Human-to-human transmission has not been demonstrated;
- Cases occur sporadically or as part of point-source outbreaks;
- Hospital or community acquired.

Pathogenicity

Virulent *Legionella* species adhere to human respiratory epithelial cells via pili (fimbriae). *Legionella* species can also survive and grow within phagocytic cells, neutralising the normal bacteria-killing mechanisms.

Associated infections

- *Central nervous system*: meningoencephalitis;
- *Respiratory*: pneumonia (community and hospital acquired);
- *Cardiovascular*: prosthetic valve endocarditis (very rare).

L. pneumophila can cause a flu-like illness with no lower respiratory symptoms, called Pontiac fever. *Legionella* may also spread to other areas of the body, including lymph nodes, brain, kidney and bone marrow.

Laboratory diagnosis

- Diagnosis is made by culture of sputum or bronchoalveolar lavage fluid on specialised media-buffered charcoal yeast extract agar (BCYE); colonies take between 2 and 7 days to grow;
- Legionellae are classified into species according to surface antigens;
- Legionellae can be detected directly in respiratory specimens by direct immunofluorescence microscopy;
- *Legionella* antigen may be detected in urine samples by immunoassay;
- Serological tests are often used to confirm the diagnosis of legionellosis; a rise in serum antibody titre may take up to 6 weeks.

Treatment and prevention

This is with clarithromycin combined, in severe cases, with rifampicin. Fluoroquinolones are also effective.

Prevention is achieved by monitoring and appropriate disinfection in man-made water systems.

Acinetobacter

Acinetobacter species share a number of common features with pseudomonads. They are short, Gram-negative bacilli, strict aerobes, and grow well on simple media with minimal nutrients. However, unlike pseudomonads, they are oxidase-negative. They occur in many environments, including hospitals, and are an important cause of healthcare-associated infection (particularly *A. baumannii*). Hospital outbreaks, most notably chest infections, occur particularly in ICUs. *Acinetobacter* species frequently acquire plasmids expressing multiple antibiotic-resistance patterns, including quinolones, many aminoglycosides and β-lactam agents. Meropenem and amikacin may be active. Some multi-resistant isolates are sensitive only to colistin.

11

Campylobacter, Helicobacter and Vibrio

Martin Skirrow[1], Cliodna McNulty[1] and Tom Elliott[2]
[1]Health Protection Agency, Gloucestershire Royal Hospital, Gloucester, UK
[2]University Hospitals Birmingham NHS Foundation Trust, Birmingham, UK

Campylobacter

Definition

Spirally curved, Gram-negative bacilli; motile with single polar flagella; non-sporing; non-capsulated; microaerophilic.

Classification

There are several species, but only *Campylobacter jejuni* and *C. coli* commonly infect humans (cause acute enterocolitis). *C. fetus*, the type species of the genus, occasionally causes systemic infection in persons with immune deficiency.

Epidemiology

Campylobacter spp. are a leading cause of acute infective diarrhoea worldwide. In most industrialised countries, they are the most common cause of acute bacterial enterocolitis. The infection is essentially a zoonosis with a wide range of reservoirs, including wild birds, poultry, cattle, sheep, pigs and pets. Modes of transmission are correspondingly varied, but broiler chickens are a major source, either through handling the raw product or eating undercooked meat. Raw milk and untreated water are established sources of infection. Transmission from infected subjects is uncommon, except from young children with uncontrolled bowel actions.

Morphology and identification

- *Campylobacter* spp. have a characteristic morphology. The long polar flagella are attached to a unique cone-shaped structure. Like the true *Vibrio* spp., *Campylobacter* spp. are among the fastest moving bacteria. It is possible to recognise them in microscopic examinations of wet preparations of faeces from patients with diarrhoea.
- For culture they require microaerobic conditions with added CO_2. Selective media containing specific antimicrobials and compounds that neutralise free radicals, such as charcoal, are essential for their isolation from faeces. They are oxidase and catalase positive, but do not metabolise

Medical Microbiology and Infection Lecture Notes, Fifth Edition. Edited by Tom Elliott, Anna Casey,
Peter Lambert and Jonathan Sandoe.
© 2011 Blackwell Publishing Ltd. Published 2011 by Blackwell Publishing Ltd.

sugars. Further biochemical tests are used for speciation.

Pathogenicity

The *Campylobacter* cell wall contains endotoxins. Cytopathic extracellular toxins and enterotoxins have also been demonstrated, but their exact role is unclear. They cause acute inflammation of the intestinal mucosa, like that caused by *Salmonella* and *Shigella* spp. Infection is self limiting and seldom lasts for more than a week. Mean incubation period is 3 days.

Associated conditions

- *Campylobacter enteritis*: this can mimic acute appendicitis; occasionally genuine appendicitis is present. It can also mimic an acute attack of ulcerative colitis.
- *Reactive arthritis and Guillain Barré syndrome*: (polyneuropathy with paralysis) are complications that may arise during the recovery phase of illness.

Laboratory diagnosis

- Culture of faeces on selective media at 42 °C under microaerophilic conditions;
- Serology for serum antibodies to *Campylobacter* spp. can be of value in culture-negative patients with suspected late sequelae and in the investigation of outbreaks.

Treatment

Rehydration. Erythromycin or ciprofloxacin indicated only for severe illness.

Helicobacter

H. pylori

Definition

Curved Gram-negative bacilli; motile; non-sporing; non-capsulated; microaerophilic.

Classification

Helicobacter spp. are in the same broad bacterial group as *Campylobacter* spp. There are many *Helicobacter* species, each adapted to a particular animal or niche. *H. pylori* is the species associated with man.

Epidemiology

H. pylori infects human gastric epithelial cells and humans are the main reservoir.

The microorganism is acquired most commonly in early childhood and usually becomes chronic, often life-long. Transmission is by the faecal-oral or oral–oral routes and is associated with close contact (intrafamilial) and poor sanitation. Thus, in developed countries, prevalence is now very low in children (<10 years, 1%), but about 25% in adults more than 50 years of age (reflecting the higher rates of transmission when they were children). Prevalence is higher in countries with poor sanitation, with 50% of over 50 year olds infected.

Morphology and identification

- *H. pylori* grows slowly at 37 °C on enriched media in a microaerophilic atmosphere (characteristic of gastric mucus).
- They have four to six mono-polar sheathed flagella (Figure 11.1) that facilitate motility through gastric mucus.
- The rapid urease test is a unique characteristic, used for laboratory identification and diagnosis of *H. pylori*.

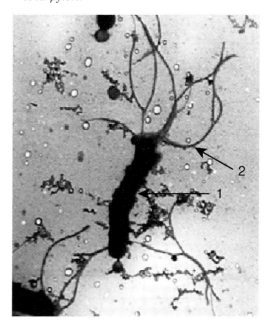

Figure 11.1 Negative-stain electronmicrograph of a single *H. pylori* (1) showing flagella (2).

Pathogenicity and associated infections

Urease is an important colonisation factor, enabling the microorganism to neutralise gastric acid through the production of ammonia from urea.

Most subjects remain asymptomatic, but *H. pylori* is the most common cause of duodenal ulceration and gastric cancer. *H. pylori* initially causes a neutrophilic gastritis, which becomes chronic ('chronic active' gastritis). *H. pylori* damages antral D cells that release somatostatin, thereby interrupting the negative feedback inhibition of gastric acid from the gastric corpus. Gastric acid thus increases, thereby inducing gastric metaplasia in the duodenum. These metaplastic cells are susceptible to *H. pylori* infection, leading to duodenitis and the risk of ulceration. Extension of *H. pylori* into the gastric corpus causes chronic active inflammation and eventually atrophy of cells, a precursor to metaplasia and cancer.

Diagnosis

- *Invasive tests*: Gastric biopsy to identify typical histopathological appearance; culture of *H. pylori* on selective medium in a microaerobic atmosphere; biopsy urease test, which detects the preformed urease produced by *H. pylori* by a rise of pH in urea broth with an indicator. The latter is a simple, rapid, inexpensive and specific test, because *H. pylori* is unique in producing a urease with a high affinity and rate of activity.
- *Non-invasive tests*: The urea breath test is highly sensitive and specific. ^{13}C- or ^{14}C-labelled urea is given to the patient; if *H. pylori* is present, the urease splits the urea, producing labelled CO_2, which is detected in expired air. The stool antigen test, also highly sensitive and specific, detects the presence of H. pylori in stools using monoclonal antibodies. Serology is less specific and is not appropriate in populations with low infection prevalence.

Treatment

Combination treatment is required due to poor antibiotic penetration into the gastric mucosa, gastric acidity and increasing antimicrobial resistance. Clearance in 80% of patients can be attained with a proton pump inhibitor, e.g. omeprazole, that reduces gastric acidity, coupled with two antimicrobials such as amoxicillin, clarithromycin, metronidazole, doxycycline, levofloxacin, rifabutin or bismuth salt.

Vibrio

Definition

Gram negative; comma-shaped bacteria; aerobic and facultatively anaerobic; grow in alkaline conditions; motile; ferment carbohydrates; oxidase-positive. The main species of medical importance are *Vibrio cholerae*, *V. parahaemolyticus*, *V. vulnificus* and *V. alginolyticus*.

V. cholerae

Classification

- *V. cholerae* strains are subdivided according to O-antigens. *V. cholerae* O1 is the cause of cholera. Other *V. cholerae* (non-O1) strains may occasionally cause diarrhoea.
- *V. cholerae* O1 has a number of biotypes, including the 'classic' strain, which was the principal cause of cholera until the mid-1960s. The 'El Tor' biotype has been responsible for most cases of cholera over the last two decades. In the 1990s, O139 caused epidemics in Southeast Asia.

Epidemiology

- Found in water contaminated with human faeces; no animal reservoirs;
- Important cause of severe infection in developing countries, where potable water and sewage systems are poor;
- Transmitted via consumption of contaminated food or water.

Morphology and identification

- *V. cholerae* is characterised by an ability to grow in alkaline conditions (pH > 8.0). Alkaline broth is used to grow the microorganism selectively from faecal samples. A special selective medium (thiosulphate–citrate–bile salt–sucrose agar) is also used. *V. cholerae* forms characteristic yellow colonies on this medium.

- Specific slide agglutination reactions for 'O' antigens distinguish *V. cholerae* from non-cholera *Vibrio* spp.
- Biochemical tests are used for confirmation.

Pathogenicity

V. cholerae produces an enterotoxin that acts on intestinal epithelial cells, stimulating adenyl cyclase activity. This results in water and sodium ions passing into the gut lumen to produce profuse, watery diarrhoea (rice-water appearance).

Associated infections

Acute enteritis.

Laboratory diagnosis

Isolation of microorganism from faeces on selective media.

Prevention

Avoidance of contaminated food; oral vaccines suitable for travellers.

Treatment

Rehydration; ciprofloxacin shortens duration of illness.

Non-cholera *vibrio* spp

V. cholerae that do not agglutinate with O1 and O139 antisera are known as non-cholera *Vibrio* spp. These microorganisms may also cause diarrhoea, which is normally much less severe than that from classic cholera. Occasionally they cause severe cellulitis and necrotising fasciitis.

V. parahaemolyticus

V. parahaemolyticus is a cause of food poisoning 12–18 hours after the ingestion of contaminated seafood, particularly oysters. The illness is characterised by vomiting and diarrhoea.

Treatment

By rehydration and a quinolone in severe cases.

12

Treponema, Borrelia and Leptospira

Susan O'Connell
Health Protection Agency Laboratory, Southampton, UK

Spirochaetes

These bacteria, in the order Spirochaetales, are thin $(0.1–0.5 \times 5.0–20.0\,\mu m)$, helical and weakly Gram-negative. *Treponema*, *Borrelia* and *Leptospira* are three genera which cause human diseases (Table 12.1). Laboratory diagnoses are based primarily on serological tests, as few spirochaetes can be cultured readily *in vitro*.

Treponema

Definition

Gram-negative spiral bacteria; motile; non-capsulated; non-sporing; non-culturable *in vitro*.

Classification

Treponema species that cause human disease are *Treponema pallidum* and *T. carateum*. *T. pallidum* subspecies *pallidum* causes syphilis, *T. pallidum* subsp *endemicum* causes bejel (endemic or non-venereal syphilis) and another subspecies, *T. pallidum* subsp *pertenue*, causes yaws. *T. carateum* causes pinta. These treponemes are morphologically and immunologically indistinguishable, but have some genomic differences that may be significant in relation to pathogenicity.

T. pallidum

Morphology and identification

The microorganism is a thin spirochaete, 0.5×10.0 µm, which cannot be grown *in vitro* and grows only slowly *in vivo*. Motile forms can be visualised in clinical specimens by dark field microscopy or with specialised staining.

Associated infection and epidemiology

Syphilis (Chapter 31).

Laboratory diagnosis

Diagnosis is principally based on serology, but microscopy can be useful in early infection.

Microscopy

Primary, secondary and congenital syphilis can be diagnosed by dark field examination for spirochaetes in fresh material from skin lesions or lymph node aspirates.

Medical Microbiology and Infection Lecture Notes, Fifth Edition. Edited by Tom Elliott, Anna Casey, Peter Lambert and Jonathan Sandoe.
© 2011 Blackwell Publishing Ltd. Published 2011 by Blackwell Publishing Ltd.

Table 12.1 Spirochaetes and associated infections

Spirochaete	Associated infections
Treponema	
T. pallidum subsp *pallidum*	Syphilis
T. pallidum subsp *pertenue*	Yaws
T. pallidum subsp *endemicum*	Bejel (endemic non-venereal syphilis)
T. carateum	Pinta
Borrelia	
B. recurrentis	Louse-borne relapsing fever
B. duttoni and others	Tick-borne relapsing fever
B. burgdorferi sensu lato	Lyme borreliosis
Leptospira	
(Several species and serovars)	Flu-like illness; meningitis; uveitis
	Weil's disease (severe multi-system disease)

Serology

Diagnosis of syphilis in most patients is based on two types of serological tests: non-specific and specific treponemal assays:

1 *Non-specific antibody tests* are commonly used, including the Venereal Disease Research Laboratory (VDRL) and rapid plasma reagin (RPR) tests. They can detect the IgM and IgG antibodies that develop against lipids released from *T. pallidum* during early stages of disease. Cardiolipin-cholesterol-lecithin, the antigen used in these assays, was initially extracted from beef heart and is not derived from treponemes, hence these tests are non-specific. False-positive results are common, occurring in the presence of other conditions including viral infections, autoimmune diseases, leprosy, tuberculosis and malaria. Positive results need confirmation by specific serological tests.

   All antibody tests will be negative at the earliest stage of infection. Cardiolipin-based tests may give positive results at a slightly earlier stage than some of the treponema-specific tests, and they are also helpful in assessing treatment response, as titres usually drop significantly and can become negative following satisfactory treatment.

2 *Specific antibody tests* are based on *T. pallidum*-derived antigens. Commonly used tests include syphilis enzyme immunoassays, the fluorescent treponemal antibody (FTA-abs) test and the *T. pallidum* particle or haemagglutination assays (TPPA, TPHA), in which latex particles or erythocytes coated with *T. pallidum* antigens are agglutinated by serum from patients with antibodies to *T. pallidum*. Positive results may reflect previous infection, because residual antibodies can remain after treatment, and can also result from other treponemal infections, e.g. yaws, pinta, as the microorganisms causing these conditions are essentially identical to *T. pallidum*.

   Specific IgM antibody tests are also used to diagnose congenital infections.

3 *Polymerase chain reaction* is being developed for diagnosis.

Treatment

Parenteral penicillin. Detailed guidelines are available for treatment and follow-up of patients and management of their sexual contacts.

T. pallidum subsp *endemicum*

This microorganism causes bejel (endemic syphilis), mainly in children in hot dry climates. Primary lesions occur as mucous patches in the mouth or angular stomatitis. A secondary stage can occur, similar to syphilis. Late infection can cause gummas and affect bone and cartilage.

Spread is by direct contact or shared feeding utensils. Laboratory diagnostic procedures and treatment are as for syphilis.

T. pallidum subsp *pertenue*

T. pertenue causes yaws, which occurs mainly in children in humid tropical regions in Central Africa, South America and the Pacific islands. It is primarily a skin disease; destructive lesions (granulomata) of the skin, lymph nodes and bone can occur.

Spread is by direct contact with infected skin lesions. Laboratory diagnostic procedures and treatment are as for syphilis.

T. carateum

T. carateum causes pinta and is found in remote parts of Central and South America. It occurs in all age groups. After a 1- to 30-week incubation period, small papules develop on the skin. These can enlarge, last for several years and result in hypopigmented lesions. Laboratory diagnosis and treatment are as for syphilis.

Borrelia

Definition

Gram-negative, spiral bacteria; motile; non-capsulated; non-sporing; require specialised media for culture; anaerobic or microaerophilic.

Borrelia species are associated with two important human infections: relapsing fever (primarily *B. recurrentis* and *B. duttoni*), and Lyme borreliosis (*B. burgdorferi* group).

B. recurrentis, B. duttoni and other relapsing fever-associated *Borrelia* species

Associated infections and epidemiology

Relapsing fever occurs worldwide; characterised by episodes of fever and spirochaetaemia, which can cause severe multi-system effects, separated by periods when the patient is apyrexial. The relapsing picture is related to the ability of *Borrelia* species to vary their outer surface protein antigenic structure as many as 30 times, thus evading specific host antibodies for some time:

- Epidemic relapsing fever is caused exclusively by *B. recurrentis* and is spread via human body lice, *Pediculus humanus*. There is no known non-human reservoir host. It is strongly associated with catastrophic events such as war or famine, resulting in overcrowding, poor hygiene and lice infestations. An untreated patient may have a relapse 7–10 days after an initial febrile episode of 3–6 days. The mortality rate in untreated infections can be 40%.
- Endemic relapsing fever is caused by many *Borrelia* species and is spread from rodent reservoir hosts via infected *Ornithodoros* soft ticks during blood meals. Multiple relapses, tending to become shorter and less severe with succeeding episodes, can occur in untreated patients. The mortality of untreated infection is about 5%.

Laboratory diagnosis

Borreliae can be identified in stained blood or buffy coat smears taken when the patient is pyrexial. Serological tests are not readily available.

Treatment

Tetracycline is the treatment of choice.

B. burgdorferi

Epidemiology

At least five genospecies of *B. burgdorferi* sensu lato cause Lyme borreliosis, which occurs mainly in forested areas of the temperate northern hemisphere. Borreliae are transmitted to humans by *Ixodes* hard ticks that have previously fed on infected mammals and birds. About 1,000 cases are reported annually in the UK.

Associated infections

Lyme borreliosis is characterised initially by a skin lesion spreading from the tick bite, but can later involve the nervous system, joints and other tissues following bloodstream spread.

Laboratory diagnosis

Two-stage IgM and IgG antibody tests. Samples giving reactions in a sensitive screening test are assessed for specificity by second-stage immuno-blot, because there is significant risk of false-positive screening results with other infections and autoimmune conditions. Tests can be negative in the first few weeks of infection, but sensitivity in late stage disease is more than 99%.

Borrelial DNA can be detected in skin and synovial fluid/biopsy samples by PCR.

Treatment

Oral doxycycline or amoxicillin; parenteral ceftriaxone for encephalomyelitis.

Prevention

Avoidance of tick bites; early removal of attached ticks.

Leptospira

Definition

Gram-negative, coiled bacteria; non-capsulated; non-sporing; motile; aerobes that grow slowly in enriched media.

Morphology and identification

Leptospires are motile microorganisms with two periplasmic flagella, each anchored at opposite ends of the microorganism. They can be grown on specially defined media enriched with serum, although prolonged incubation may be required.

The genus *Leptospira* has numerous species and intraspecies serovars; only some are pathogenic to human beings, principally the *L. interrogans* serovars Icterohaemorrhagiae, Canicola, Pomona, and *L. borgpetersenii* serovar Hardjo.

Epidemiology

- Occurs worldwide, particularly following periods of high rainfall and flooding;
- More prevalent in tropical and subtropical regions;
- Maintained in nature through chronic renal infection in animals, e.g. rats (serovar Icterohaemorrhagiae), dogs (Canicola), cows (Hardjo) and pigs (Pomona);
- Human infections occur mainly through exposure to water contaminated with infected urine;
- Microorganisms can enter through broken skin, mucous membranes or conjunctiva;
- At-risk groups include sewer workers, farmers and those involved in water sports. About 50 cases/year are notified in the UK.

Associated infections

Leptospirosis ranges from a mild flu-like illness, uveitis and meningitis to the potentially life-threatening Weil's disease, with jaundice and renal damage.

Laboratory diagnosis

Blood or urine can be cultured in specialised media but takes several weeks. Serology using microagglutination (MAT) and other techniques is available from reference laboratories.

Treatment and prevention

- Treatment is with penicillin or doxycycline.
- Rodent control measures help to prevent infection. Groups at risk should be made aware of the illness and appropriate prevention measures.

13

Gram-negative anaerobic bacteria

Peter Lambert
Aston University, Birmingham, UK

The Gram-negative anaerobic bacilli include the genera *Bacteroides*, *Prevotella*, *Porphyromonas*, *Fusobacterium* and *Leptotrichia*. Unlike the Gram-positive anaerobic clostridia, they do not form spores. Gram-negative anaerobes form a major component of the normal flora of humans.

Definition

Gram-negative bacilli; non-motile; non-sporing; strict anaerobes; grow on complex media; some species capsulate.

Bacteroides, *Prevotella* and *Porphyromonas*

The genus *Bacteroides* has undergone major taxonomic revision and now consists of the genera *Bacteroides*, *Prevotella* and *Porphyromonas*. The *Bacteroides* genus contains many species, the most important being *B. fragilis*. *Prevotella* also includes many species, including *Prevotella melaninogenica*, *intermedia* and *nigrescens*. *Porphyromonas* has fewer species, including *P. gingivalis*, which is associated with advanced periodontal disease.

Epidemiology

Species of *Bacteroides* and related genera make up the largest component of the bacterial flora of the human intestine, and are an important part of the normal flora of the mouth and genito-urinary tract. They protect against colonisation and infection by more pathogenic bacteria; they can also cause infections.

Morphology and identification

Occasionally form short filaments. Some species have a polysaccharide capsule. Visible colonies appear only after 48 hours of incubation. Some *Porphyromonas* and *Prevotella* species produce a pigment that results in black colonies.

Associated infections

- *Gastrointestinal*: intra-abdominal abscesses, peritonitis (often in mixed infections with coliforms);

- *Skin and soft tissue*: abscesses and surgical wound infection;
- *Central nervous system*: brain abscesses.

Prevention

Postoperative, intra-abdominal infections can be prevented by good surgical technique and prophylactic antibiotics.

Treatment

Metronidazole and clindamycin are effective antibiotics against almost all Gram-negative anaerobic bacteria; most species are sensitive to penicillin but some, particularly *B. fragilis*, are resistant because of β-lactamase production.

Fusobacterium

Fusobacterium species are spindle-shaped, with pointed ends. They are often nutritionally demanding. The genus is classified into various species, *F. necrophorum* and *F. nucleatum* being the most important in human infections.

Fusobacteria are commensals of the oral cavity. They are one of the causative microorganisms, along with other anaerobes, of acute ulcerative gingivitis (primarily *F. nucleatum*) and other oral infections. *F. necrophorum* may occasionally cause severe sepsis with metastatic abscesses.

Leptotrichia

Leptotrichia species are long, slightly curved bacilli with pointed ends. The genus consists of a single species, *L. buccalis*, which is part of the normal oral flora and may be associated with oral infections such as Vincent's angina.

Gram-negative anaerobic cocci

The role of Gram-negative anaerobic cocci in disease is not clear. However, *Veillonella* spp. are thought to be a component of mixed anaerobic infections. They are commonly found in supragingival dental plaque and have been occasionally implicated in cases of osteomyelitis and endocarditis.

14

Chlamydiaceae, *Rickettsia*, *Coxiella*, Mycoplasmataceae and Anaplasmataceae

Jonathan Sandoe
Leeds Teaching Hospitals NHS Trust and University of Leeds, Leeds, UK

Chlamydiaceae

Definition

Chlamydiaceae are obligate intracellular bacteria with a unique biphasic life cycle.

Classification

The family Chlamydiaceae contains two genera, *Chlamydia* and *Chlamydophila*. The former contains one human pathogen *Chlamydia trachomatis*, the latter includes the pathogens *Chlamydophila psittaci* and *Chlamydophila pneumoniae*. Classification is based on antigens, morphology of intracellular inclusions and disease patterns (Table 14.1). All chlamydiaceae share a common group antigen but may be distinguished by species-specific antigens.

Morphology and identification

Chlamydiaceae have two distinct morphological forms:

1 The elementary body (EB): an infectious extracellular particle (300–400 nm).
2 The reticulate body (RB): an intracellular noninfectious particle (800–1,000 nm).

They multiply in the cytoplasm of host cells after a well-defined developmental cycle:

- EBs bind to specific host cell receptors and enter by endocytosis. Target cells include conjunctival, urethral, rectal and endocervical epithelial cells.
- Intracellular EBs remain within phagosomes and replicate. Lysosomal fusion with the phagosome-

Medical Microbiology and Infection Lecture Notes, Fifth Edition. Edited by Tom Elliott, Anna Casey, Peter Lambert and Jonathan Sandoe.
© 2011 Blackwell Publishing Ltd. Published 2011 by Blackwell Publishing Ltd.

Table 14.1 Classification and common infections of *Chlamydiaceae*

Species	Serotypes	Natural host	Transmission	Common infections
C. trachomatis	A–C	Humans	Hands/eyes/flies	Trachoma, conjunctivitis
C. trachomatis	D–K	Humans	Sexual	Cervicitis, urethritis
			Genito-ocular	Conjunctivitis
			Sexual	Proctitis
			Perinatal	Pneumonia
C. trachomatis	L1, L2, L3	Humans	Sexual	Lymphogranuloma venereum; Genital ulcers
C. psittaci	Many	Birds and some mammals	Aerosol	Pneumonia
C. pneumoniae	1	Humans	Aerosol	Acute respiratory infection

containing EBs is inhibited, probably by chlamydial cell-wall components.

- After about 8 h, EBs become metabolically active and form RBs that synthesise DNA, RNA and protein, utilising host cell adenosine triphosphate (ATP) as an energy source.
- RBs undergo multiple divisions and the phagosome becomes an 'inclusion body' (visible by light microscopy).
- After about 24 h, the RBs reorganise into smaller EBs and, after a further 24–48 h, the host cell lyses and infective EBs are released.

C. trachomatis

Epidemiology

- *C. trachomatis* is the most common cause of sexually transmitted infection in the developed world.
- The majority of *C. trachomatis* infections are genital and sexually acquired.
- Trachoma is the leading cause of preventable blindness in the world.
- Asymptomatic infections can occur in both men and women.
- *C. trachomatis* can be divided into different serotypes ('serovars'): A–C, D–K, and L1, L2 and L3.
- *C. trachomatis* serotypes D–K are found worldwide.
- Lymphogranuloma venereum (LGV) serotypes L1–3 occur primarily in Africa, Asia and South America.

- Eye infections probably result from autoinoculation with infected genital secretions.
- Similarly, neonates can be infected during birth from an infected mother.

Pathogenesis

C. trachomatis gains access via disrupted mucous membranes and can infect mucosal columnar or transitional epithelial cells, resulting in severe inflammation. In LGV, the lymph nodes, which drain the site of the primary infection, are involved.

Associated infections

- *Eye*: 'Trachoma' caused by serotypes A–C; adult inclusion conjunctivitis, a milder disease than trachoma, caused by serotypes D–K and associated with genital infections; neonatal conjunctivitis: *C. trachomatis* can be acquired at birth from an infected mother, associated with serotypes D–K.
- *Respiratory*: Neonatal pneumonitis: usually presents 3–12 weeks after birth; often associated with neonatal conjunctivitis; acquired through maternal transmission during birth.
- *Genitourinary*: LGV is a sexually transmitted infection with genital ulcers and suppurative inguinal adenitis; urethritis and cervicitis are associated with serotypes D–K

Complications include pelvic inflammatory disease and perihepatitis in women, and epididymitis and Reiter's syndrome in men.

Laboratory diagnosis

- Chlamydiaceae do not grow on bacterial culture media.
- Cell culture: swabs from the affected site, collected in a special transport medium, are inoculated into tissue culture. Growth of *C. trachomatis* is recognised by Giemsa staining, showing intracellular bodies, or by immunofluorescence staining with specific antisera. This test is largely confined to specialist laboratories.
- Direct antigen detection can be made by immunofluorescence or enzyme-linked immunosorbent assay (ELISA) methods. Both techniques utilise labelled specific antibodies to *C. trachomatis*.
- Serology: antibodies to *C. trachomatis* may be detected by complement fixation or micro-immunofluorescence tests, but this has limited value because it is difficult to distinguish between past and current infections.
- Nucleic acid amplification tests to detect either chlamydial DNA or RNA, using polymerase chain reaction (PCR) or ligase chain reaction, or chlamydial ribosomal RNA, using transcription-mediated amplification, are now widely used. These are performed on urine and vaginal swabs. They are more sensitive than culture and non-invasive.

Treatment

- *Urogenital infection*: doxycyline or azithromycin;
- *Trachoma*: for individual or sporadic cases, doxycycline (azithromycin for children, breast-feeding or pregnant women). Eyelid deformities may need surgery.
- *Neonatal conjunctivitis*: erythromycin.

C. psittaci

C. psittaci causes infection in birds (e.g. parrots and budgerigars) and domestic animals.

Epidemiology

Transmission to humans is via inhalation, usually of dried bird guano. Pet shop workers, bird fanciers and poultry farm workers are at particular risk of developing psittacosis.

Associated infections

Respiratory: flu-like illness, pneumonia.

Laboratory diagnosis

By serology, including immunofluorescence or complement fixation test. Culture of *C. psittaci* is also possible, but is performed only in laboratories with high-level containment facilities.

Prevention

Treat infected birds; quarantine.

Treatment

A tetracycline (e.g. doxycycline) is the drug of choice; erythromycin is an alternative.

C. pneumoniae

This was originally designated TWAR (Taiwan-associated respiratory disease) agent, but is now called *C. pneumoniae* and is a significant cause of atypical pneumonia.

Infection is spread via direct human contact, with no apparent animal reservoir. It is associated with respiratory infections, including pharyngitis, sinusitis and pneumonia (which can be severe, particularly in elderly people). Diagnosis is by serology for antibodies against *C. pneumoniae* (detection of *C. pneumoniae* DNA by PCR is being developed); treatment includes either a tetracycline or erythromycin.

Rickettsia

Definition

Rickettsiaceae cause a number of important human infections, including typhus and the related spotted fevers.

They are small, Gram-negative bacilli (0.2–1 μm diameter); obligate intracellular pathogens; utilise ATP from host cell; grow only in tissue culture. The genus contains a number of species that cause human infection (Table 14.2).

Epidemiology

Rickettsial infections are zoonoses with a variety of animal reservoirs and insect vectors.

Associated infections

Epidemic or louse-borne typhus, murine typhus, scrub typhus and spotted fevers.

Table 14.2 Vectors and infections associated with *Rickettsia*

Species	Principal host/reservoir	Vector	Disease
R. typhi	Rats	Fleas	Murine typhus
R. prowazekii	Humans/squirrels	Lice	Epidemic or Louse-borne typhus
R. tsutsugamushi	Rats	Mites	Scrub typhus
R. akari	Mice	Mites	Rickettsial pox
R. rickettsii[a]	Dogs	Ticks	Rocky mountain spotted fever

[a]Tick-borne spotted fevers in areas of the world outside the USA carry a variety of names and are caused by Rickettsiae very similar to *R. rickettsii* (e.g. Boutonneuse fever caused by *R. conorrii* occurs in the Mediterranean region).

Laboratory diagnosis

This is by serology. The Weil–Felix test detects cross-reacting antibodies to Rickettsiae, which agglutinate certain strains of *Proteus* (OX-19 and OX-2). The test is non-specific and has now been superseded by more specific serological tests based on purified rickettsial antigens (immunofluorescence assays and ELISA).

Treatment and prevention

Treatment is with tetracycline or chloramphenicol. Infection can be prevented by avoidance of the various vectors. A vaccine to *R. prowazekii* is available.

Coxiella

A pleomorphic coccobacillus with a Gram-negative cell wall (0.4–0.7 μm). Spores are produced prolonging survival. This is an obligate intracellular animal pathogen (commonly cattle, sheep; goats) that occasionally infects humans via tick bites or inhalation of dried, contaminated matter. At-risk groups include farmers, vets and abattoir workers. Urine, faeces, milk and birth products may be a source. Outbreaks can occur.

Coxiella burnetii causes Q-fever (non-specific illness of fever, severe headache, chills, severe malaise, myalgia and later pneumonitis), endocarditis, hepatitis and neurological infections. Contact with animals gives a clue to the diagnosis. Laboratory diagnosis is by serology (complement fixation, ELISA and immunofluorescence tests). Treat with a tetracycline. For endocarditis, treatment is prolonged and valve replacement may be needed. A vaccine is being developed for prevention.

Mycoplasmataceae

Definition

Small (0.15–0.25 μm), Gram-negative microorganisms; pleomorphic with no cell wall; grow slowly on enriched media; aerobic or facultatively anaerobic.

The family Mycoplasmataceae consists of two genera: *Mycoplasma* (69 species) and *Ureaplasma* (2 species). Only a few species have been identified as human pathogens, including: *Mycoplasma pneumoniae*, *M. hominis*, *M. genitalium*, *M. fermentans* and *Ureaplasma urealyticum*.

Epidemiology

M. pneumoniae infection is common worldwide and is an important cause of acute lower respiratory tract infections; epidemics can occur. Immunity to *M. pneumoniae* is short-lived. Infection is spread by respiratory secretions. *M. hominis* and *U. urealyticum* colonise the genitourinary tracts.

Associated infections

- *Respiratory*: pharyngitis; community-acquired pneumonia (*M. pneumoniae*)
- *Central nervous system*: meningitis, encephalitis, transverse myelitis (*M. pneumoniae*)
- *Genitourinary* (debated): urethritis, pelvic inflammatory disease (*U. urealyticum*, *M. hominis*, *M. genitalium*: urethritis)

Laboratory diagnosis

- *Culture*: mycoplasmas and ureaplasmas can be grown on enriched media; penicillin is often added to inhibit other microorganisms. Although *M. pneumoniae* can be isolated from sputum after incubation for up to 3 weeks, diagnosis is normally by serology. *M. hominis* grows after about 4 days, producing colonies with a 'fried egg' appearance. *U. urealyticum* requires urea for growth and forms small colonies.

• *Serology*: *M. pneumoniae* infections can be diagnosed by serological tests (complement fixation test or enzyme immunoassays) for IgG (4-fold rise in titres is indicative of current infection) or IgM.

Treatment

Macrolides (e.g. erythromycin) or tetracycline.

Anaplasmataceae

The family Anaplasmataceae contains two medically important genera of small (0.5 μm) Gram-negative bacteria, *Anaplasma* and *Ehrlichia*. They are obligate intracellular pathogens, usually transmitted via tick bites, which have a tropism (affinity) for monocytes or granulocytes. Infections caused by these microorganisms occur in the distribution of their tick vectors and have been identified in Europe, the Americas, Africa and Asia. Clinical manifestations are usually non-specific with fever, general malaise, headache, myalgia; severe multisystem disease can occur and is more common in immunocompromised patients. Treatment is with a tetracycline.

Basic virology

Peter Mackie
Leeds Teaching Hospitals NHS Trust, Leeds, UK

Virus structure (Figure 15.1)

Size and shape

Electron microscopy (approx. $\times 50,000$ magnification) is the most useful way to determine the shape and size of viral particles. Viruses range in size from 20 to 300 nm in diameter and many have unique shapes that aid identification. All viruses have one of two symmetrical shapes: icosahedral (with two-, three- or five-fold axis of symmetry) or helical.

Genome

Viruses contain either deoxyribonucleic acid (DNA) or ribonucleic acid (RNA). Nucleic acids represent the main component of the virus core and are associated with core proteins. Viral nucleic acids range from 1.5×10^6 daltons (parvoviruses) to 200×10^6 daltons (poxviruses) and may be single stranded or double stranded, circular or linear, a single molecule or in segments, and have positive or negative polarity. Positive sense-RNA is similar to messenger RNA (mRNA) and can be translated by the host cell. Negative sense viral RNA must be converted to positive sense by an RNA polymerase.

Capsid

A protein coat encloses the genome and core proteins, consisting of capsomeres (capsid subunits).

Envelope

Lipid bilayer membrane surrounding the capsid of some viruses (enveloped viruses); the envelope carries glycoproteins, which form projections or spikes. This lipid layer is acquired as the virus buds through the host cell's cytoplasmic membrane.

Virion

This term describes the complete infectious virus particle; in some cases the particles may lack nucleic acids (empty particles) or carry defective genomes (defective particles), which can interfere with normal replication (defective interfering particles).

Virus cultivation

Viruses are obligate intracellular parasites and can therefore replicate only in living cells. Viruses utilise the host cell metabolism to assist in the synthesis of viral nucleic acid, proteins and

Medical Microbiology and Infection Lecture Notes, Fifth Edition. Edited by Tom Elliott, Anna Casey,
Peter Lambert and Jonathan Sandoe.
© 2011 Blackwell Publishing Ltd. Published 2011 by Blackwell Publishing Ltd.

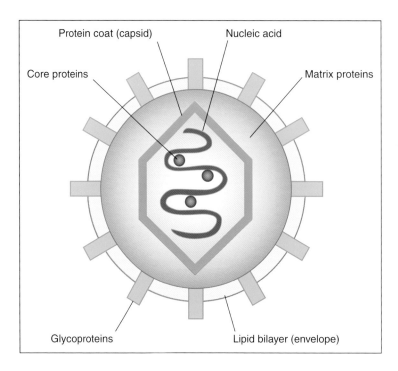

Protein coat (capsid)

Nucleic acid

Core proteins

Matrix proteins

Glycoproteins

Lipid bilayer (envelope)

Figure 15.1 An enveloped virus.

progeny virions. The host cell range of viruses may be narrow or wide. Clinical virologists use three or four different cell lines to isolate medically important viruses in the laboratory.

Many different groups of viruses may be grown in cell cultures. The use of embryonic eggs and laboratory animals for virus culture is reserved for specialised investigations. Cell culture lines for virus cultivation are often derived from tumour tissues, which can be maintained in the laboratory for many years by a process of sub-culturing (continuous cell lines). Cells may also be obtained directly from animal species (e.g. rhesus monkey kidney cells). Such primary cell lines are useful to culture fastidious viruses, but are difficult to maintain and ethical issues have restricted their use.

Virus replication in cell cultures may be detected using a bench-top microscope by observing:

- *Cytopathic effect (CPE)*: some viruses can be recognised by their effect on the appearance of the inoculated cell layer, e.g. necrosis, lysis, 'rounding', 'ballooning' or the formation of multinucleated giant cells (syncitia).
- *Haemadsorption*: viruses expressing haemagglutinins on the cell's surface may be recognised by adsorption of human group 'O' red blood cells. On low power microscopy, clumps of red blood cells can be seen attached to virally infected cells. If no virus is present, then red blood cells remain dispersed in liquid media. This technique is useful if no CPE is observed (e.g. cells infected with influenza viruses do not produce a CPE, but do haemadsorb).
- *Immunofluorescence*: the appearance of virus-encoded proteins on the surface, nucleus, or cytoplasm of infected cells may be detected by immunofluorescence techniques (IFT). IFT utilises antibodies, which have been chemically labelled with a fluorescent dye, that are specific to viral proteins. Examination of cell cultures with a microscope (using an ultraviolet light source) enables visualisation of fluorescing cells to show infection has taken place. If no fluorescing cells are seen, then infection has not taken place.

Cell culture techniques for diagnostic purposes have been used for over 50 years. However, this procedure has largely been replaced in diagnostic laboratories by more rapid and sensitive molecular based technology, such as real-time polymerase chain reaction (PCR) for DNA viruses and reverse-transcription PCR (RT-PCR) for RNA viruses.

Viral infection of host cells

Viral replication in host cells involves the following steps:

1 *Attachment* (or 'adsorption') of the viral capsid (naked viruses) or of envelope components (enveloped viruses) to cell surface molecules (receptors); this involves specific interaction between viral glycoproteins (e.g. the haemagglutinin of influenza virus) and host cell surface components (e.g. *N*-acetylneuraminic acid for influenza virus). Many viruses have highly specific receptors, which limits the range of cell types that can be infected;
2 *Penetration* of the virus into the host cell (often by receptor-mediated endocytosis);
3 *Uncoating* follows, which involves the enzymatic removal of viral protein coat and liberation of nucleic acid and attached core proteins;

4 *Production* of virus-specific mRNA, in order to direct the host cell ribosome to produce viral proteins (core, capsid). The mechanisms for virus-specific mRNA production depend on the viral genome type:
   (a) RNA or DNA;
   (b) single or double stranded;
   (c) positive sense or negative sense.
   Examples are shown in Figure 15.2. The mechanisms for replication of viral nucleic acid also depend on viral genome type; examples are given in Figure 15.3;
5 *Morphogenesis and maturation* occur with assembly of components (nucleic acid and proteins) to form sub-viral particles (pre-core, core particles) and viral particles (virions, empty particles);
6 *Release* of the virus is by bursting of infected cells (lysis) or by budding through the plasma membrane. Lysis results in cell death but budding does not necessarily kill cells, allowing viral particles to be shed for extended periods, e.g. in hepatitis B infection the host cell remains viable

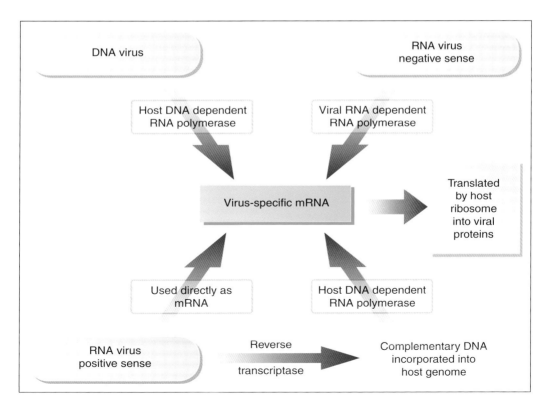

Figure 15.2 Synthesis of virus-specific mRNA.

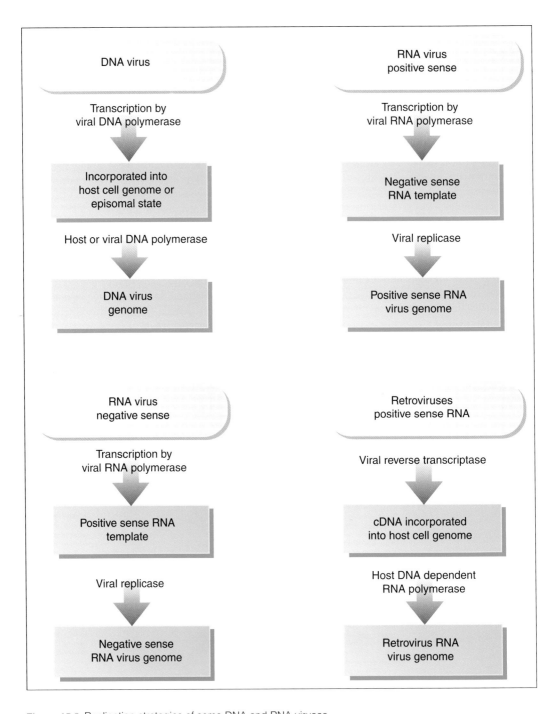

Figure 15.3 Replication strategies of some DNA and RNA viruses.

and continues to release virus particles or subviral antigens at a slow rate. These persistent infections act as a continuing source of new infectious viruses.

During latent infections, the virus does not undergo replication. Viral nucleic acid may remain in the host-cell cytoplasm (e.g. episomal Epstein-Barr virus (EBV) DNA) or become incorporated into the host genome (e.g. human immunodeficiency virus, (HIV)). A trigger is required to activate viral replication, transcription and translation. This trigger is often associated with periods of immunosuppression in the host, e.g. during chemotherapy, organ transplantation, HIV infection or from an inherited disease.

Antiviral drugs are designed to interfere with one or more of the above replication steps (Chapter 22).

Epidemiology

- *Incubation period:* the interval from first acquiring the infection to onset of illness; *Generation time:* average period between infection and transmission of the virus. This period is normally less than the incubation period, as infections are transmitted before the onset of illness (e.g. patients are infectious 48 hrs before a chickenpox rash appears);
- *Transmission of viruses:* two major patterns exist:
  (a) viruses circulate within a single species (e.g. influenza B only within human); and
  (b) viruses that cross the species barrier (e.g. rabies and influenza A viruses).

- *Person-to-person route:* either by horizontal route including respiratory droplets (>2 μm, e.g. respiratory syncitial virus (RSV)), aerosol (<2 μm) produced by coughing and sneezing (e.g. influenza), gastrointestinal (e.g. norovirus); vertical route, such as mother to child transmission (e.g. HIV), placental-foetal (e.g. cytomegalovirus (CMV)), at delivery of new born (e.g. herpes simplex virus (HSV)).

Virus classification

The official taxonomy of viruses is based on four characteristics:

1 Nature of the nucleic acid in the virion;
2 Symmetry of the capsid;
3 Presence or absence of an outer lipid envelope;
4 Dimensions of the virion and capsid.

For convenience viruses can also be classified according to the following:

- Disease or organ system involved (Table 15.1);

Table 15.1 Viral classification according to disease or organ system involved

Organ system involved (disease)	Examples of clinically important viruses
Systemic infections	Measles virus, rubella virus, varicella-zoster virus (VZV), enteroviruses, retroviruses
Central nervous system	Polio- and other enteroviruses; rabies virus, arthropod-borne viruses, herpes simplex virus (HSV), measles virus, mumps virus, retroviruses, cytomegalovirus (CMV)
Respiratory tract (common cold, tracheitis, bronchitis, bronchiolitis, pneumonia)	Influenzavirus, parainfluenzavirus, respiratory syncytial virus (RSV), human metapneumovirus (hMPV), adenovirus, rhinoviruses, (enteroviruses), CMV
Eye (conjunctivitis, retinitis)	HSV, adenovirus, CMV
Skin and mucous membranes (rash, warts)	HSV, papillomavirus, chickenpox virus, measles virus, rubella virus, parvovirus
Liver (hepatitis)	Hepatitis viruses A–E, yellow fever virus, rubella virus, CMV, EBV
Salivary glands	Mumps virus, CMV
Gastrointestinal tract (gastroenteritis)	Rotaviruses, adenoviruses, astroviruses, norovirus, sapoviruses

Note: this classification is clinically oriented and not virus systematic. The same clinical symptoms can be caused by numerous viruses, and one virus can cause different clinical syndromes.

Table 15.2 Classification of virus families according to nucleic acid and virion structure

Nucleic acid type	Symmetry of nucleocapsid	Envelope	Virus family	Example of virus
DNA SS linear	Icosahedral	No	*Parvoviridae*	Human parvovirus
DNA DS circular	Icosahedral	No	*Papovaviridae*	BK virus
DNA DS linear	Icosahedral	No	*Adenoviridae*	adenovirus
DNA DS linear	Icosahedral	Yes	*Herpesviridae*	HSV
DNA DS linear	Complex	Yes	*Poxviridae*	Orf virus
DNA DS circular	Icosahedral	Yes	*Hepadnaviridae*	HBV
RNA SS linear	Icosahedral	No	*Picornaviridae*	Rhinovirus, ECHO (Enteric cytopathic human orphan) virus
RNA SS linear	Icosahedral	No	*Caliciviridae*	norovirus
RNA SS linear	Icosahedral	Yes	*Togaviridae*	Rubella virus
RNA DS	Icosahedral	No	*Reoviridae*	rotavirus
RNA SS	Complex	Yes	*Flaviviridae*	yellow fever virus
RNA SS	Complex	Yes	*Arenaviridae*	Lassa virus
RNA SS	Icosahedral	Yes	*Coronaviridae*	SARS (severe acute respiratory syndrome) virus
RNA SS	Icosahedral	Yes	*Retroviridae*	HIV type 1
RNA SS	Helical	Yes	*Orthomyxoviridae*	influenza A virus
RNA SS	Helical	Yes	*Bunyaviridae*	La Crosse virus
RNA SS	Helical	Yes	*Paramyxoviridae*	RSV

DS, double stranded; SS, single stranded

- Nucleic acid type/virion structure (virus families; Table 15.2);
- Replication strategy (Figure 15.3).

Detection of virus infections

Detection of virus can be direct (detection of all or part of the virus particle) or indirect (detection of a host response to infection, usually specific antibody):

- *Direct detection:* utilises light microscopy (CPE); electron microscopy (visualisation of virions); particle agglutination test (particles coated with virus-specific antibodies are mixed with a clinical sample, e.g. detection of rotavirus in stool extracts); IFT (e.g. detection of RSV in exfoliated respiratory cells); serology (use of antibody to detect viral antigens, (e.g. hepatitis B surface antigen in serum); nucleic acid detection (e.g. real-time PCR and RT-PCR. These are the major diagnostic methods of active viral infections).
- *Indirect detection:* by serology (including complement fixation test, haemagglutination inhibition test, or enzyme-linked immunosorbent assay (ELISA)).

Major virus groups

Peter Mackie
Leeds Teaching Hospitals NHS Trust, Leeds, UK

DNA viruses (Table 16.1)

Table 16.1 Classification of virus families according to nucleic acid and virion structure

CLASSIFICATION OF VIRUS FAMILIES

Nucleic acid type	Symmetry of nucleocapsid	Envelope	Virus family
DNA SS linear	Icosahedral	−	*Parvoviridae*
DNA DS circular	Icosahedral	−	*Papovaviridae*
DNA DS linear	Icosahedral	−	*Adenoviridae*
DNA DS linear	Icosahedral	+	*Herpesviridae*
DNA DS linear	Complex	+	*Poxviridae*
DNA DS circular	Icosahedral	+	*Hepadnaviridae*
RNA SS linear	Icosahedral	−	*Picornaviridae*
RNA SS linear	Icosahedral	−	*Caliciviridae*
RNA SS linear	Icosahedral	+	*Togaviridae*
RNA DS	Icosahedral	−	*Reoviridae*
RNA SS	Complex	+	*Flaviviridae*
RNA SS	Complex	+	*Arenaviridae*
RNA SS	Icosahedral	+	*Coronaviridae*
RNA SS	Icosahedral	+	*Retroviridae*
RNA SS	Helical	+	*Orthomyxoviridae*
RNA SS	Helical	+	*Bunyaviridae*
RNA SS	Helical	+	*Paramyxoviridae*
RNA SS	Helical	+	*Rhabdoviridiae*

DS, double stranded; SS, single stranded; −, absent; +, present.

Medical Microbiology and Infection Lecture Notes, Fifth Edition. Edited by Tom Elliott, Anna Casey, Peter Lambert and Jonathan Sandoe.
© 2011 Blackwell Publishing Ltd. Published 2011 by Blackwell Publishing Ltd.

Herpesviruses

The herpesviruses comprise a large family of enveloped, double-stranded DNA viruses. Following infection, all herpesviruses establish a latent infection that persists for life. Reactivation with the production of progeny virus may occur at intervals and produce recurrent symptoms or signs. The viruses have a comparatively complex genome coding for several enzymes involved in nucleic acid metabolism.

Herpesviruses (Family – *Herpesviridae*) include the following species:

- herpes simplex virus (HSV, type 1 and type 2);
- varicella-zoster virus (VZV);
- cytomegalovirus (CMV);
- Epstein–Barr virus (EBV);
- human herpesviruses (HHV), types 6–8.

Herpes simplex virus (HSV)

Virus

Enveloped DNA viruses, 100–300 nm in diameter. There are two serotypes: HSV-1 and HSV-2, which share 50% nucleic acid sequence identity.

Epidemiology

HSV is distributed worldwide. Antibodies to HSV-1 are acquired early in childhood and 90% of adults show serological evidence of past infection (seropositive). Antibodies to HSV-2 are acquired mainly between 14 and 40 years of age.

Pathogenesis

Spread is by direct contact (sexual activity is the main route of HSV-2 transmission). The incubation period is variable (2–12 days). HSV enters mucosal surfaces or a break in the skin, replicates productively in epithelial cells at the site of inoculation and spreads to adjacent tissue. There are local IgA, IgM and IgG responses, but the virus avoids elimination as its DNA establishes latent infection in sensory ganglia. Reactivation is associated with various stimuli (stress, immunocompromised status or bacterial infection). Infections are either primary or recurrent (by the same type), with the former being clinically more severe.

Associated diseases

- *Skin and soft tissues*: herpes labialis 'cold sores' (HSV-1, less commonly HSV-2), skin lesions;
- *Genitourinary*: herpes genitalis (HSV-2 and HSV-1);
- *Ocular*: kerato-conjunctivitis, retinitis;
- *Respiratory*: pneumonitis;
- *Gastrointestinal*: oesophagitis;
- *Central nervous system*: meningitis (mainly HSV-2), encephalitis (mainly HSV-1, particularly in neonates and immunocompromised patients).

Microbiological diagnosis

- *Swab*: base of a skin/mucosal lesion, place in virus transport medium and test by real-time PCR;
- *Cerebrospinal fluid* (*CSF*): required if encephalitis or meningitis is suspected;
- Older less sensitive diagnostic tests include: electron microscopy of vesicle fluid; direct fluorescent antibody staining of exfoliated cells around vesicular lesions; isolation of virus in cell culture;
- *Serology* (e.g. enzyme-linked immunosorbent assay) is generally not helpful for the diagnosis of these infections.

Treatment

Aciclovir, valaciclovir, famciclovir, foscarnet, cidofovir (Chapter 22)

Varicella-zoster virus (VZV)

Virus

Enveloped DNA virus, 100–300 nm in diameter.

Epidemiology

VZV has a worldwide distribution. Infections are acquired early in childhood and 90% of adults are seropositive. The incidence of chickenpox has fallen dramatically in countries such as the USA, where childhood immunisations include a varicella vaccine.

Pathogenesis

Spread is by respiratory droplets or direct contact with vesicle fluid. The incubation period is 2 weeks with a range of 7–23 days. The virus enters via the respiratory tract, viraemia follows and a generalised rash occurs (chickenpox). Virus then becomes latent in the sensory ganglia; a variety of stimuli (immunosuppression) may result in reactivation with vesicles in various dermatomes (shingles).

Associated diseases

- *Skin and soft tissue*: chickenpox (primary infection); shingles (recurrent infection);
- *Respiratory*: pneumonitis can complicate chickenpox;
- *Central nervous system*: encephalitis can complicate chickenpox;
- *Ocular*: 'shingles' can affect the eye – ophthalmic zoster; retinitis;
- *Foetal*: congenital varicella syndrome;
- *Multiple organs*: Disseminated VZV infection (all body system involvement) can occur in immunocompromised individuals and neonates, with devastating consequences if untreated.

Diagnosis

- *Swab*: skin/mucosal lesion and place in virus transport medium for testing by real-time PCR;
- *CSF*: required if encephalitis or meningitis is suspected;
- *Clotted blood*: VZV IgM for evidence of recent infection, VZV IgG indicates past infection and immunity;
- Less sensitive testing includes electron microscopy of vesicle fluid; direct fluorescent antibody staining of vesicular material; isolation in cell culture.

Treatment

Aciclovir, valaciclovir, famciclovir, foscarnet.

Prevention

- *Passive*: zoster immunoglobulin (ZIG) for protection of contacts with no evidence of past infection (seronegative) and at risk of serious VZV

infection, i.e. pregnant women and immunocompromised patients;
- *Active*: live attenuated vaccine given in early childhood (US) and for healthcare workers in contact with vulnerable patient groups.

Cytomegalovirus (CMV)

Virus

Enveloped DNA virus, 200 nm in diameter.

Epidemiology

CMV has a worldwide distribution. In the developing world 90% of adults are seropositive. In the developed world only 60–70% of adults are CMV seropositive.

Pathogenesis

Spread is by contact with infected urine, secretions (oropharyngeal) and through intrauterine and perinatal transmission (vaginal secretions and breast milk); the virus may also be acquired by blood transfusion, haematopoetic stem cell transplantation or by organ transplantation. The incubation period is 4–8 weeks. The primary infection is often asymptomatic. CMV remains latent in various myeloid cell types and can cause low level persistent infection in salivary glands and kidneys. Recurrent infection in immunocompromised individuals following solid organ or stem cell transplants is common.

Associated diseases

- *Blood*: infectious mononucleosis-like syndrome in immunocompetent patients (fever, pharyngitis, lymphadenopathy);
- *Multiple organs*: disseminated infection occurs in immunocompromised individuals (e.g. transplant recipients, HIV infected patients) leading to pneumonitis, gastritis, hepatitis or retinitis;
- *Foetal*: congenital infections occur in less than 1% pregnancies and are associated with an increased risk of impaired intellectual development and hearing loss.

Diagnosis

- *EDTA-blood and urine*: (whole blood) for CMV DNA by real-time PCR. This will give a result that indicates the viral load (copies/mL) in the sample and can be monitored over time.

- *Other methods include*: isolation in cell culture; serology (IgM for active disease, IgG for immune status and IgG avidity to differentiate recent or past infection). Histopathologists examine tissue biopsy samples by staining for typical intra-nuclear inclusion bodies. ('Owl's eye' inclusion bodies).

Treatment

Ganciclovir, foscarnet and cidofovir (Chapter 22). In immunocompromised patients, frequent monitoring of CMV load by PCR assists in the decision to use antiviral drugs before the disease becomes established (pre-emptive therapy).

Epstein–Barr virus (EBV)

Virus

Enveloped DNA virus, 150–200 nm in diameter.

Epidemiology

EBV has a worldwide distribution. The proportion of the population who are seropositive increases with age, reaching more than 90% in older adults. Two peaks of infection occur: 1–6 and 14–20 years.

Pathogenesis

Spread is by contact with infected saliva; the primary site of infection is the epithelium of the pharynx. B lymphocytes become infected and EBV may lie dormant in these cells. The incubation period is 30–50 days. Atypical monocytes seen in a blood-film ('infectious mononucleosis') are EBV-specific cytotoxic T lymphocytes essential for the control of EBV proliferation in the host.

Associated diseases

- *Blood*: glandular fever syndrome ('infectious mononucleosis'), glandular fever may be complicated by widespread EBV infection in a few patients (hepatitis, myocarditis and meningo-encephalitis).
- *Lymphoid tissue*: EBV is implicated in the pathogenesis of several tumours, including Burkitt's lymphoma, nasopharyngeal carcinoma and post-transplant lympho-proliferative disease (PTLD).

Diagnosis

- *Serum*: detection of EBV specific IgM by enzyme immunoassay; detection of heterophile antibodies ('Paul–Bunnell test' – antibodies that appear early in EBV infection and cross-react with sheep or horse erythrocytes, resulting in agglutination);
- *Peripheral blood smear*: detection of atypical mononuclear cells by microscopy;
- *EDTA-blood*: real-time PCR for EBV specific DNA is useful when an antibody response may not be elicited, e.g. following transplantation or in HIV patients who have a low CD4 cell count. EBV levels should be monitored in immunocompromised patients to assess the risk of PTLD.

Treatment

No effective antiviral treatment available. Rituximab, a monoclonal antibody specific for CD20 on B-lymphocytes has been used to control EBV infections in transplant patients; there is currently no licence for this use in the UK.

Human herpesvirus (HHV) 6 and 7

Viruses

Enveloped DNA viruses, 150–200 nm. The two viruses show 90% DNA sequence homology. HHV-6 isolates are classified into two closely related groups: variants A and B. No disease has been clearly associated with HHV6-A.

Epidemiology

Worldwide distribution with initial infection occurring early in childhood; 90% of children are seropositive for HHV6 by 2 years of age and for HHV7 by 5 years of age.

Pathogenesis

Infection can result from direct contact with saliva, via blood products and via organ transplantation. Viruses infect mainly T lymphocytes where they establish latent infection. Other cell targets include macrophages, natural killer cells and astrocytes.

Associated disease

- *Skin and soft tissues*: roseola infantum (exanthem subitum);
- *Central nervous system*: febrile convulsions in infants and young children meningitis, encephalitis;

- *Gastrointestinal*: hepatitis in immunocompromised patients;
- *Respiratory*: pneumonitis can occur in immunocompromised patients, particularly haemopoietic stem cell (HSCT) transplant recipients.

Diagnosis

- *EDTA-blood*: detection of virus specific DNA by real-time PCR. Results are given as a viral load, e.g. 3,000 copies/ml, which can be monitored for rise or fall in levels over time.

Treatment

Antipyretics are often used in symptomatic children. Antiviral drugs are not indicated for immunocompetent patients.

Ganciclovir, foscarnet and cidofovir have been used in immunocompromised patients.

Human herpesvirus (HHV) 8

Virus

Enveloped DNA virus 150–200 nm.

Epidemiology

This virus is endemic in Africa and some parts of Italy, Greece, Spain and Brazil. The prevalence is more than 40% in adults. Higher rates are seen in cohorts of men who have sex with men (MSM) in the developed world and in association with HIV infection.

Pathogenesis

Transmission in endemic areas is through close contact with infected saliva. In non-endemic areas, sexual transmission is important. Accidental transmission from receiving infected blood products and after organ transplantation also occurs.

Associated disease

- *Skin and soft tissue*: Kaposi's sarcoma, rare forms of B-cell lymphomas seen in association with HIV infection (body cavity-associated lymphoma, Castleman's disease).

Diagnosis

- *EDTA-blood*: detection of virus specific DNA by real-time PCR;

- *Serum*: serology, detection of antibodies by IFT and EIA.

Treatment

No established antiviral treatment.

Adenoviruses

Virus

Non-enveloped double-stranded DNA virus, 70–100 nm in diameter. There are 51 human adenovirus serotypes.

Epidemiology

Adenoviruses are endemic worldwide. Infection is spread either by the faecal-oral route, inhalation of respiratory droplets and aerosols or by direct inoculation of virus from contaminated fingers into the eye. Epidemics have been observed among closed communities, such as boarding schools and military recruits. Frequent infection occurs in transplant recipients. These infections arise because of a damaged immune system permitting unrestricted viral replication, which results in disseminated infections.

Pathogenesis

The incubation period is 2–15 days. Receptors for adenoviruses are found on a wide range of cell types and vary between serotypes. Some serotypes are more invasive than others. For example, adenovirus types 40 and 41 are associated only with gastroenteritis (Chapter 28), whilst other species are associated with urinary tract infections and types 8, 19 and 37 with eye infections.

Associated diseases

- *Respiratory tract*: pharyngitis, pharyngoconjunctival fever, pneumonia (infants, young children and military recruits);
- *Ocular*: conjunctivitis;
- *Gastrointestinal*: gastroenteritis in infants and young children;
- *Genitourinary*: haemorrhagic cystitis;
- *Multiple organs*: common/severe in transplant recipients.

Diagnosis

- *EDTA-blood*: detection of virus specific DNA by real-time PCR;
- *Throat swabs*: in virus transport medium for investigation of acute infection by real-time PCR;
- *Eye swabs*: for diagnosis of 'red eye' conjunctivitis, this may occur in small outbreaks;
- *Faeces*: 1 g faecal fluid for PCR;
- *Urine*: 1 mL in sterile container for PCR.

Other less sensitive laboratory methods include: adenovirus isolation in cell culture; direct detection of viral antigen in respiratory secretions by immunofluorescence (nasopharyngeal aspirate (NPA) required) or in stool samples by EIA; detection by electron microscopy (faeces and urine); detection of viral antibody by serology (e.g. complement fixation test).

Treatment

Mainly symptomatic care in otherwise healthy patients

Cidofovir is used in immunocompromised patients who may be susceptible to life-threatening disseminated infections.

Parvoviruses

Virus

Small, round, non-enveloped DNA viruses of diameter 18–25 nm; single serotype: human parvovirus B19 or erythrovirus.

Epidemiology

Parvoviruses are endemic worldwide. Infection is common in children aged between 4 and 10 years. About 40% of children are seropositive by the age of 15 years. In the elderly, more than 90% have detectable antibodies to parvovirus, indicating past exposure and often asymptomatic infection.

Pathogenesis

The incubation period is up to 17 days. Transmission is by respiratory secretions and blood products. The virus replicates in rapidly dividing erythroid progenitor cells.

Associated diseases

- *Skin and soft tissues*: erythema infectiosum or fifth disease is characterised by fever, chills and myalgia, followed by a maculopapular rash at around 17 days.
- *Musculoskeletal*: arthropathy is more common in adults, particularly women.
- *Blood*: aplastic crisis can occur in patients with chronic haemolytic anaemias (e.g. thalassaemia, spherocytosis). Chronic infection can cause pure red cell aplasia in immunocompromised patients.
- *Foetal*: hydrops foetalis, spontaneous abortions and intrauterine death may result from infections in pregnancy.

Diagnosis

- *Clotted blood*: EIA to detect parvovirus specific IgM indicating recent infection or specific IgG for evidence of past infection and subsequent immunity;
- *EDTA-blood*: real-time PCR to detect parvovirus DNA in peripheral blood PCR is a more appropriate test than serology for immunocompromised patients.

RNA viruses (Table 16.1)

Influenza viruses

Virus

Enveloped single-stranded RNA virus of 80–120 nm diameter; segmented genome (8 segments); there are 3 types, A, B and C, determined by the nucleoprotein; type A infects humans and animals, whereas types B and C infect humans only. The envelope contains two glycoproteins: haemagglutinin (HA), which attaches the virus to cellular receptors and neuraminidase (NA), which mediates the release of newly formed viruses from infected cells. Variations in HA and NA determine subtypes (in humans: H1, H2, H3, N1, N2). Nomenclature is based on type, origin, strain, year of isolation and subtype e.g.:

A/PR/8/34/H1N1

Type	Host	Origin	Strain No.	Year	Subtype
A	Human	Puerto Rico	8	1934	H1N1

Epidemiology

Antigenic variation ('drift' and 'shift') is an important factor in global epidemiology:

* *Antigenic 'drift'*: minor antigenic changes in HA and NA as a result of sequential point mutations (affects types A, B and C).
* *Antigenic 'shift'*: major antigenic changes occur in HA and NA as a result of genetic reassortment with animal viruses (affects type A only).

Antigenic drift leads to frequent epidemics, while antigenic shift results in a change in subtype and leads to pandemics.

Pathogenesis and immune response

Spread by respiratory droplets and aerosols; infects the upper respiratory tract; incubation period of 1–4 days; antibody in serum (IgM) and secretions (IgA) appears about day 6. HA is an important virulence determinant.

Associated disease

* *Upper respiratory tract*: influenza C causes mild respiratory illness mainly in children, otitis media;
* *Lower respiratory tract*: primary viral pneumonia, secondary bacterial pneumonia;
* *Central nervous system*: Reye's syndrome, encephalitis.

Diagnosis

* *Combined throat and nasal swab*: for reverse transcription PCR (RT-PCR), but virus isolation in tissue culture or embryonated eggs is still used in reference laboratories; antigen detection by immunofluorescence (requires NPA) or EIA; point-of-care tests utilising immunochromatography; or,

* *Clotted blood*: serology (complement fixation test, haemagglutination inhibition test).

Treatment

For patients at risk of severe influenza infection, use oseltamivir or zanamivir (Chapter 22). It is important to determine whether currently circulating strains of influenza A are susceptible to these agents. Resistance to oseltamivir has been seen frequently in recent epidemics.

Prevention

Inactivated trivalent vaccines have an efficacy of 60–80%, provided that vaccine components and current wild-type viruses are sufficiently similar. The constituents of the vaccine are reviewed each year and include two of the most recent influenza A strains and one influenza B strain (hence trivalent). Antiviral prophylaxis is used to limit the spread of infection in certain situations (e.g. to reduce the transmission of a new pandemic strain when vaccine is not available).

Paramyxoviruses

Virus

Spherical or pleomorphic enveloped RNA viruses, 150–300 nm in diameter, non-segmented genome.

> **BOX 16.1 The four genera included in the *Paramyxoviridae* family**
>
> **Pneumovius** (respiratory syncytial virus [RSV]; metapneumovirus).
>
> **Paramyxoviruses** (parainfluenzaviruses types 1–4).
>
> **Rubulavirus** (mumps virus).
>
> **Morbillivirus** (measles virus).

Respiratory syncytial virus (RSV)

Virus

Two major serotypes: A and B.

Epidemiology

RSV has a worldwide distribution; seasonal activity during winter months in temperate climates and throughout the year in warmer climates. Infects more than 50% of infants aged less than 1 year, and by 3 years of age all children have experienced an RSV infection.

Pathogenesis

Transmission is via respiratory droplets or fomites; incubation period 2–8 days; infects epithelium of upper respiratory tract and then spreads to lower respiratory tract, causing bronchiolitis. IgA, IgG and IgM responses are not protective against recurrent infections and IgE may play a role in the pathogenesis of disease.

Associated diseases

- *Lower respiratory tract*: bronchiolitis. Complications include pneumonia, exacerbation of asthma. Severe disease occurs in pre-term infants, infants with underlying pulmonary or cardiac disease and all immunocompromised patients.

Diagnosis

- *Nasopharyngeal aspirate or combined throat and nasal swabs*: detection of viral RNA by reverse transcriptase real-time PCR (RT-PCR); isolation in cell culture; antigen detection by immunofluorescence (requires nasopharyngeal aspirate) or EIA; point-of-care tests utilising immunochromatography or serology (complement fixation test).

Treatment

Generally symptomatic care.
  Aerosolised ribavirin can be used for infants and adults at risk of severe RSV infection (e.g. RSV infection recently following an allogeneic haematopoetic stem cell transplant).

Prevention

Palivizumab is an RSV specific humanised mouse monoclonal antibody indicated for use in children at risk of life-threatening RSV infection. Monthly injections are required during the annual RSV epidemic period. Recipients of palivizumab are normally premature infants with chronic lung disease. Attempts to develop an RSV vaccine have so far been unsuccessful.

Parainfluenza viruses

Virus

Four serotypes.

Epidemiology

Type 3 causes annual epidemics during spring and summer, type 1 bi-annual outbreaks during winter. Fifty per cent of infants are infected by 1 year of age.

Pathogenesis

Transmission is by respiratory droplets and fomites; incubation period around 2–8 days. Replication occurs in nasopharyngeal epithelium followed by spread to tracheobronchial tree. Humoral immune response is not protective and recurrent infections are common.

Associated diseases

- *Upper respiratory tract*: croup, otitis media;
- *Lower respiratory tract*: bronchiolitis, pneumonia. Severe disease occurs in immunocompromised children and adults.

Diagnosis

- *Nasopharyngeal aspirate or combined throat and nasal swab*: detection of viral specific RNA by RT-PCR; isolation in cell culture; antigen detection by immunofluorescence (requires NPA)

Treatment

Symptomatic; aerosolised ribavirin in severely immunocompromised patients.

Prevention

No vaccine available.

Measles virus

Virus

Single serotype.

Epidemiology

Measles virus has worldwide distribution, but prevalence is low where uptake of MMR vaccination is more than 85%. Infections depend on the state of immunity and size of the population. Rapid epidemics occur when the virus is introduced into isolated, susceptible communities.

Pathogenesis

Transmission is via large droplets and aerosol; incubation period 10–12 days to prodromal symptoms and 10–21 days to appearance of rash. Infection starts in epithelium of upper respiratory tract followed by replication in local draining lymph nodes, spreads to viscera and skin via the blood. IgA, IgG and IgM responses lead to life-long immunity.

Associated diseases

- *Upper respiratory tract*: characterised by a febrile illness with a rash and pharyngitis, conjunctivitis, otitis media;
- *Lower respiratory tract*: complications include severe pneumonia;
- *Central nervous system*: encephalitis, subacute sclerosing panencephalitis (SSPE).

Severity of illness increases in adults and immunocompromised patients.

Diagnosis

- *Clotted blood*: detection of measles specific IgM;
- *Nasopharyngeal aspirate*: measles RT-PCR;
- *CSF*: for measles IgG levels (SSPE) and RT-PCR to detect current infection.

Treatment

Symptomatic care

Prevention

Live attenuated virus vaccine (part of MMR) is used in the childhood immunisation schedule. The vaccine is more than 95% effective after 2 doses. The first immunisation is given at the age of 15 months (to avoid failure as a result of the presence of maternal measles antibody); earlier administration is given in developing countries, because of the high measles mortality rate in children less than 1 year old. A second MMR vaccine should be given prior to the start of school aged 5 years (UK).

Mumps

Virus

Single serotype.

Epidemiology

Mumps virus has a worldwide distribution. High incidence in children between 4 and 10 years of age; peak activity between January and May in temperate climates.

Pathogenesis

Transmission is via large droplets and fomites; incubation period 16–18 days. Infection starts in the epithelium of upper respiratory tract followed by replication in local draining lymph nodes and spread to viscera by blood. IgA, IgG and IgM responses lead to life-long immunity.

Associated diseases

- *Upper respiratory tract*: characterised by a febrile illness, with upper respiratory tract symptoms and swollen parotid salivary glands;
- *Endocrine organs*: pancreatitis, oophoritis, orchitis;
- *Central nervous system*: meningitis, encephalitis, which can result in deafness.

Diagnosis

- *Clotted blood*: detection of mumps specific IgM by EIA.

Treatment

Symptomatic care.

Prevention

Live attenuated virus vaccine is available as the monovalent form (mumps only), or in combination with the rubella and measles vaccine (MMR). See measles section for timing of vaccine.

Rhinoviruses

Viruses

Members of the *Picornaviridae* family of viruses. Icosahedral, non-enveloped RNA viruses 28–30 nm in diameter.

The picornavirus families are a diverse group of human pathogens, including the enteroviruses and rhinoviruses. There are more than 100 serotypes of human rhinoviruses, divided in to 3 groups: A, B and C.

Epidemiology

Rhinoviruses are endemic worldwide. In temperate climates, two peaks of infection are documented in autumn and early spring.

Pathogenesis

Transmission is by inhalation of droplets and aerosols containing virus or by exposure to the virus in respiratory secretions during close contact. The incubation period is 2–4 days. Replication takes place in the nasal mucosa, with the release of several pro-inflammatory cytokines, leading to characteristic symptoms of the common cold.

Associated disease

- *Upper respiratory tract*: cause of the common cold syndrome (30–60% of cases, Chapter 25). Complications: acute otitis media, severe respiratory illness in infants with bronchopulmonary dysplasia and immunocompromised patients, exacerbation of asthma;
- *Lower respiratory tract*: recent evidence suggests that group C rhinoviruses are associated with more serious lower respiratory tract infections

Diagnosis

- *Nasopharyngeal aspirate or combined throat and nasal swabs*: detection of rhinovirus specific RNA by RT-PCR; isolation in cell culture

Treatment

Symptomatic care.

Coronaviruses

Virus

Enveloped RNA viruses 120 nm in diameter.

Surface projections look like a crown under electron microscopy, hence the name – coronaviruses. Three major strains: human coronaviruses (HCoV) 229E and OC43 and severe acute respiratory syndrome coronavirus (SARS-CoV).

Epidemiology

HCoV have a worldwide distribution and infections occur throughout the year, affecting all age groups equally. A SARS-CoV epidemic started in 2002 in southern China, from where it spread to Hong Kong, Vietnam, Singapore, Canada, Taiwan, Thailand and other parts of the world. The epidemic ended in 2003, affecting 8,500 patients (95% in Asia) with a mortality rate of 9.5%.

Pathogenesis

The incubation period is 2–5 days for HCoV and 2–10 days for SARS-CoV. Transmission is by respiratory droplets, aerosols and possible faecal-oral route for SARS-CoV. Replication takes place in the epithelial cells of the respiratory tract and gut with development of strain-specific antibody. Asymptomatic shedding in faeces is common.

Associated infection

- *Upper respiratory tract*: common cold syndrome: HCoV is responsible for 25% of cases;
- *Lower respiratory tract*: pneumonia;
- *Gastrointestinal tract*: diarrhoea.

Diagnosis

- *Throat and combined nasal swab*: real-time RT-PCR, growth in cell culture, electron microscopy;
- *Clotted blood*: serology (IFA, EIA and immunoblot).

Treatment

Symptomatic care.

Control

No specific vaccine.

Enteroviruses

Viruses

> **BOX 16.2 Genera include:**
>
> **Polioviruses** (types 1, 2, 3)
> **Coxsackie A viruses** 23 types, (types 1–22, 24)
> **Coxsackie B viruses** 6 types, (types 1–6)
> **Echoviruses** 31 types, (types 1–9, 11-27, 29-33)
> **Enteroviruses** 4 types, (types 68–71).

Members of *the Picornaviridae* family of viruses. cosahedral, non-enveloped RNA viruses, 28–30 nm in diameter
  Enteroviruses include five genera (Box 16.2).

Epidemiology

Enteroviruses have worldwide distribution. Infections occur in infancy in developing countries and in early childhood in developed countries.

Pathogenesis

The incubation period is from 2–40 days; normal habitat and primary site of replication are the upper respiratory tract and intestinal tract (hence 'enteroviruses'; followed by viraemia and infection of target organs, i.e. CNS (brain, meninges and spinal cord) or muscle tissue (heart, skeletal muscle) and skin. Long-lasting local IgA and humoral IgM/IgG response develops after natural infection. Transmission is primarily via faecal-oral route.

Associated diseases

- *Upper respiratory tract*: pharyngitis, herpangina, 'hand, foot and mouth disease', conjunctivitis;
- *Central nervous system*: poliomyelitis, aseptic meningitis, encephalitis;

- *Heart*: myocarditis, pericarditis;
- *Neonate*: severe systemic infection.

Diagnosis

- *Throat swab, and/or faeces and/or CSF*: detection of specific RNA by RT-PCR; isolation in cell culture. Serology is generally not helpful.

Prevention and control

Both live (Sabin) and killed (Salk) vaccines are available and used successfully by the World Health Organization (WHO) in its poliomyelitis eradication programme. Only four countries in the world are NOT free of poliomyelitis. The inactivated vaccine has been used in the UK since 2006.

Treatment

Symptomatic care.

Rubella virus (Chapter 40)

Virus

Enveloped RNA virus, diameter 60 nm with a single serotype.

Epidemiology

Rubella virus has worldwide distribution. Prior to the introduction of MMR vaccination, rubella was a frequent childhood infection. In the developing world, 25% of women of child-bearing age are susceptible to rubella.

Pathogenesis

Transmission is by large droplets. The incubation period is 13–20 days. Primary replication occurs in epithelial cells of the upper respiratory tract and the cervical lymph nodes followed by a viraemic phase. The rash coincides with the appearance of serum antibody. Lifelong immunity follows natural infection. Primary infection during the first 12 weeks of pregnancy often leads to generalised foetal infection and congenital rubella syndrome (cataracts, deafness, cardiac abnormalities, hepatosplenomegaly, purpura or jaundice).

Associated disease

- *Upper respiratory tract*: rubella is usually characterised by a mild illness with upper respiratory
tract symptoms, rash, lymphadenopathy and
transient arthralgia;
- *Central nervous system*: encephalitis, post-
infectious encephalopathy;
- *Neonates*: congenital rubella syndrome if infection occurs in first 12 weeks of pregnancy.

Diagnosis

- *Clotted blood*: for acute infection, specific IgM
antibody is determined by EIA; specific IgG indicates current immune status (e.g. ante-natal
screening);
- *Foetal blood*: to detect evidence of intrauterine infection by RT-PCR and cell culture (see
Chapter 40 for further details).

Treatment

Symptomatic care.

Proven infection during the first 3 months of
pregnancy is an indication for therapeutic abortion.

Human normal immunoglobulin in cases of
persistent infection in immunocompromised
patients.

Prevention and control

Live attenuated MMR vaccine is used. Immunisation programmes exist in most developed countries. Women found to have no rubella antibodies
in their ante-natal screening blood, should receive
MMR immunisation after the delivery of the baby
(post-partum).

Rotaviruses

Virus

RNA virus, 75 nm in diameter with wheel-like
structure. Segmented genome (11 segments).

Five groups (A–E), and within group A at least
two subgroups (I, II) and various serotypes (including G and P types); G1–G4 viruses cause over
90% of human infections.

Epidemiology

Rotaviruses occur worldwide with different serotypes co-circulating, usually affecting children of
less than 2 years, with a winter peak in temperate
climates.

Pathogenesis

Infection is via the faecal-oral route, with an incubation period of 1–2 days. Virus replication occurs
in the epithelium of the small intestine and results
in the release of large numbers of particles in
human faeces (1×10^{11} particles/gram). There are
local (IgA) and humoral (IgM/IgG) serotype-spe-
cific and cross-reactive immune responses, which
confer limited protective immunity.

Associated disease

- *Gastrointestinal*: self-limiting diarrhoea and vomiting lasting 4–7 days; mild-to-severe dehydration can occur (depending on strain). In resource
poor countries, there is a significant infant mortality rate associated with these infections.

Diagnosis

- *Faeces*: clarified faecal extract is tested by an
antigen (virus protein) capture assay; reverse-
transcription PCR; point-of-care-tests based on
immunochromatography.

Treatment

Rehydration with oral rehydration fluid.

Prevention and control

Increased personal and water hygiene helps control
outbreaks. Rotavirus vaccine is now universally
used as part of the childhood schedule in the USA.

Norovirus and sapoviruses

Viruses

Small non-enveloped RNA viruses, diameter
27–35 nm.

Members of the *Caliciviridae* family, which show a characteristic cup-shaped depression on surface of particle when viewed by electron microscopy.

Epidemiology

Noroviruses and sapoviruses have a worldwide distribution. Outbreaks occur year round but more frequently during winter months in temperate climates. Outbreaks associated with contaminated water supplies and food. More than 30% of children are seropositive by 3 years of age, and more than 80% are seropositive in early adulthood. Norovirus infections are the most common cause of gastroenteritis outbreaks in hospitals and also often associated with homes for the care of the elderly. Such outbreaks result in ward closures and restrict hospital admission during the busiest winter months.

Pathogenesis

Transmission by faecal-oral route, possibly aerosol due to projectile vomiting; incubation period is 16–48 h. Virus replication takes place in epithelial cells of the villi of the small intestine. Norovirus infection does not confer lasting protective immunity, because of frequent mutation in the virus.

Associated diseases

- *Gastrointestinal*: gastroenteritis characterised by projectile vomiting and diarrhoea lasting for 12–60 h.

Diagnosis

- Detection in stool by electron microscopy, EIA and RT-PCR.

Treatment

Symptomatic care.

Prevention

No vaccine available. Strict source isolation of infected patients is required to limit nosocomial infections.

Hepatitis viruses (includes DNA and RNA viruses) (Chapter 29)

Hepatitis A virus (HAV)

Virus

Member of *Picornaviridae* family of viruses, genus *Hepatovirus*. Small non-enveloped RNA virus 28–32 nm (previously enterovirus 72); only one serotype.

Epidemiology

Most infections in endemic areas (developing world) occur before 5 years of age and the majority are asymptomatic. In the developed world, most clinical cases occur in adults. Common source outbreaks result from contamination of drinking water and food. Infections acquired frequently by travellers from non-endemic to endemic areas. Antibody prevalence in young adults is 30–60%, higher in lower socioeconomic groups.

Pathogenesis

Transmission is via the faecal-oral route. The incubation period is 2–6 weeks (mean 30 days). All age groups are susceptible to hepatitis A infection and disease severity increases with age. In most cases, there is complete recovery and a specific antibody response persists lifelong. There is no chronic disease or carrier state.

Associated disease

- *Liver*: Acute hepatitis.

Diagnosis

- *Clotted blood*: serology (EIA), testing for specific HAV IgM (acute infection) or IgG (immune status);
- *EDTA-blood*: reverse-transcription PCR is carried out at a few reference laboratories to confirm difficult to interpret serology results.

Treatment

Symptomatic care.

Prevention

A killed HAV vaccine is available and recommended for high risk groups.

Hepatitis B virus (HBV)

Virus

Member of the *Hepadnaviridae* family of viruses. DNA virus, 42 nm in diameter, consisting of:

- Core: DNA, partially circular genome;
- Nucleocapsid (hepatitis B core antigen, HBcAg); 'e' antigen (HBeAg) is a cleavage product of the core antigen found on infected cells or free in serum;
- Envelope (hepatitis B surface antigen, HBsAg);
- Also exists as 22 nm spherical or filamentous particle consisting of hepatitis B surface antigen, HBsAg.

Epidemiology

Hepatitis B virus has a worldwide distribution, with more than 360 million carriers (prevalence in north and mid-Europe and North America 0.1–0.5%; southern Europe 2–5%; Africa and Southeast Asia 6–20%).

Pathogenesis

- Transmission is via exposure to blood and blood products containing the virus, by sexual intercourse and vertically at birth (this is the main route of transmission in Asia and Africa);
- Incubation period of 6 weeks–6 months;
- Viral replication in liver results in lysis of hepatocytes by cytotoxic T cells in those who mount an effective immune response;
- Hepatic damage is reversed in 8–12 weeks in ≥90% cases; 2–10% become chronic carriers (persistence of HBsAg for >6 months);
- 95% of newborns of carrier mothers become carriers if untreated;
- The four phases of chronic infection include:
  - immune tolerance (usually infections acquired at birth);
  - immune clearance (many patients clear HBe antigen and covert to HBe antibody positivity);
  - inactive carrier (HBe antibody positive with low levels of virus present in blood);
  - hBeAg-negative chronic hepatitis B (HBe antigen negative, HBe antibody positive & HBV DNA detected).

Not all patients go through each of the four phases.

Associated diseases

- *Liver*: acute, chronic carrier or rarely fulminant (rapidly progressive, with liver failure); cirrhosis; hepatocellular carcinoma.

Diagnosis

- *Clotted blood*: serological tests are made by immunoassays detecting HBsAg, HBeAg and antibodies to HBcAg (IgM and IgG), anti-HBeAg and anti-HBsAg;
- *EDTA-blood*: for quantitative nucleic acid detection to determine viral load and genotype assessment.

Prevention

HBV vaccines and/or HBV immunoglobulin (HBIG) for post-exposure prophylaxis and babies born to carrier mothers.

Treatment

Lamivudine, adefovir, entecavir, telbivudine, clevudine and tenofovir.

Hepatitis C virus (HCV)

Virus

RNA virus, 40–50 nm in diameter; Member of the *Flaviviridae* family of viruses.

There are six main genotypes, which respond differently to antiviral treatment.

Epidemiology

HCV occurs worldwide. Antibody prevalence varies between less than 1% in the USA and Western Europe and 2% in southern Italy, Spain and central Europe. Higher prevalence rates, up to 20%, are detected in Egypt. There is high prevalence of infection among injecting drug users in most parts of the world.

Associated diseases

- *Liver*: HCV has a similar pathogenesis to HBV; infections are followed by chronic hepatitis in 60–80% of cases; cirrhosis, hepatocellular carcinoma.

Diagnosis

- *Clotted blood*: serology by EIA to detect HCV antibodies, antigens and by RT-PCR;
- *EDTA-blood*: to determine genotype and viral load.

Prevention

Since 1991, routine testing of all blood and organ donors for HCV antibody has been undertaken, to prevent transmission by transfusion or transplantation.

Treatment

Pegylated interferon-α, ribavirin.

Delta agent ('hepatitis D virus', HDV)

Virus

Defective RNA virus; 36 nm in diameter, which replicates only in HBV-infected cells.

Epidemiology

Worldwide distribution; high prevalence in the Mediterranean area, Africa, South America, Japan and the Middle East.

It has similar transmission and affects the same risk groups to HBV.

Associated disease

- *Liver*: infections are either a co-infection with HBV or a superinfection of chronic HBV infection leading to aggravation of HBV disease.

Diagnosis

- *Clotted blood*: serology (EIA) can be used to detect HDV antibody and HDV antigen; nucleic acid detection methods are available in hepatitis reference facilities.

Prevention

HBV vaccination and subsequent immunity to HBV reduces the risk of acquiring the delta agent.

Hepatitis E virus (HEV)

Virus

Non-enveloped, positive-strand RNA virus, it represents the only species in the *Hepeviridae* family. There are 4 known genotypes that infect certain mammals including man.

Epidemiology

Endemic in Indian subcontinent, Southeast Asia, Middle East, North Africa and Central America.

Common source outbreaks caused by contaminated water or food are common. In developed countries, sporadic cases are detected among travellers returning from endemic areas. More recently strains (genotypes 3 and 4) of hepatitis E have been detected in domestic animals in industrialized countries and are implicated in zoonotic infections.

Pathogenesis

Transmission by the faecal-oral route and rarely by blood transfusion in endemic countries

Incubation period is up to 6 weeks. Specific IgG and IgM antibodies are produced.

Associated diseases

- *Liver*: acute self-limiting hepatitis with no evidence of chronic infection;
- High mortality rate (10–20%) in pregnant women has been observed in India.

Diagnosis

- *Clotted blood*: serology (detection of IgG and IgM antibodies by EIA); nucleic acid detection in reference laboratories.

Treatment

Symptomatic care.

Prevention

Vaccine under development.

Human retroviruses

Human immunodeficiency virus (HIV) (Chapter 41)

Virus

A member of the *Lentivirinae* subfamily of the *Retroviridae* family. Enveloped RNA viruses with 100–150 nm in diameter virion.

Replicates through DNA intermediates utilising the RNA-directed DNA polymerase (reverse transcriptase)

There are two types: HIV-1 and HIV-2 (40% sequence homology). HIV-1 is divided into three groups: M (11 subtypes A–K), and O and N groups. Group M subtypes include 95% of the global virus isolates and have worldwide distribution, whereas groups O and N are confined to parts of West and Central Africa. Generally HIV isolates, even from a single individual, show a high level of variation. The term quasi-species is used to describe this pool of diverse and changing viruses present in an individual.

Epidemiology

There has been worldwide spread of HIV since 1981. Estimates of prevalence worldwide vary greatly. By the end of 2010, 60 million people worldwide were estimated to be living with HIV (25 million in Africa and 7.5 million in Asia); 20 million people have died of HIV since the epidemic started in 1981.

The main risk groups for HIV infection are:

- men who have sex with men (MSM);
- intravenous drug users;
- people with haemophilia and blood transfusion recipients before 1985;
- sexually promiscuous individuals;
- children born to HIV-infected mothers;
- heterosexual contacts of HIV-infected individuals.

Pathogenesis and immune response

Transmission is mainly through sexual intercourse, via blood or blood products or from mother to child during delivery and/or breast feeding. HIV directly infects and kills cells that are essential for an effective immune response. The virus attaches to the cellular receptor CD4 and chemokine coreceptor CCR5 or CXCR4. By infecting the key cells of the adaptive immune response, this explains the main clinical feature of disease as being profound immune suppression. This results in early impairment of various CD4-cell functions followed by a decrease in CD4-cell numbers. A humoral antibody response against most HIV-specific proteins develops. In later stages, deficiency of both the humoral and the cellular immune responses leads to the development of AIDS.

Associated diseases

- *Immune system*: Acquired immunodeficiency syndrome (AIDS) is characterised by severe disease resulting from generalised infections with bacteria including: mycobacteria, viruses (e.g. HSV, CMV and VZV), fungi (e.g. *Pneumocystis, Candida, Aspergillus and Cryptococcus*),

protozoa including *Toxoplasma* and with associated tumours (Kaposi's sarcoma, lymphomas).

Diagnosis

- *Clotted blood*: detection of HIV-specific antibody and antigen by passive particle agglutination tests (PPAT), fourth generation EIA and western blotting (WB).
- *EDTA-blood*: molecular techniques for detecting HIV, quantifying viral load; typing and drug resistance genotyping have become a significant part of patient diagnosis and clinical management.

Treatment

Five classes of drugs are available:

1. nucleoside reverse transcriptase inhibitors (e.g. zidovudine, lamivudine);
2. non-nucleoside reverse transcriptase inhibitors (e.g. nevarapine and delavirdine);
3. protease inhibitors (e.g. indinavir, atazanavir);
4. fusion inhibitors (enfuvirtide);
5. integration inhibitors (raltegravir).

A combination of three drugs (highly active antiretroviral therapy or HAART) is the accepted standard form of treatment. Antiretroviral drug resistance is a continuing problem and patients require follow-up to monitor HIV load and CD4 counts.

Prevention and control

- There is no antiviral cure.
- No effective vaccine has been developed; there are problems as a result of viral variability, latency and evasion to immune response.
- Testing of all blood and organ donors prevents transmission from those sources.
- Information campaigns, needle exchange programmes and condom use.
- Post-exposure prophylaxis with HAART is recommended after sexual exposure or exposure in healthcare settings.

Human T-cell lymphotropic viruses (HTLV-I and HTLV-II)

Virus

Members of the delta-retroviruses genus of the *Retroviridae* family.

The RNA genome is less variable than that of HIV; HTLV-II shows 60–70% sequence homology with HTLV-I.

Epidemiology

HTLV-I is endemic in Japan, the Caribbean, Melanesia, part of sub-Saharan Africa and Brazil. HTLV-II is endemic among Native American Indians in North, Central and South America. A high proportion of intravenous drug users in North America are seropositive.

Pathogenesis

Transmission is by blood exposure, sexual intercourse and from mother to child through breast-feeding. HTLV-I can immortalise T lymphocytes *in vitro* and can transactivate T cells *in vivo*, but no oncogenes have been identified. No similar characteristics have been proved for HTLV-II. Most infected individuals remain asymptomatic carriers for life. Only 2–4% of infected people develop adult T-cell leukemia and lymphoma (ATLL) after many decades of infection. HTLV-I can invade the CNS and the resulting inflammatory immune response is responsible for the pathogenesis of HTLV-associated myopathy (HAM).

Associated diseases

- *Blood*: adult T-cell leukemia and lymphoma;
- *Central nervous system*: HTLV-associated myopathy;
- *Eye*: uveitis.

Diagnosis

- *Clotted blood*: detection of HTLV-I-specific antibody is made by EIA, particle agglutination assays and western blotting;
- *EDTA-blood*: nucleic acid detection methods.

Prevention and control

Testing of all blood donors is undertaken in countries, such as the USA and the UK.

Treatment

No antiviral drugs are available.

Human papillomavirus (HPV)

Virus

Non-enveloped DNA virus, 55 nm in diameter with over 100 genotypes recognised.

Epidemiology

HPV occurs worldwide.

Pathogenesis

Transmission is by close direct contact, sexual intercourse and perinatal transmission through the birth canal. Infects and replicates in squamous epithelium on both keratinised and mucosal surfaces. Infection results in persistent and latent infection, which can result in malignant transformation.

Associated disease

- *Skin and soft tissue*: warts (e.g. plantar warts) and other skin conditions (epidermodysplasia verruciformis), genital warts (e.g. condyloma acuminata) and cervical, penile and anal carcinoma; laryngeal papillomatosis in young children.

Diagnosis

- *Genital swabs and biopsy samples*: real-time PCR for limited number of high risk genotypes.

Therapy

Suspicious areas of dysplasia are subject to surgery or cauterisation or cryotherapy and laser therapy; interferon, imiquimod and podophyllum are indicated for the treatment of genital warts.

Prevention

Two HPV vaccines are currently available against HPV-16 and -18. These HPV types can cause cervical and other types of genital cancer. The current strategy in economically developed countries is to immunise younger women prior to the age of sexual activity. Prevenar 13 has now superseded Prevanar 7.

Rabies virus

Virus

Member of the *Rhabdoviridae* family

It is a bullet-shaped RNA virus (75–180 nm). Several genotypes (include classic rabies, European, Australian bat rabies and rare African genotypes). All known to cause disease in humans, but the most common source is classic rabies.

Epidemiology

Rabies virus has a wide animal reservoir (e.g. foxes, skunks, racoons, bats) and is enzootic in terrestrial mammal species worldwide. Some parts of the world are considered free from rabies, i.e. Ireland, New Zealand. The UK used to be free from rabies but recently three isolations of bat rabies were made, including a fatal case in a Scottish bat conservationist. Human infections occur mostly in Asia, Africa and South America and dogs are the cause of more than 90% of these infections.

Pathogenesis

Infection mainly occurs through the bite of a rabid animal and rarely after corneal transplant from infected patients. Incubation period can be as short as 4 days to 19 years, but is generally 20–90 days. Multiplication takes place in muscle cells and at neuromuscular junctions. The virus migrates along peripheral nerves to the CNS. Replication in the CNS (mainly basal ganglia, pons, and medulla) causes nerve cell destruction and inclusion bodies (Negri bodies). Finally, migration occurs from the CNS along peripheral nerves to different tissues, including peripheral nerves, skeletal and cardiac muscles and salivary glands.

Associated disease

- *Central nervous system*: paraesthesiae; anxiety; hydrophobia; paralysis; coma. Mortality rate is 100%.

Diagnosis

- *Clotted blood and CSF*: detection of virus specific RNA by RT-PCR; serology (rabies antibodies in blood and CSF);
- *Animal brain*: investigated at specialist veterinary reference laboratory using histological and molecular procedures;
- *Hair follicles*: detection of viral antigens by immunofluorescence,

Therapy and control

Pre-exposure prophylaxis: immunisation of at-risk groups (veterinary personnel, laboratory workers, travellers to endemic areas) – 3 doses (0, 7, 28 days) of rabies vaccine followed by a booster dose 1 year later.

Post-exposure prophylaxis: 5 doses of vaccine (0, 3, 7, 14, 28 days), plus 1 dose of rabies immunoglobulin.

Spread can be controlled by quarantine of animals in the UK and immunisation of domestic animals, such as dogs and cats in endemic areas.

Basic mycology and classification of fungi

Elizabeth Johnson
Health Protection Agency Mycology Reference Laboratory, Bristol, UK

Characteristics

Fungi are eukaryotic microorganisms, distinct from plants in not containing chlorophyll and are classified in a kingdom of their own. Fungi have macroscopic fruiting bodies (mushrooms and toadstools) or are microscopic (moulds and yeasts). Although many fungi are capable of causing disease in a sufficiently immunocompromised patient, only a few species cause human disease on a regular basis. Fungi are non-motile; they may grow as single cells (yeasts) or multi-septate, branching filamentous hyphae. An intertwined network of hyphae is a mycelium.

Classification

The classification of fungi is based largely on their method of sexual reproduction. Those that do not reproduce sexually were previously referred to as 'fungi imperfecti'. Those that reproduce sexually may be self-fertile or require strains of an opposite type to allow sexual fusion to occur. The fungi that cause human disease can be broadly split into yeasts, moulds or dimorphic fungi, which have both yeast and mould forms, depending on growth temperature (Table 17.1).

Fungal infections

Fungal infections can be divided clinically into three groups: superficial, sub-cutaneous and deep mycoses. Most deep mycoses are opportunist infections occurring in immunocompromised patients. Tables 17.2 and 17.3 outline some superficial and deep mycoses, respectively.

Laboratory diagnosis

- *Direct microscopy* of clinical material from deep or superficial sites; the characteristic morphology of fungal elements facilitates identification.
- *Culture*: fungi can be grown on most routine media, but may require prolonged incubation. Antibiotic-containing selective media (e.g. Sabouraud's glucose agar), which inhibit bacterial growth, are often used. Incubation at both 37°C and 28°C facilitates the isolation of common filamentous fungi and yeasts.

Medical Microbiology and Infection Lecture Notes, Fifth Edition. Edited by Tom Elliott, Anna Casey, Peter Lambert and Jonathan Sandoe.
© 2011 Blackwell Publishing Ltd. Published 2011 by Blackwell Publishing Ltd.

Table 17.1 Groups of fungi that cause human disease

Group	Comment	Examples
Yeasts	Have round or oval cells that multiply by budding or grow predominantly as yeasts that bud; but may also form pseudohyphae or even true hyphae in some species	*Cryptococcus neoformans* *Candida albicans*
Filamentous fungi	Grow as hyphae and produce a mycelium; produce asexual spores (conidia or sporangiospores), which may be single or multi-celled. Conidia can be produced in long chains on aerial hyphae (conidiophores), as wet masses on phialides (a conidiogenous cell that produces conidia without increasing in length) or as budding aleuriospores (a spore produced as a result of the expanding of the ends of conidiophores or hyphae).	*Aspergillus* spp. *Fusarium* spp. *Trichophyton* spp.
	Sporangiospores are produced in sporangia on aerial hyphae known as sporangiophores	*Rhizopus* spp. *Mucor* spp.
Dimorphic fungi	Have two forms of growth: filamentous at 28 °C (saprophytic phase) and yeast like at 37 °C (parasitic phase)	*Blastomyces, Histoplasma capsulatum, Penicillium marneffei*

- *Serology*: serological tests both for antibody and antigen detection are available for the diagnosis of some fungal infections (e.g. cryptococcosis, candidiasis and aspergillosis), but these may lack specificity and sensitivity. Testing for beta-glucan has a good negative predictive value.

Examples of fungal pathogens

Cryptococcus

- *C. neoformans, C. grubii* and *C. gattii* are encapsulated yeasts that cause cryptococcal meningitis. The first two are found worldwide, whilst *C. gattii* is associated with Eucalyptus and is most common in Australia and parts of Africa. Their natural habitat is soil, particularly soil contaminated with pigeon droppings, which due to the presence of high molecular weight nitrogenous compounds, act as a natural selective medium.

- *Cryptococcal species* have polysaccharide capsules that can be visualised in clinical specimens, such as cerebrospinal fluid, by mixing the fluid with Indian ink. They can be isolated from sputum, bronchoalveolar lavage fluid, tissue biopsies and other clinical specimens, or the capsular antigen can be detected by sensitive and specific latex agglutination tests on CSF or serum.

Table 17.2 Superficial mycoses

Fungi	Type of fungus	Principal infections	Epidemiology
Candida albicans	Yeast	Oral thrush, vaginitis, cutaneous candidiasis Worldwide	
Dermatophytes *Epidermophyton* *Microsporum* *Trichophyton*	Filamentous	Tinea (ringworm) of skin, nail and hair	Worldwide
Malassezia furfur	Yeast	Pityriasis versicolor	Worldwide, most common in the tropics

Table 17.3 Deep mycoses

Fungi	Type of fungus	Principal infections	Epidemiology
Aspergillus fumigatus	Filamentous	Lung infection, disseminated aspergillosis	Worldwide
Candida albicans	Yeast	Oesophagitis, endocarditis, candidaemia with disseminated candidiasis	Worldwide
Cryptococcus neoformans	Yeast	Meningitis	Worldwide
Histoplasma capsulatum	Dimorphic	Lung infection	USA
Coccidioides immitis	Dimorphic	Lung infection	Central/South America
Blastomyces dermatidis	Dimorphic	Lung infection	Africa, America
Paracoccidioides brasiliensis	Dimorphic	Lung infection	South America
Rhizopus arrhizus	Filamentous	Rhinocerebral infection, lung infection, (zygomycosis or mucormycosis)	Worldwide disseminated infection
Fusarium	Filamentous	Lung, sinus, fungaemia	Worldwide
Scedosporium	Filamentous	Lung, disseminated	Worldwide

- Infection is thought to be acquired by inhalation of yeast cells, which become desiccated and are blown on air currents. Human infections are rare; most occur in immunocompromised individuals, including those with HIV.
- Primary infection occurs in the lungs and is usually asymptomatic. Acute pneumonia may occur with fungaemia and infection in various organs, particularly the brain and meninges. Treatment of cryptococcal meningitis is with amphotericin and flucytosine in combination, followed by fluconazole.

Candida

- The genus *Candida* contains a large number of species, about eight of which are regularly found causing infection. *C. albicans* remains the most frequently isolated pathogen, although infection with *C. glabrata* appears to be increasing and *C. parapsilosis* and *C. tropicalis* are also frequently encountered. *C. albicans* is a commensal of the mouth and gastrointestinal tract.
- Superficial *Candida* infections are common and include vaginal and oral candidiasis (thrush), skin and nail infections, which can arise in warm, moist areas such as skin folds or because hands are immersed in water for long periods, and as a

complication of antibiotic therapy that temporarily reduces the bacterial flora.
- Invasive *Candida* infections usually arise from the patients own commensal flora following surgery, use of broad spectrum antibiotics or intravascular catheters and can affect any organ of the body. Candidaemia may result in abscesses in various organs (e.g. brain, liver, spleen). These infections occur primarily in immunocompromised patients. Endophthalmitis is another potential consequence of candidaemia.
- *Candida* can also colonise prosthetic materials, e.g. intravascular catheters and peritoneal dialysis catheters, resulting in bloodstream infection and peritonitis, respectively. *Candida* spp. are a rare cause of endocarditis.

Laboratory diagnosis

By direct microscopy of appropriate clinical material for oval Gram-positive cells, some of which may be budding or producing pseudohyphae (a string of elongated cells produced as a result of budding in some yeasts); culture; and serology for *Candida* antibodies or antigen in patients with deep-seated infections. Budding yeast and pseudomycelia (a mycelium-like mass of pseudohyphae) may also be seen with appropriate stains in histopathological specimens.

Treatment

Topical with an azole, nystatin or amphotericin; parenteral therapy is with fluconazole, flucytosine, itraconazole, voriconazole, posaconazole, caspofungin, anidulafungin, micafungin or amphotericin B.

Malassezia species

- *M. furfur* is part of the normal human flora. In skin scrapings, it can be seen as yeast cells, which bud on a broad base and short, unbranched curved hyphae.
- It causes pityriasis versicolor, a superficial scaly skin infection with depigmentation.
- *Malassezia* spp. are yeasts, which can also cause deep infections, *M. pachydermatis* for example causes infection particularly in neonates receiving parenteral nutrition.

Diagnosis

By microscopy of skin scales showing yeast cells or from blood culture onto a lipid rich medium.

Treatment

Topical or oral with azole antifungals.

Aspergillus

- The genus *Aspergillus* contains a number of species, including *A. fumigatus* species complex (the most frequent human pathogens) and *A. niger*.
- It is a common saprophyte worldwide, frequently found in soil and dust. Outbreaks of aspergillosis in immunocompromised patients have occurred because of construction work adjacent to hospitals, which can result in the release of large numbers of spores.
- *A. niger* is common cause of otitis externa.
- *A. fumigatus* infections are acquired by inhalation of spores (conidia) (Figure 17.1), resulting in diffuse lung infection in immunocompromised patients or, occasionally, a large mycelial mass (aspergilloma), which can develop in pre-existing lung cavities.
- Infection can also spread to other sites, including adjacent blood vessels and sinuses, or become disseminated to the liver, kidneys and brain (Figure 17.2). The fungus also causes chronic infections of the external auditory canal.

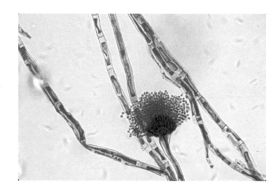

Figure 17.1 Microscopy of fruiting body (conidiophore) of *Aspergillus fumigatus* stained with lactophenol cotton blue.

- *Aspergillus* infections are most frequent in immunosuppressed patients, e.g. patients with leukaemia, solid organ or stem cell transplant recipients and patients with AIDS.
- *Aspergillus* is also associated with allergic alveolitis, which occurs in atopic patients with recurrent exposure to aspergillus spores; symptoms include fever, cough and bronchospasm.
- Patients with cystic fibrosis are frequently colonised with *Aspergillus* species, which may develop into acute bronchopulmonary aspergillosis (ABPA) or more invasive disease.

Laboratory diagnosis

Direct microscopic examination of appropriate samples for branching septate, hyphae; culture (Figure 17.3); serology, although antibody

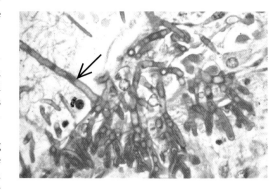

Figure 17.2 Invasive *Aspergillus* hyphae in brain tissue

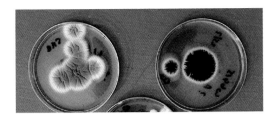

Figure 17.3 *Aspergillus fumigatus* (left) on Sabouraud's agar. Strains produce green colonies with white periphery. *Aspergillus niger* (right) demonstrating dense black colonies with white periphery.

detection is of limited value in immunocompromised patients, antigen detection for galactomannan or β-glucan may be useful and *Aspergillus*-specific PCR for the detection of circulating genomic fragments is helpful in some patients. *Aspergillus* may also be seen in histopathological specimens and is the gold standard confirmation of infection.

Treatment

Amphotericin B, itraconazole, voriconazole, posaconazole or echinocandins.

Dermatophytes

The dermatophytes are a group of related filamentous fungi, also referred to as the ringworm fungi, which infect the keratinised tissues; skin, hair and

nails. Three clinically important genera have been described (Table 17.4) (Figures 17.4 and 17.5).

Epidemiology

The natural habitat is humans, animals or soil; human infection results from spread from any of these reservoirs. Dermatophyte infections are found worldwide, with different species predominating in various climates.

Laboratory diagnosis

- Skin scrapings, hair or nail clippings from active lesions are examined microscopically in 20–30% potassium hydroxide on a glass slide; the presence of hyphae confirms the diagnosis. Optical brighteners, such as calcofluor or blankophor, can enhance the detection of fungal elements when viewed under a fluorescence microscope. Occasionally, the dermatophyte species can be identified by typical morphology.
- Samples can be cultured on Sabouraud's medium at 28 °C. Subsequent species identification is based on growth rate, colony appearance and microscopic morphology.
- Infected hair may fluoresce under ultraviolet light (Wood's light) and is characteristic of certain infections, e.g. *Microsporum canis*.

Treatment

Depends on the site and severity of infection. Options include topical imidazoles (e.g. clotrimazole,

---

Table 17.4 **Clinically important genera of dermatophytes**

Genera	Infection
Epidermophyton	*E. floccosum*, the only species. It infects the skin (tinea corporis), nails (tinea unguium), groin (tinea cruris) and feet (tinea pedis) (Plate 36)
Microsporum	*M. audouini* causes epidemic ringworm of the scalp (tinea capitis) in children. *M. canis*, which predominantly affects cats and dogs, occasionally causes ringworm in children
Trichophyton	*T. mentagrophytes* var. *interdigitale* is the most common cause of tinea pedis
	T. rubrum causes severe recurrent skin and nail infections *T. violaceum* is a common cause of tinea capitis in Asian subcontinents, North America and the West Indies
	T. tonsurans is an increasingly common cause of scalp ringworm, especially in the Afro-Caribbean population

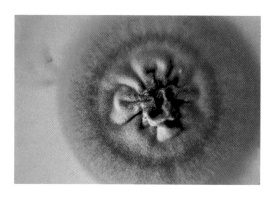

Figure 17.4 Colony of *Epidermophyton floccosum* illustrating its undulating surface.

miconazole); oral griseofulvin, itraconazole, fluconazole or terbinafine.

Mucormycosis

The term 'mucormycosis' (or 'zygomycosis') refers to infections caused by a variety of filamentous fungi, most of which are currently classified in the sub-phylum *mucoromycotina*. Medically important species include *Rhizopus arrhizus* and *Lichtheimia corymbifera* (previously *Absidia corymbifera*).

Epidemiology

Mucoraceous fungi are found worldwide, in soil and decaying organic matter. Infections occur primarily in uncontrolled diabetic or immuno-compromised individuals following inhalation of spores, but wound infections are also seen. As with *Aspergillus*, hospital outbreaks of infection

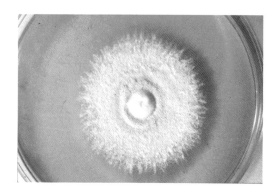

Figure 17.5 Colony of *Trichophyton mentagraphytes* illustrating its powdery white surface.

have occurred in association with building work or contaminated fomites.

Risk factors

Diabetes mellitus, burns, neutropenia.

Infection

- *Pulmonary*: an often fatal infection of immuno-compromised patients may result in disseminated infection (e.g. brain, liver, gastrointestinal tract).
- *Rhinocerebral*: an infection of the nasal sinuses may spread rapidly to involve the face, orbit and brain. It occurs particularly in uncontrolled diabetes mellitus and is often fatal if treatment is delayed.
- Necrotic tissue from burns.

Laboratory diagnosis

Microscopy and culture of appropriate specimens are undertaken (including tissue from necrotic lesions, sputum, bronchoalveolar lavage (BAL)). On microscopic examination, this group of fungi are characterised by the formation of broad, ribbon-like, hyphae with few septae and are fast growing in culture often filling all the air-space inside petri dishes. Tissue should not be homogenised, as this will decrease the chances of isolation of viable fungi.

Treatment

Amphotericin B, especially higher doses of lipid formulations and posaconazole, plus urgent débridement of necrotic tissue in rhinocerebral infection and stabilisation of underlying predisposing factors.

Fusarium and *Scedosporium* species

Environmental fungi found as plant pathogens or in polluted water, usually acquired by inhalation or aspiration of polluted water:

- Infection with *Fusarium* species is predominantly seen in neutropenic patients and mimics invasive aspergillosis. Skin lesions occur in 60–70% of infected patients.
- *Scedosporium* species can infect otherwise healthy individuals following aspiration of

polluted water during near-drowning accidents, also infects neutropenic individuals.
- Infection with either is primarily pulmonary but can become disseminated.

Laboratory diagnosis

Microscopy and culture of appropriate specimens. Blood culture is often positive in *Fusarium* infection. Identification in culture depends on examination of the form of spores and spore production. Branching, septate hyphae resemble those of *Aspergillus.*

Treatment

Voriconazole, posaconazole.

Coccidioides immitis and *C. posadasii*

C. immitis and *C. posadasii* are closely related dimorphic fungi found in the soil in hot arid areas of southwest USA, and Central and South America.

Infection

This follows inhalation of arthrospores (a spore produced by fragmentation of a hypha at the septum) and is often subclinical. A mild, self-limiting pneumonia (Valley fever), often accompanied by a maculopapular rash, occurs in some patients. Severe progressive disseminated disease (e.g. meningitis, osteomyelitis) may occur, principally in immunosuppressed patients. Pulmonary infection may occur in AIDS patients who have lived in or travelled through endemic regions but otherwise healthy individuals are also at risk.

Laboratory diagnosis

Direct microscopy for the presence of endospore-containing spherules and culture of appropriate specimens (this is classified as a higher-risk pathogen and culture should be attempted only in specialised centres because of the risk of infection); serology (e.g. complement fixation and immuno-precipitation) for IgM and IgG antibodies is available at specialist laboratories.

Treatment

Amphotericin, itraconazole and fluconazole.

Blastomyces dermatitidis

B. dermatitidis is a dimorphic fungus found in the soil in North and South America, and Africa. Humans are probably infected by inhalation.

Infections

Primary pulmonary infection may be complicated by haematogenous spread to involve the skin (granulomatous ulcers), bone and joints, brain and other organs.

Laboratory diagnosis

Microscopy and culture of appropriate specimens are undertaken in specialised containment facilities. As this fungus is dimorphic, yeast cells are seen in samples from infected patients and at high temperatures (37 °C) *in vitro*, whilst a mycelial form is found in the environment and when cultured at lower temperatures. Serology is available at specialist laboratories, but is of limited value.

Treatment

Amphotericin B or itraconazole.

Histoplasma capsulatum

H. capsulatum is a dimorphic fungus found world-wide, but infections occur most commonly in North, Central and South America. The natural habitat is soil, particularly in sites enriched with bird or bat droppings (e.g. caves).

Infections

Infection is acquired by inhalation of conidia, which germinate in the lung to produce budding yeast cells. Pulmonary infection is normally self-limiting, but chronic pulmonary disease with cavitations (similar to tuberculosis) may occur in patients with underlying lung disease. Disseminated histoplasmosis (liver, bone, brain, skin) may occur, particularly in immunocompromised patients.

Laboratory diagnosis

Microscopy of stained blood films or histological sections of tissue (oval yeast forms seen within mononuclear phagocytes); culture, using specialised containment facilities. As this fungus is dimorphic, yeast cells are seen in samples from infected patients and at high temperatures (37 °C) *in vitro*, whilst a mycelial form is found in the environment and when cultured at lower temperatures; serology (e.g. complement fixation test).

Treatment

Amphotericin, itraconazole or fluconazole.

Paracoccidioides brasiliensis

A high risk pathogen, which is a dimorphic fungus found in the soil in Central and South America. *P. brasiliensis* causes pulmonary infection and mucocutaneous lesions, including ulceration of the mucous membranes of the nasal and oral pharynx, which may progress to destruction of the palate and nasal septum. Disseminated infections occur with haematogenous spread to various sites, including the spleen, liver, bone and brain.

Laboratory diagnosis

Direct microscopy of pus, sputum or tissue biopsy; culture; serology (e.g. immunodiffusion test for precipitating antibodies).

Treatment

Itraconazole, or amphotericin plus sulphadiazine.

Pneumocystis jirovecii (previously named *P. carinii*)

Classification

A unicellular fungus; forms endospores and cysts.

Epidemiology

Worldwide distribution; transmission is probably by inhalation, but understanding of the epidemiology is incomplete. One theory suggests that *P. jirovecii* colonises the lungs of many individuals and infection in immunocompromised individuals represents reactivation. Extrapulmonary infection at other sites occurs rarely.

Clinical conditions

Opportunist lung infection is seen in immunocompromised individuals and severely malnourished children; extra-pulmonary infections occur rarely (e.g. heart, liver, kidneys and eyes). In HIV infection, risk of pneumonia increases if CD4 cell count is less than 200 mm^3.

Diagnosis

By direct examination of bronchial biopsies, washings or bronchoalveolar aspirates or open lung biopsies. Cysts are identified by induced sputum, histopathological stains or specific fluorescein-labelled antibodies.

Treatment

Co-trimoxazole.

Prevention

Prophylaxis required for certain immunocompromised patients (e.g. AIDS patients, after transplantation); use of co-trimoxazole or nebulised pentamidine.

Parasitology: protozoa

Peter Chiodini
The Hospital for Tropical Diseases and The London School of Hygiene and Tropical Medicine,
London, UK

Classification

Parasites include:

1 *Protozoa*: unicellular eukaryotic microorganisms;
2 *Helminths*: multicellular microorganisms with organ systems.

Protozoa

Classification

Protozoa are classified into four groups according to their structure (Tables 18.1 and 18.2).

Amoebae

Classification

Many amoebae are human commensals (e.g. *Entamoeba coli* and *Endolimax nana*). *Entamoeba histolytica* is an important human pathogen. Some free-living amoebae, e.g. *Naegleria fowleri* and *Acanthamoeba* species, are opportunistic human pathogens.

Structure/physiology

Amoebae are unicellular microorganisms, with a simple two-stage life cycle:

1 *Trophozoite*: actively motile pleomorphic feeding stage;
2 *Cyst*: infective stage.

Division occurs by binary fission of the trophozoite or production of multiple trophozoites in a multinucleated cyst. Amoebae are motile via the formation of pseudopods. Cyst formation occurs under adverse conditions.

Entamoeba histolytica

Epidemiology

E. histolytica has worldwide distribution, primarily in subtropical and tropical regions. Infected cases (symptomatic or asymptomatic carriers) act as a reservoir. Spread is usually via water or food contaminated with cysts, and occasionally via oral-anal sex.

Pathogenesis

Cysts are ingested and gastric acid promotes release of the trophozoite in the small intestine. Trophozoites multiply and may cause necrosis and ulceration in the large intestine. Invasion through the gut wall into

Medical Microbiology and Infection Lecture Notes, Fifth Edition. Edited by Tom Elliott, Anna Casey, Peter Lambert and Jonathan Sandoe.

Table 18.1 Classification of medically important parasites

Subkingdom	Associated organisms
Protozoa	Amoebae
	Ciliates
	Sporozoa
	Flagellates
Helminths	Nematodes (roundworms)
	Cestodes (tapeworms)
	Trematodes (flukes)

the peritoneal cavity, and bloodstream spread to other organs (primarily the liver) may occur.

Clinical manifestations

Intestinal amoebiasis, ranging from mild diarrhoea (often bloody) to severe colitis with systemic symptoms. Chronic infection can mimic inflammatory bowel disease (intermittent diarrhoea with abdominal pain and weight loss). Liver abscesses and, less commonly, lung and brain abscesses are found.

Laboratory diagnosis

Microscopy of freshly passed stools for the presence of trophozoites. Cysts may not be seen in acute dysentery. Multiple stool specimens should be examined. For cyst passers, it is important to distinguish cysts of *E. histolytica* from those of non-pathogenic amoebae. Serological tests (e.g. indirect fluorescent antibody test (IFAT)) are the diagnostic method of choice for amoebic liver abscess. Serology is also helpful in the diagnosis of amoebic dysentery, but is less valuable in endemic areas, because antibodies persist for months or years. Serology is almost always positive in amoebic liver abscesses.

Treatment

Intestinal amoebiasis and hepatic amoebiasis are treated with metronidazole. Asymptomatic carriage may be treated with diloxanide.

Table 18.2 Medically important protozoa

Microorganism	Principal infections
Amoebae	
Entamoeba histolytica	Dysentery; invades intestine, with ulceration; may spread to other organs, including liver and lungs
Naegleria	Amoebic meningoencephalitis
Acanthamoeba	Granulomatous amoebic encephalitis
Ciliates	
Balatidium coli	Diarrhoea
Sporozoa	
Cryptosporidium species	Diarrhoea
Isospora belli	Diarrhoea
Toxoplasma gondii	Glandular fever syndrome
	Congenital infections, with central nervous system defects; encephalitis in immunocompromised individuals
Plasmodium species	Malaria
Flagellates	
Giardia intestinalis	Diarrhoea; malabsorption
Trichomonas vaginalis	Urogenital infections
Trypanosoma species	Sleeping sickness; Chagas disease
Leishmania species	Visceral leishmaniasis
	Cutaneous leishmaniasis

Prevention

Stop food and water contamination with human faeces. Chlorination of water is not sufficient to kill cysts; filtration is required for cyst removal. Boiling water kills cysts.

Free-living amoebae

Infection may follow swimming in water contaminated with *Naegleria* and *Acanthamoeba* species.

Naegleria fowleri

This is a rare cause of meningoencephalitis. Infection follows swimming in fresh water contaminated with *N. fowleri*. The amoebae colonise the nasopharynx and then invade the central nervous system (CNS) via the cribriform plate. Cerebrospinal fluid (CSF) examination shows polymorphs and motile amoebae. Infection is frequently fatal, although some cases have been treated successfully with amphotericin B.

Acanthamoeba species

This is a very rare cause of granulomatous encephalitis in immunocompromised patients. Eye infections, particularly keratitis and corneal ulceration, may result from contact lens-cleaning solutions contaminated with *Acanthamoeba* species. Diagnosis of eye infections may be made by culture of corneal scrapings. Treatment is with topical miconazole, propamidine isethionate, and neomycin in combination or with propamidine plus polyhexamethylene biguanide (or chlorhexidine). Corneal grafting may be needed to restore normal vision.

Ciliates

The only species pathogenic to humans is *Balantidium coli*, a common pathogen of pigs.

Pathogenesis

B. coli produces proteolytic cytotoxins, which facilitate tissue invasion and intestinal mucosal ulceration.

Epidemiology

B. coli is found worldwide, with pigs and cattle as important reservoirs. Infection is via the faecal-oral route, with occasional outbreaks following contamination of water supplies. Person-to-person spread may occur. *B. coli* cysts are ingested and trophozoites form, which invade the mucosa of the large intestine and terminal ileum.

Clinical manifestations

An asymptomatic carrier state can occur. *B. coli* causes gastrointestinal infection; symptoms include abdominal pain and watery diarrhoea containing blood and pus. Mucosal ulceration is rarely followed by invasive infection.

Laboratory diagnosis

Microscopy for trophozoites and cysts in faeces.

Treatment

Tetracycline or metronidazole.

Sporozoa

Classification

The Sporozoa include the Coccidia (*Cryptosporidium* species, *Isospora belli*, *Toxoplasma gondii*) and *Plasmodium* species. They undergo asexual (schizogony) and sexual (gametogony) reproduction, and have a variety of hosts, including humans.

Cryptosporidium hominis

Structure and life cycle

Mature oocysts containing sporozoites are ingested. The sporozoites are released and attach to the intestinal epithelium and mature (schizogony). Sexual forms develop (gametogeny) and a fertilised oocyst is produced, which is passed in the faeces.

Laboratory diagnosis

Microscopy of faecal specimens by a modified acid-fast stain for the presence of oocysts. PCR for species identification and typing.

Isospora belli

I. belli causes diarrhoea and malabsorption, especially in immunocompromised patients. Treatment is co-trimoxazole.

Toxoplasma gondii

Structure and life cycle (Figure 18.1)

Cats are the definitive host. Asexual and sexual cycles result in oocyst formation. Oocysts release sporozoites, which then multiply in the host as tachyzoites and disseminate via the bloodstream, particularly to muscle and brain. Multiplication at these sites leads to tissue damage. Tissue cysts containing bradyzoites also develop.

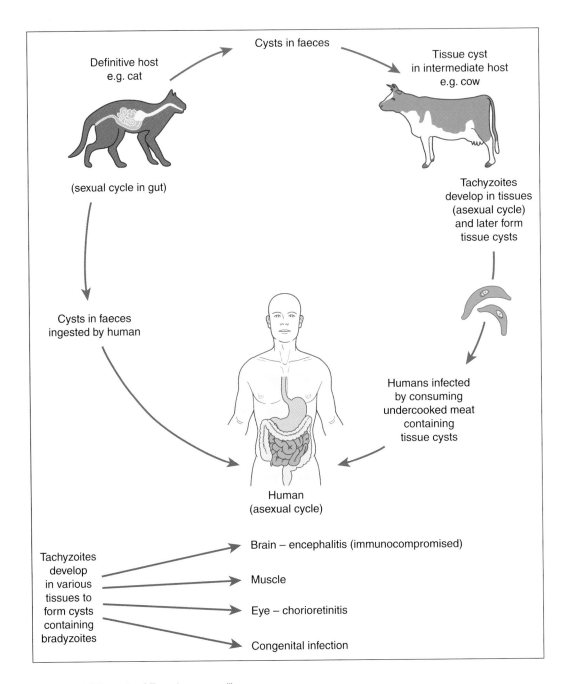

Figure 18.1 Life cycle of *Toxoplasma gondii*.

Epidemiology

Human infection with *T. gondii* is common, occurring worldwide. A wide variety of animals carry the microorganism. Humans become infected from:

- ingestion of undercooked meat containing tissue cysts;
- ingestion of oocysts from cat faeces;
- transplacental transmission (maternal infection in pregnancy);
- cardiac transplantation, the recipient receives a heart containing *Toxoplasma* cysts;
- reactivation caused by immunosuppression, e.g. AIDS.

Clinical manifestations

- Most infections are asymptomatic.
- *In immunocompetent hosts*: glandular fever-like syndrome;
- *In immunocompromised hosts*: myocarditis, choroidoretinitis, meningoencephalitis;
- *Congenital infection*: choroidoretinitis, hydrocephalus and intracerebral calcification.

Diagnosis

- Serology (e.g. ELISA): by demonstration of rising IgG antibodies in paired sera, or IgM antibodies to differentiate between active and previous infection. Serology in AIDS is not useful, because IgG antibodies do not distinguish between reactivated and latent infection.
- PCR (polymerase chain reaction) detection of parasite DNA in blood, CSF or amniotic fluid may be useful.
- MRI (magnetic resonance imaging) of the brain shows characteristic multiple, dense, ring-enhancing lesions with contrast.

Histology

By examination of appropriate biopsies for tachyzoites or tissue cysts.

Treatment

Pyrimethamine, plus sulphonamide and folinic acid. Indefinite suppressive treatment in AIDS.

Prevention

Cooking meat. Avoiding contact with cat faeces.

Plasmodium

Plasmodia are causative of malaria and are parasites of erythrocytes with two hosts:

1 Mosquitoes, where sexual reproductive stages (gametogony) take place;
2 Humans or other animals, where asexual reproductive stages occur (schizogony).

There are several species of plasmodia, which vary in detailed life cycle and clinical features, and can be separated morphologically (some are outlined in Table 18.3).

Life cycle

All plasmodia share a common life cycle (Figure 18.2), but with some important variations:

1 Anopheles mosquitoes bite humans and infectious plasmodia (sporozoites) are introduced into the bloodstream.
2 The sporozoites are carried to liver parenchymal cells, where asexual reproduction (schizogony) occurs in the liver to form merozoites (preerythrocytic cycle, 7–28 days).
3 Liver hepatocytes rupture, liberating merozoites, which attach to and penetrate erythrocytes. Note: *P. vivax* and *P. ovale* have a dormant hepatic phase, with sporozoites becoming

Table 18.3 Species of malaria infecting humans

Species	Fever cycle (h)	Clinical condition
Plasmodium falciparum	36–48	Malignant tertian malaria
Plasmodium malariae	72	Quartan malaria
Plasmodium ovale	36–48	Benign tertian malaria
Plasmodium vivax	36–48	Benign tertian malaria
Plasmodium knowlesi	24	Quotidian malaria

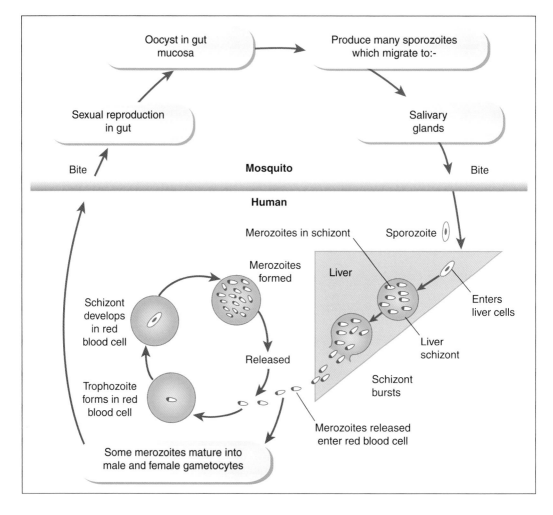

Figure 18.2 Life cycle of *Plasmodium falciparum*.

hypnozoites that do not divide and can result in relapse months, very occasionally years, after the initial disease.

4 Asexual reproduction occurs in the erythrocytes; merozoites are released and infect further erythrocytes. Some merozoites develop within erythrocytes into male and female gametocytes. *P. falciparum* may be associated with high levels of parasitaemia (up to 30% or more of circulating erythrocytes); lower levels (<5%) are found with other species.

5 The mosquito bites a host and ingests mature male and female gametocytes.

6 The sexual reproductive cycle occurs in the mosquito's digestive system. Sporozoites form, migrate to salivary glands and are inoculated into a new host.

Epidemiology

• In tropical and subtropical areas, plasmodia are dependent on the correct conditions for breeding of anopheles mosquitoes. *P. falciparum* is responsible for more than 80% of cases in tropical areas.

• In endemic areas, repeated infections or exposure results in relative immunity and less severe disease. Visitors to endemic areas are more severely affected.

Table 18.4 Clinical comparison of the types of malaria

Characteristic	P. vivax	P. ovale	P. malariae	P. falciparum	P. knowlesi
Incubation period (days)	10–17 Sometimes prolonged for months to years	10–17	18–40	8–11	9–12
Duration of untreated infection	5–7 years	12 months	20 + years	6–17 months	Not fully documented
Anaemia	+ +	+	+ +	+ + + +	+ +
Central nervous system involvement	+	±	+	+ + + +	+ +
Renal involvement	±	+	+ + + +	+	+

± to + + + +, less likely to very common.

- Transmission via contaminated blood transfusions or needle sharing can rarely occur.

Clinical features

- *The incubation period* is variable (10–40 days, but may be prolonged).
- *Fever/sweats*: symptoms are related to release of toxins when schizonts burst and so intervals between bouts of pyrexia are dependent on the erythrocytic cycle of the *Plasmodium* species (Table 18.3).
- *Anaemia*: this is caused by erythrocyte haemolysis. It is most severe with *P. falciparum* malaria and may result in haemoglobinuria ('blackwater fever').
- *Cerebral malaria*: *P. falciparum* schizonts sequester and contribute to blocking of capillaries in the brain; the resultant hypoxia causes confusion and eventually coma, with a high mortality.
- A clinical comparison of the types of malaria is given in Table 18.4.

Laboratory diagnosis

Thick and thin blood films are taken. The typical morphology of the parasite within the erythrocytes allows the differentiation of the *Plasmodium* species (Figure 18.3). PCR is sometimes required to identify the species present.

Treatment

- Chloroquine is the treatment of choice for malaria caused by *P. vivax, P. ovale, P. malariae*

and uncomplicated *P. knowlesi* infections. Supplementary treatment with primaquine is important to destroy the liver hypnozoite stages of *P. vivax* and *P. ovale*, provided the glucose 6 phosphate dehydrogenase (G6PD) is normal.
- Uncomplicated falciparum malaria is treated with quinine plus doxycycline or artemether with lumefantrine or atovaquone with proguanil.
- Given the complexity of the epidemiology of drug resistance, specialist advice should be taken when treating patients with falciparum malaria. Uncomplicated *P. knowlesi* is treated with chloroquine. If severe, treat as for severe falciparum malaria.

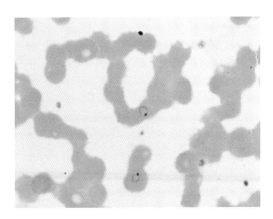

Figure 18.3 *Plasmodium falciparum* malaria parasites in a blood film.

Prevention

This is important for travellers to endemic areas. Avoidance of mosquito bites is necessary (e.g. covering exposed limbs, use of mosquito nets and repellants). Prophylactic anti-malarials may be taken. The exact regimen is dependent on whether resistance is present in the area being visited; examples include atovaquone plus proguanil; doxycycline; mefloquine; and chloroquine plus proguanil.

Flagellates

Classification

Human pathogenic flagellates include *Giardia intestinalis* (gastrointestinal tract), *Trichomonas vaginalis* (genital tract), *Trypanosoma* species (blood/tissues) and *Leishmania* species (blood/tissues).

Giardia intestinalis

Pathogenesis and life cycle

Cysts are ingested and gastric acid stimulates the release of trophozoites in the small intestine, which then multiply by binary fission. Trophozoites attach to the intestinal villi by a sucking disc. Inflammation of the epithelium may occur, but invasion is rare. Trophozoites divide by binary fission. Cyst formation occurs as the microorganisms move through the colon.

Epidemiology

Giardia occurs worldwide. Transmission is via ingestion of contaminated water or food, or direct person-to-person spread via the faecal-oral route.

Clinical manifestations

Asymptomatic carriage is common. Active infection causes diarrhoea and malabsorption occasionally. Chronic infection may cause failure to thrive in children.

Laboratory diagnosis

Stool microscopy for cysts and trophozoites. If clinical suspicion is high and stool examination is negative, duodenal aspiration or biopsy may be helpful.

Treatment

Tinidazole or metronidazole.

Prevention

The cysts resist routine levels of chlorination. Water can be decontaminated by boiling or filtration.

Trichomonas vaginalis

Structure

T. vaginalis is a pear-shaped protozoan with four flagella. No cyst stage has been recognised.

Epidemiology

It has a worldwide distribution, with sexual intercourse being the primary method of transmission.

Pathogenesis/clinical conditions

T. vaginalis is a parasite of the human urogenital system; there are no animal reservoirs. Infection results in a watery vaginal discharge, although extensive inflammation and erosion of the epithelium can occur. Males are usually asymptomatic carriers; however, occasionally, urethritis and prostatitis can occur.

Laboratory diagnosis

This is by microscopy of vaginal or urethral discharge for trophozoites or isolation in special media.

Treatment

Metronidazole for affected patients and sexual partner(s).

Trypanosoma species

Trypanosomes are haemoflagellates living in the blood and tissue of human hosts. The life cycle involves two hosts: blood-sucking insects and mammals. It causes two diseases:

1 African trypanosomiasis (sleeping sickness) caused by *T. brucei gambiense* and *T. brucei rhodesiense* and transmitted by the tsetse fly:
2 American trypanosomiasis (Chagas disease) caused by *T. cruzi*, and transmitted by reduviid bugs.

Trypanosoma brucei gambiense (West African sleeping sickness)

Life cycle

1 The infective stage (trypomastigote) is present in the salivary glands of the tsetse fly. The trypomastigote has a flagellum and an undulating membrane along the length of the body allowing motility.
2 Trypomastigotes enter the host via insect bites and reach the lymphatic system, blood and CNS. Non-flagellate forms (amastigotes) develop in some tissues (e.g. heart and muscle).
3 Tsetse flies feed on the infected host and take in trypomastigotes, which multiply in the intestine; epimastigotes subsequently form in the salivary glands and develop into infective trypomastigotes.
4 The tsetse fly remains infective for life.

Epidemiology

Limited to West and Central Africa. Asymptomatic humans are the main reservoirs, though animals may become infected.

Clinical condition

The incubation period is 2–3 weeks. A nodule or chancre at the site of the bite is very rare in West African trypanosomiasis. The parasite enters the bloodstream and results in lymphadenopathy, irregular fever and myalgia. CNS involvement (sleeping sickness) may occur with lethargy and encephalitis, leading to convulsions, hemiplegia, coma and occasionally death.

Diagnosis

Microscopy of thick and thin blood films, lymph node aspirates and CSF for trypomastigotes; serology (e.g. IFAT).

Treatment

Eflornithine, suramin or pentamidine for blood stage infection. Eflornithine, if there is CNS involvement.

Prevention

Vector control, insect repellents, and insecticide-impregnated clothing.

Trypanosoma brucei rhodesiense (East African sleeping sickness)

Life cycle

The life cycle is similar to that of *T. brucei gambiense*, with trypomastigote and epimastigote stages. Transmission is by the tsetse fly.

Epidemiology

It is found in East Africa. Domestic and game animals are the main reservoirs. Asymptomatic human carriers are not normally a source of infection.

Clinical conditions

It has a shorter incubation than *T. brucei gambiense*. A chancre at the site of the bite is more commonly seen. The illness is more severe and progresses rapidly and may involve the heart, kidney and CNS. Mortality is greater than for the West African form.

Diagnosis and prevention

As above.

Treatment

Suramin. Melarsoprol under steroid cover if CNS involvement.

Trypanosoma cruzi (Chagas disease)

Life cycle

1 The life cycle is similar to other trypanosomes, except when the infected bug bites humans, trypomastigotes are released simultaneously in the faeces; these enter the wound after scratching.
2 Spread is via the lymphatic and blood systems and results in invasion of many organs, including the liver, heart, muscles and brain.
3 Within host cells, trypomastigotes transform into amastigotes, which multiply by binary fission and form either further amastigotes or trypomastigotes; the latter are ingested by a feeding insect, multiply in the intestine and are then passed in the faeces.

Epidemiology

T. cruzi is found in North, Central and South America. Reservoirs are humans and domestic animals.

Clinical disease

Chagas disease may be asymptomatic, acute or chronic. An oedematous swelling may form at the site of the bite. Acute infection results in high fever, erythematous rash, oedema and myocarditis. Chronic disease may develop years after the initial infection. Microorganisms proliferate in various organs, including the brain, spleen, liver, heart and lymph nodes, resulting in lymphadenopathy, hepatosplenomegaly, myocarditis and cardiomegaly. Granulomata and cysts may form in the brain. Chronic gastrointestinal disease produces symptoms resembling achalasia or Hirschsprung's disease. Cardiac disease is the most common presentation, including congestive cardiac failure, conduction abnormalities and aneurysm formation. Transplacental transmission may occur in chronically infected women. Transmission by blood transfusion has occurred.

Laboratory diagnosis

Microscopy of biopsies of affected tissues; thick blood films for trypomastigotes in the acute phase; serological tests (e.g. ELISA and IFAT) for chronic disease; PCR amplification of parasite DNA from blood or body fluids.

Treatment

Benznidazole or nifurtimox; supportive measures for complications.

Prevention

Insecticides; avoidance of insect bites, sleeping under netting; improvement in living conditions. Blood for transfusion should be screened for antibodies to *T. cruzi*.

Leishmania species

Leishmania species are obligate, intracellular parasites transmitted to mammalian hosts by sand flies. An estimated 12 million people are infected worldwide.

Classification

There are three main types of human disease: visceral (*Leishmania donovani* complex), cutaneous (*L. tropica*, *L. major*) and mucosal (*L. braziliensis*) (Table 18.5).

Life cycle

1 A promastigote stage is present in the saliva of infected sand flies and is inoculated into the bite site.

Table 18.5 Syndromes caused by *Leishmania* species

Microorganism	Reservoir	Clinical condition	Location	Average incubation period
L. donovani complex	Humans or dog	Visceral leishmaniasis (kala-azar)	Mediterranean Indian subcontinent South America Africa South Asia	3 months
L. tropica	Humans or dog	Cutaneous leishmaniasis (oriental sore)	Africa Asia Middle East	1–2 months
L. major	Rodents		Mediterranean	
L. braziliensis	Sloths and related species	Mucosal leishmaniasis	Central and South America	A few weeks to months

2 Promastigotes lose their flagella, enter the amastigote stage, are engulfed by tissue macrophages, and carried via the reticuloendothelial system to the bone marrow, spleen and liver. Amastigotes multiply, resulting in tissue damage.

3 Amastigotes are taken up by the sand fly during feeding, develop into promastigotes, multiply in the mid-gut and then migrate to the salivary glands.

Visceral leishmaniasis

This is caused by *L. donovani* complex. The infection occurs in India, China, southern Russia, Africa, the Mediterranean basin and Latin America.

Clinical conditions

Fever, weight loss and diarrhoea are present, with hepatosplenomegaly and renal involvement. Darkening of the skin, mainly the face and hands (kala-azar), malabsorption and anaemia may occur. Untreated, visceral leishmaniasis is fatal. Those who are treated and recover are unlikely to relapse unless their cell-mediated immunity is suppressed (e.g. AIDS).

Diagnosis

Histological examination of appropriate tissue biopsies; splenic aspirate, bone marrow or lymph nodes for amastigotes; serology. PCR amplification of parasite DNA increases sensitivity. Serology (e.g. direct agglutination test).

Treatment

Liposomal amphotericin B is the agent of choice. Sodium stibogluconate is an alternative.

Cutaneous leishmaniasis

Caused by *L. tropica* and *L. major* in southern Europe, Asia and Africa, and by *L. mexicana* complex in Latin America.

Clinical conditions

Cutaneous disease with a papule at the bite site, followed by necrosis of epidermis and ulceration. Infections remain localised, although lesions may be multiple.

Diagnosis

Histological examination for amastigotes or DNA detection in smears or biopsy material. Serology is unhelpful in cutaneous leishmaniasis.

Treatment

Sodium stibogluconate.

Mucosal leishmaniasis

Caused by *L. braziliensis* complex in Latin America.

Clinical conditions

Infection mainly involves the mucous membranes of the upper respiratory tract (palate, nose) and related tissue, with ulceration, tissue destruction and a resulting disfigurement.

Diagnosis

Histological examination or DNA detection in biopsies.

Treatment

Sodium stibogluconate or amphotericin B.

Parasitology: helminths

Peter Chiodini
The Hospital for Tropical Diseases and The London School of Hygiene and Tropical Medicine, London, UK

Nematodes

The common nematodes of medical importance are listed in Table 19.1.

Ascaris lumbricoides (roundworm)

Structure and life cycle (Figure 19.1)

- Adult worms are cylindrical; the female is up to 35 cm long and the male up to 30 cm long.
- After ingestion of an infective egg, larval worms are released into the duodenum, and penetrate the intestinal wall to reach the bloodstream, passing via the liver and heart to the pulmonary circulation. These larval worms pass into the alveoli, migrate via the bronchi, trachea and pharynx, are swallowed and return to the small intestine.
- Male and female worms mature and mate in the intestine; up to 200,000 eggs per day are produced by the female and passed in stools.

Epidemiology

Ascaris lumbricoides is found throughout the world, but particularly in areas of poor sanitation where faecal-oral transmission may occur. Eggs can survive for long periods (several years), making *Ascaris* the most common pathogenic helminth worldwide.

Clinical manifestations/ complications

Victims are asymptomatic when the worm load is light. Vomiting and abdominal discomfort may occur. Complications include:

- pneumonitis (following larval migration in the lungs);
- intestinal obstruction with mature worms (children);
- malnutrition in children;
- perforation of the intestine and hepatic abscesses (rare).

Laboratory diagnosis

Stool microscopy for the presence of fertilised or unfertilised eggs. An adult worm is occasionally passed in faeces or vomit. Larvae are sometimes found in sputum in the lung migration phase.

Treatment and prevention

Treatment is with mebendazole, albendazole or piperazine. Surgical or endoscopic relief of intestinal obstruction. Control is by improved sanitation and avoidance of food contaminated with human faeces.

Medical Microbiology and Infection Lecture Notes, Fifth Edition. Edited by Tom Elliott, Anna Casey, Peter Lambert and Jonathan Sandoe.
© 2011 Blackwell Publishing Ltd. Published 2011 by Blackwell Publishing Ltd.

Table 19.1 Medically important nematodes

Microorganism	Notes on disease/infection
Ascaris lumbricoides (roundworm)	Larval worms migrate via bronchi; adult worms may cause intestinal obstruction in children
Enterobius vermicularis (pin- or threadworm)	Perianal itching
Trichinella spiralis	Periorbital oedema; myalgia; fever
Toxocara canis	Larvae migrate to liver and lungs (visceral larva migrans) or eyes (ocular visceral migrans)
Trichuris trichiura	Anaemia, intestinal irritation

Enterobius vermicularis (pin worm)

Structure and life cycle (Figure 19.2)

- The female worm (10 mm × 0.4 mm) has a pointed tail; the male worm (3 mm × 0.2 mm) has a curved end. Infection follows ingestion of an embryonated egg.
- Larvae hatch in the small intestine and migrate to the large intestine, where they mature into adults in approximately 1 month.
- The male fertilises the female, which migrates to the perianal area and lays eggs, which become infective within hours.
- Perianal irritation leads to scratching; eggs contaminate hands, particularly nails, resulting in autoinfection or transmission to a new host.

Epidemiology

This is a common parasitic infection, with 500 million cases worldwide, mainly in temperate

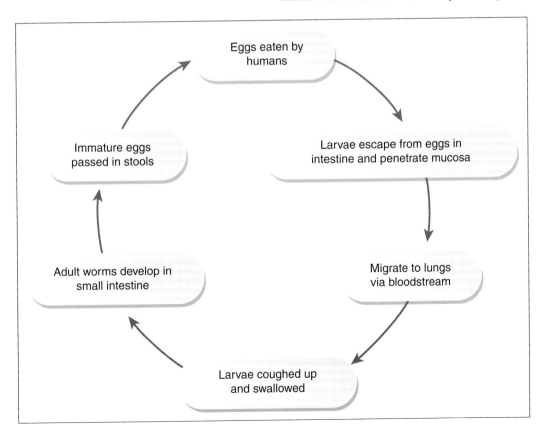

Figure 19.1 Life cycle of *Ascaris lumbricoides*.

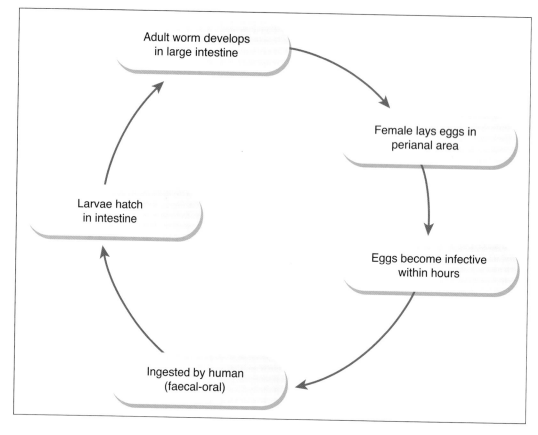

Figure 19.2 Life cycle of *Enterobius vermicularis*.

regions. Person-to-person or environment-to-person spread is responsible for transmission.

Clinical manifestations and complications

Individuals are frequently asymptomatic. Patients allergic to worm secretions may experience perianal pruritus. In heavily infected females, worm migration into the vagina may occur.

Laboratory diagnosis

By microscopy; the best method is a Sellotape slide applied around the perianal region to pick up eggs. Adult worms may be found in stool specimens.

Treatment and prevention

Mebendazole is given to treat the entire family simultaneously. Reinfestation may occur, because eggs may survive in the environment for 3 weeks. Improved personal hygiene is advised, including cutting of fingernails and regular washing of bedclothes and towels.

Toxocara canis and *Toxocara cati*

Structure and life cycle

- *T. canis* and *T. cati* are parasites of dogs and cats, respectively. Male and female worms develop in the intestine and produce eggs that are ingested by other dogs or cats and the cycle continues.
- Humans are an unintentional host; on ingestion, the eggs hatch into larval forms, which can penetrate the intestinal mucosa and migrate to various organs, particularly the lung, liver and eyes. Larvae are unable to develop further and granuloma formation results.

Epidemiology

It is associated with infected dogs and cats; worldwide distribution.

Clinical manifestations and complications

Toxocariasis may result in pneumonitis, hepatosplenomegaly, eosinophilia and retinal granuloma, which may present with retinal detachment.

Laboratory diagnosis

Serology by ELISA. Biopsies of the liver or other affected organs may show eosinophilic granulomata, but are not usually needed for diagnosis.

Treatment

Often unnecessary; albendazole for visceral larva migrans; steroids are also used in severe cases. Laser photocoagulation may kill larvae in the eye.

Prevention

Young pets should be treated routinely ('deworming'); avoid contact with animal faeces.

Trichuris trichiura (whipworm)

Structure and life cycle

- Ingested eggs develop into larvae in the small intestine, which then migrate to the large intestine and mature into adult worms. The fertilised female worm produces eggs.
- Eggs are excreted and mature in the soil.

Epidemiology

Trichuris trichiura has a wide distribution in the tropics and subtropics, particularly in areas with poor sanitation. No animal reservoir has been identified.

Clinical manifestations and complications

Patients are often asymptomatic, but heavy worm infection may produce abdominal distension and diarrhoea with weight loss; anaemia and eosinophilia. Bloody diarrhoea (the Trichuris Dysentery Syndrome) and anal prolapse are seen occasionally.

Laboratory diagnosis

Microscopy of stools to look for characteristic eggs.

Treatment

Mebendazole or albendazole.

Prevention

Good personal hygiene and adequate sanitation can help to prevent infection.

Ancylostoma duodenale and *Necator americanus* (hookworm)

Structure and life cycle

- Infective larvae penetrate intact skin, enter the circulation and are carried to the lungs; after maturation, larvae are expectorated and swallowed, and develop into adult worms in the small intestine.
- The adult worms lay eggs, which are excreted and, in hot humid conditions, develop rapidly into infective larvae that may infect a new host by penetration of exposed skin, particularly bare feet.

Epidemiology

Found primarily in subtropical and tropical regions.

Clinical manifestations and complications

- There may be a rash at the entry site (ground itch); occasionally pneumonitis occurs during the larval migration.
- Adult worms produce gastrointestinal symptoms, including epigastric pain. Bloody diarrhoea may occur in infants.
- Chronic anaemia may result from blood loss, particularly in malnourished individuals.

Laboratory diagnosis

Stool microscopy for eggs.

Treatment and prevention

Mebendazole for treatment; preventive measures include improved sanitation and wearing of shoes to prevent soil contact in endemic areas.

Strongyloides stercoralis

Structure and life cycle

- *Strongyloides stercoralis* is similar to hook-worms, except that the eggs hatch into larvae in the intestinal mucosa before being passed in the faeces. The larvae mature directly into infective larvae that are able to penetrate skin, or enter a non-parasitic cycle outside the human host.
- A special feature of *Strongyloides* is that larvae may also reinfect the host by penetrating the intestinal mucosa (autoinfection); this is more common in immunocompromised patients.
- Infection may be quiescent for up to 30 years and then reactivate when the immune system is compromised (e.g. organ transplantation), resulting in disseminated infection.

Epidemiology

They are found in warm, moist environments, similar to hookworm.

Clinical manifestations

Pneumonitis, diarrhoea, malabsorption and gut ulceration may occur. Immunosuppressed patients may develop severe infection affecting multiple organs.

Laboratory diagnosis

Stool microscopy for larvae; sampling of proximal small intestine with string capsules or by endoscopic aspiration may be needed in low-level infections. In disseminated infection, filariform larvae may be found in stool, duodenal contents, sputum and bronchial washings. Serology; 85% sensitive in uncomplicated infection, but there are cross-reactions with other intestinal nematode infections.

Treatment

Ivermectin.

Prevention

As for hookworm.

Trichinella spiralis

Structure and life cycle

- Human infection occurs accidentally, because this parasite is found primarily in carnivorous animals. Humans may become affected after ingestion of encysted larvae in undercooked meat, particularly pork.
- Larvae are released in the small intestine, where they mature into adult worms that produce further larvae. The larvae penetrate the intestinal wall and are released into the circulation, becoming encysted in various tissues, particularly striated muscle.
- The life cycle is completed in animals that are infected after ingestion of striated muscle containing encysted larvae.

Epidemiology

Worldwide distribution; associated with eating pork or the meat of wild carnivores.

Clinical manifestations

Trichinosis presents with muscle pain, tenderness and peri-orbital oedema. Encephalitis and pneumonitis may occur. Infection is occasionally fatal, usually as a result of myocarditis.

Laboratory diagnosis

Eosinophilia, the presence of encysted larvae in implicated meat or biopsied muscle from the patient, and serology can be used.

Treatment

Mebendazole kills adult worms but has no effect on encysted larvae; albendazole can also be used in the early stages; steroids plus mebendazole or albendazole are used in severe allergic reactions or myocarditis.

Prevention

Meat should be cooked thoroughly.

Wuchereria bancrofti and *Brugia malayi* (filarial worms)

These are transmitted by mosquitoes.

Structure and life cycle

- Infective larvae are introduced after a bite from an infected mosquito; they migrate via the lymphatics to regional lymph nodes.
- Adult worms mature in the lymphatics, fertilisation occurs and microfilariae are produced. These enter the circulation and are ingested by feeding mosquitoes.
- In the mosquito, larvae migrate via the stomach to the mouthparts to complete the cycle.

Epidemiology

The worms are found in tropical and subtropical Africa, Asia and South America.

Clinical manifestations and complications

Early signs include flu-like illness, lymphangitis and lymphadenopathy. Chronic infection results in blockage of the lymphatics with peripheral oedema, and eventually limb fibrosis (elephantiasis).

Laboratory diagnosis

By detection of microfilariae in blood films (taken at night as microfilariae show nocturnal periodicity) and serology.

Treatment

Diethylcarbamazine.

Prevention

Mosquito control; avoiding bites.

Loa loa

Structure and life cycle

- *Loa loa* is similar to *Wuchereria bancrofti*. The insect vector is *Chrysops*, the mango fly.
- In humans, larvae mature and migrate subcutaneously. Fertilisation results in microfilariae, which pass into the bloodstream and are ingested by feeding flies.

Epidemiology

Loa loa infection is found in tropical Africa.

Clinical manifestations

There is swelling where the worms migrate subcutaneously. Adult worms may be seen migrating under the conjunctiva, hence the name 'eye-worm'.

Laboratory diagnosis

By detection of microfilariae in blood and serology.

Treatment and prevention

Treatment is with diethylcarbamazine or ivermectin under steroid cover. Albendazole is preferred in patients with high microfilarial counts. Prevention is by protection from insect bites.

Onchocerca volvulus

Infection follows a bite from black flies which breed near fast-flowing rivers. Larvae develop into adult worms in subcutaneous nodules. *Onchocerca volvulus* is found in Africa and central and South America. Chronic infection results in atrophic skin and may cause blindness as a result of microfilariae migrating to the eyes. Diagnosis is by skin biopsy or slit-lamp examination of the anterior chamber of the eye for microfilariae. Bites can be reduced by clothing and insect repellents. Annually administered ivermectin effectively controls disease and decreases transmission of the parasite. Ivermectin is also used for individual case management.

Cestodes

Tapeworms are ribbon like and up to 30 feet in length. A head or scolex is present and some species also have a crown of hooklets, facilitating attachment. Segments of tapeworms are called proglottids. All tapeworms are hermaphrodites, with both male and female reproductive organs present in each segment. Food is absorbed from the host intestine through the body wall. Most tapeworms have complex life cycles, with intermediate hosts. Clinically important cestodes are listed in Table 19.2.

Table 19.2 Clinically important cestodes

Cestode	Common name	Reservoir for larvae	Definitive host for adult worm
Taenia solium	Pork tapeworm	Pigs	Humans
Taenia saginata	Beef tapeworm	Cattle	Humans
Diphyllobothrium latum	Fish tapeworm	Crustacea, fish	Humans, cats, dogs
Echinococcus granulosus	Hydatid cyst	Herbivores	Canines
Hymenolepis nana	Dwarf tapeworm	Rodents, humans	Rodents, humans

Taenia solium

Structure and life cycle (Figure 19.3)

Humans ingest pork containing larvae (cysticerci) and the larvae develop in the small intestine into the adult form. The worm produces proglottids which mature sexually, producing eggs (Figure 19.4) that pass in the faeces. Pigs ingest the eggs and larval forms develop that disseminate via the circulation to muscle to produce cysticerci.

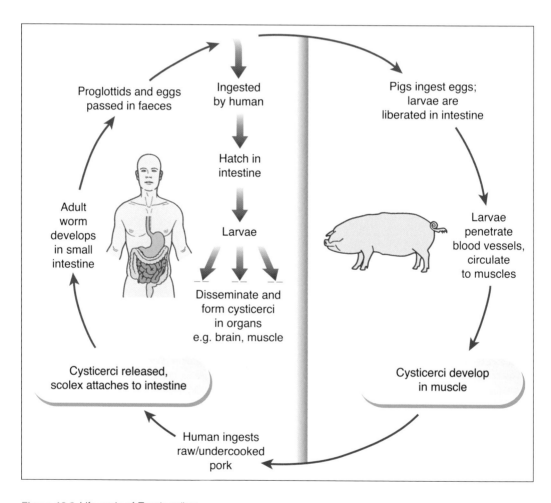

Figure 19.3 Life cycle of *Taenia solium*.

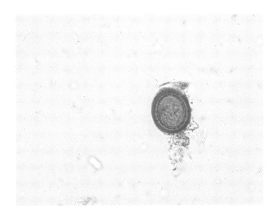

Figure 19.4 An egg of the tapeworm *Taenia* in faeces.

Epidemiology

Tapeworm infection is related to eating under-cooked pork. Cysticercosis (see below) is contracted by ingesting eggs of the pork tapeworm. It is common in Africa, India, Southeast Asia and Central America.

Clinical manifestations

Abdominal discomfort and diarrhoea.

Diagnosis

Stool microscopy for proglottids and eggs; serology for cysticercosis (but not for the intestinal worm).

Treatment and prevention

Treatment of the adult tapeworm is with praziquantel or niclosamide. Pork should be cooked thoroughly and improved sanitation is important for prevention.

Cysticercosis

Humans may become infected with the larval stage of *T. solium* after ingestion of eggs from human faeces. Larvae penetrate the intestinal wall, enter the circulation and are carried to muscles, the brain, lungs and occasionally eyes. The inflammatory response to the presence of these larvae in human tissues eventually results in calcification. Infection is often subclinical, but may present with neurological or ophthalmic manifestations.

Diagnosis

Muscle or brain radiograph may show calcified cysts; computed tomography (CT) or MRI is often diagnostic; histology; serology (immunoblot).

Treatment

Albendazole or praziquantel, but is not necessary if cysts are not viable. Steroids and anticonvulsants may be necessary to control symptoms if CNS cysts are degenerating. Obstructive hydrocephalus may need surgery.

Taenia saginata

Structure and life cycle

The life cycle is similar to *Taenia solium*, with infection resulting from ingestion of cysticerci present in insufficiently cooked beef. Human faeces contaminated with eggs are ingested by cattle and cysticerci develop in beef.

Epidemiology

Worldwide distribution.

Clinical manifestations

Abdominal discomfort or no symptoms.

Laboratory diagnosis

Proglottids and eggs are detected by stool microscopy.

Treatment and prevention

Treatment with praziquantel or niclosamide. Improved sanitation aids prevention. Beef should be cooked thoroughly.

Diphyllobothrium latum (fish tapeworm)

Structure and life cycle

There are two intermediate hosts: freshwater crustaceae and freshwater fish. Infection occurs in humans after ingestion of infected freshwater fish. The adult worm develops in the intestine, attaching to the mucosa via lateral grooves. Proglottids develop and produce eggs. In fresh water, the eggs develop into larvae, which infect crustacea. Fish eat the crustacea and larvae develop that are infective for humans.

Epidemiology

Infection occurs in temperate climates, particularly Scandinavia.

Clinical manifestations

Usually asymptomatic. Mild diarrhoea and occasionally intestinal obstruction. Megaloblastic anaemia and vitamin B_{12} deficiency can occur.

Treatment and prevention

Praziquantel is the drug of choice. Avoid eating raw or undercooked fish.

Echinococcus granulosus (dog tapeworm)

Structure and life cycle

- The adult tapeworms are found in canines, normally dogs or foxes. In the canine intestine, the adult tapeworms produce eggs, which are passed in the faeces.
- Herbivores, the normal intermediate hosts, ingest the eggs and larvae develop in various organs, resulting in cyst formation. Carnivores become infected after consuming contaminated carcasses.
- Human infection occurs when humans become the accidental intermediate host. Eggs are ingested, and larvae develop and penetrate the intestinal wall; hydatid cysts develop, principally in the liver. These cysts accumulate fluid and enlarge over several years; a germinal layer lines the cyst, which produces larval tapeworms (protoscoleces).

Epidemiology

Echinococcus granulosus is associated with sheep farming in Europe, Australasia, South America and the USA. Human infection follows ingestion of water or vegetation contaminated with eggs.

Clinical manifestations

Cysts in the liver grow over many years, resulting in hepatomegaly. Cysts in the lung, bone and brain may result in various clinical presentations.

Diagnosis

CT or ultrasonography may be diagnostic; microscopy of cyst contents; serology.

Treatment and prevention

Treatment is by a combination of medical treatment with albendazole and resection of cysts. An alternative is treatment with albendazole plus aspiration under ultrasound guidance and injection of ethanol into the cyst to act as a scolicidal agent. Avoid ingestion of contaminated food.

Hymenolepis nana

This is a common, often asymptomatic infection occurring particularly in Asia. *Hymenolepis nana* is a small (2–5 cm) worm. Eggs are produced in the small intestine and may reinfect the same host or spread to other hosts by the faecal-oral route. Heavy infection may result in diarrhoea, abdominal discomfort and weight loss. Treatment is with praziquantel.

Trematodes

Trematodes (flukes) are flatworms with oral and ventral suckers. Most flukes are hermaphrodites, containing both male and female reproductive organs in a single body. Schistosomes differ in having separate male and female worms.

All flukes require an intermediate host for completion of their life cycle. The intermediate hosts are molluscs, in which the sexual reproduction cycle occurs. Some flukes need a further intermediate host. The medically important trematodes are summarised in Table 19.3.

Fasciola hepatica (sheep liver fluke)

Structure and life cycle

- *F. hepatica* is a parasite of herbivores (sheep, cattle) and occasionally humans.
- Human infection starts with ingestion of watercress or similar vegetation contaminated with encysted metacercariae, which excyst in the du-

Table 19.3 Medically important trematodes (flukes)

	Common name	Intermediate host	Source of human infection	Definitive host
Fasciola hepatica	Sheep liver fluke	Snail	Aquatic plants (e.g. watercress)	Sheep, cattle
Opisthorchis sinensis (formerly *Clonorchis sinensis*)	Chinese liver fluke	Snail, freshwater fish	Uncooked fish	Dogs, cats, humans
Paragonimus westermani	Lung fluke	Snail, crayfish	Uncooked crabs, crayfish	Humans
Schistosoma species	Blood flukes	Snail	Water contact	Humans

odenum. The larval flukes migrate through the duodenal wall, across the peritoneal cavity and into the bile ducts via the liver. They mature into adult worms and produce eggs that are passed in faeces.

- Snails become infected and act as intermediate hosts. Cercariae (infective larvae) develop and contaminate watercress, where they encyst to form metacercariae.

Epidemiology

F. hepatica occurs worldwide, especially in sheep-rearing areas.

Clinical manifestations

Migration of the larval worm in the liver causes tender hepatomegaly. Worms in the bile duct may cause biliary obstruction.

Laboratory diagnosis

Stool microscopy for eggs.

Treatment and prevention

Triclabendazole. Avoid eating watercress grown in areas frequented by sheep and cattle.

Opisthorchis sinensis (Chinese liver fluke; formerly known as Clonorchis sinensis)

Structure and life cycle

O. sinensis has a similar life cycle to *F. hepatica*, except there are two intermediate hosts. Eggs are eaten by a snail and then hatch to release miracidia, which develop into cercariae after a process of multiplication. Free-swimming cercariae leave the snail and enter freshwater fish by penetrating under scales where they develop into metacercariae. Humans become infected by eating contaminated raw fish. Larval forms penetrate the duodenum, migrate to the bile duct and develop into adult worms.

Epidemiology

O. sinensis is found in China, Japan, Korea and Southeast Asia.

Clinical manifestations

People are usually asymptomatic, but severe infections can result in hepatomegaly, biliary obstruction and jaundice.

Laboratory diagnosis

Stool microscopy for eggs.

Treatment and prevention

Praziquantel is the drug of choice. Avoid eating uncooked fish. Improved sanitation is important in prevention.

Paragonimus westermani (lung fluke)

Structure and life cycle

- Embryonated eggs in water produce miracidia, which penetrate snails and develop into cercariae. The latter infect crabs and crayfish.

- Humans become infected by eating infected crabs or crayfish. The larvae hatch in the duodenum, migrate through the intestinal wall, cross the peritoneal cavity and eventually reach the lungs via the diaphragm.
- The worms reside within fibrous cysts in the lungs and produce eggs that then appear in the sputum or, when swallowed, in faeces.

Epidemiology

P. westermani is found in Asia, Africa, India and South America.

Clinical manifestations

Adult flukes in lungs may result in cough and chest pain; lung fibrosis may develop. Larval migration can also cause disease in other organs, particularly the brain.

Laboratory diagnosis

Microscopy of sputum and faeces for eggs. Serology.

Treatment and prevention

Praziquantel. Avoid eating uncooked freshwater crabs and crayfish; improve sanitation.

Schistosomes

Schistosomes associated with human infection (schistosomiasis) include *Schistosoma mansoni*, *S. japonicum* and *S. haematobium* (Table 19.4).

Schistosomiasis is an important infection with over 200 million people infected worldwide.

Structure and life cycle (Figure 19.5)

- Schistosomes have separate male and female worms.
- Infective cercariae penetrate the skin, enter the circulation, and develop into male and female worms in the veins of the intestine (*S. mansoni, S. japonicum*) or bladder (*S. haematobium*). The female worm produces eggs (Figure 19.6) that penetrate the intestinal or bladder wall and are passed in faeces or urine. Ova reach fresh water, hatch into larvae and infect snails. An asexual cycle results, with formation of cercariae that are released into water.

Clinical manifestations

- Skin penetration may result in local dermatitis (Swimmers' itch).
- Egg release is associated with haemorrhage, normally minor, into the bladder (haematuria) or intestine (blood in faeces).
- Egg entrapment in the bladder or intestinal wall may result in a chronic inflammatory reaction with subsequent fibrosis:
  o fibrosis and calcification of the bladder wall; obstruction of ureters, resulting in hydronephrosis and renal failure; malignant change in bladder;
  o fibrosis of the portal tracts, resulting in portal hypertension.

Table 19.4 Diagnosis of schistosome infection

Schistosoma species	Location in human	Epidemiology	Laboratory diagnosis
S. mansoni	Inferior mesenteric vein	Endemic in Africa, Middle East and South America	Stool for eggs with lateral spine Serology
S. japonicum	Superior and inferior mesenteric vein	China, Philippines	Stool for eggs Serology
S. mekongi	mesenteric veins	Laos and Cambodia	Stool for eggs Serology
S. haematobium	Inferior pelvic system	Egypt and Middle East	Urine for eggs with terminal spine Serology

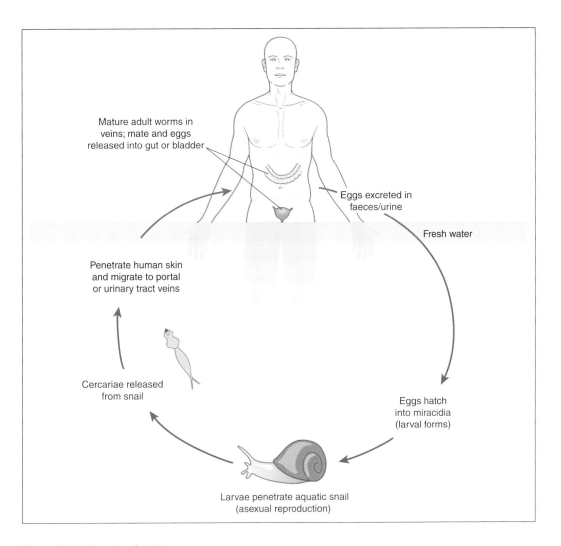

Mature adult worms in veins; mate and eggs released into gut or bladder

Eggs excreted in faeces/urine

Fresh water

Penetrate human skin and migrate to portal or urinary tract veins

Cercariae released from snail

Eggs hatch into miracidia (larval forms)

Larvae penetrate aquatic snail (asexual reproduction)

Figure 19.5 Life cycle of schistosomes.

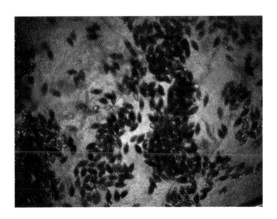

Figure 19.6 *Schistosoma haematobium* eggs in bladder.

- Egg deposition may occur in other organs, e.g. the liver (fibrosis, portal hypertension), lungs, spinal cord and brain.

Laboratory diagnosis

Table 19.4 gives details of laboratory diagnosis of schistosomes.

Treatment and prevention

Praziquantel for all species. Prevention is by improvement of sewage disposal; education and the use of molluscicides.

Part 2

Antimicrobial agents

Antibacterial agents

Peter Lambert
Aston University, Birmingham, UK

Definitions

Antimicrobial agent

Substance with inhibitory properties against microorganisms, but with minimal effects on mammalian cells (includes antibiotics and synthetic compounds).

Antibiotic

Substance produced by microorganisms that inhibits the growth of (bacteriostatic) or kills (bactericidal) other bacteria. The term 'antibiotic' is often incorrectly used to include all antimicrobial agents, some of which are synthetic, e.g. sulphonamides, trimethoprim, metronidazole and fluoroquinolones.

Semi-synthetic antimicrobials

Antibiotics chemically altered to improve properties, e.g. stability, activity, spectrum of activity and pharmacokinetics.

Mechanism of action

How an antimicrobial exerts its effects.

Interactions between antimicrobials

- Antimicrobials used in combination may be:
  additive: combined effect equal to the sum of the individual agents;
- *Synergistic*: combined effect greater than achieved with addition; e.g. gentamicin plus penicillin; or
- *Antagonistic*: drugs inhibit the action of each other.

Empirical therapy

Refers to the antimicrobial regimen used when a clinical diagnosis of infection has been made and delay in initiating therapy to await microbiological results would be inappropriate. (e.g. cefotaxime for meningitis).

Directed therapy

Directed antimicrobial regimens are prescribed to target a specific pathogen (or pathogens), usually informed by the results of microbiological investigations (e.g. benzylpenicillin for a penicillin-susceptible pneumococcal pneumonia or flucloxacillin for a meticillin-susceptible *S. aureus* septic arthritis).

Medical Microbiology and Infection Lecture Notes, Fifth Edition. Edited by Tom Elliott, Anna Casey,
Peter Lambert and Jonathan Sandoe.
© 2011 Blackwell Publishing Ltd. Published 2011 by Blackwell Publishing Ltd.

Monotherapy

Treatment with an antimicrobial on its own.

Combination therapy

Concurrent treatment with two or more antimicrobials.

Resistance

The ability of a microorganism to avoid the harmful effects of an antimicrobial by destroying it, transporting it out of the cell, or undergoing changes that block its effects.

Susceptibility

The level of vulnerability of a microorganism to an antimicrobial.

Principles of antimicrobial therapy

- The need for antimicrobial therapy should be carefully considered; mild infections often do not require treatment.
- Viral infections are not affected by antibacterial agents; many common infections are caused by viruses (e.g. upper respiratory tract infections, see Chapter 25).
- The need for urgent *empirical* therapy should be assessed; for patients with severe sepsis, appropriate antimicrobial therapy should be started as soon as possible.
- In some patients, particularly in the absence of severe sepsis when the diagnosis is unclear, it may be appropriate to delay antimicrobial therapy pending a definitive clinical or microbiological diagnosis.
- Appropriate microbiological sampling should be undertaken prior to commencing antimicrobials.
- Selection of an antimicrobial(s) should take into account the patient's allergy, drug and medical history.
- Selection of *empirical* antimicrobial(s) should take into account the likely pathogen(s) and their usual antimicrobial sensitivity pattern.

- The appropriate route of administration should be determined by pharmacokinetics, severity of infection (intravenous antimicrobials are usually required for severe infections) and patient factors (e.g. ability to swallow).
- An appropriate dose should be prescribed; this is influenced by site and severity of infection and patient factors (e.g. renal and hepatic function).
- Length of treatment depends on the severity and type of infection. For many infections, treatment can be stopped when symptoms are resolved/resolving. Exceptions include infective endocarditis, osteomyelitis.
- Combination therapy may be required:
  - to give enhanced bacterial killing (e.g. infective endocarditis treatment, Chapter 35);
  - to broaden the spectrum of antimicrobial cover, (e.g. cefuroxime and metronidazole may be used to treat abdominal sepsis to cover coliform microorganisms and anaerobes, respectively);
  - to prevent development of resistance, (e.g. tuberculosis therapy);
  - to overcome antimicrobial degradation by bacterial enzymes (e.g. co-amoxiclav contains amoxicillin plus the β-lactamase inhibitor clavulanic acid in the same preparation, piperacillin plus tazobactam is another example).
- When *empirical* antimicrobial therapy has been used, the accuracy of the initial diagnosis should be reviewed regularly and treatment altered to *directed* therapy or stopped as appropriate (e.g. when microbiological results become available).
- Antimicrobials should only be used to prevent infections (prophylaxis) when there is proved effectiveness. Prophylactic antimicrobials are used most frequently for preventing infection after certain types of surgery.

Mechanism of action of antimicrobial agents

Antimicrobials kill or inhibit the growth of microorganisms by interfering with vital structures and processes. Selectivity of action depends upon key differences in these between microbial and mammalian cells. The targets for antimicrobial action are shown in Box 20.1 and Table 20.1.

Table 20.1 Sites of action of different antimicrobial agents

Site of action	Examples of antimicrobials
Cell wall	Penicillins
	Cephalosporins
	Carbapenems
	Monobactams
	Glycopeptides
Cell membrane	Polymyxins
	Daptomycin
Protein synthesis	Aminoglycosides
	Tetracyclines
	Macrolides
	Chloramphenicol
	Lincosamides
	Oxazolidinones
	Mupirocin
	Pleuromutilins
DNA synthesis and function	Sulphonamides
	Trimethoprim
	Quinolones
	Nitroimidazoles
RNA synthesis	Rifampicin

Resistance to antimicrobial agents

Patients do not become resistant to antimicrobial agents, bacteria do.

Resistance mechanisms

Alteration of the target site

- Alteration of the target site can reduce or eliminate binding of the antimicrobial.
- Typically affects antimicrobials that act on the ribosome (e.g. macrolides), RNA polymerase (rifampicin) or topoisomerases (quinolones).
- Resistance occurs when a spontaneous bacterial mutant arises from within a previously sensitive bacterial population; in the presence of the antimicrobial the resistant mutant is 'selected out', i.e. can persist and multiply.
- For example, alteration of transpeptidases (the targets of the β-lactams) results in the microorganism becoming resistant to all β-lactam antimicrobials (e.g. MRSA has acquired additional genes, which encode transpeptidases that are not affected by β-lactam antimicrobials).

Destruction/inactivation of antimicrobial

- Mediated by bacterial enzymes;
- *β-lactamases* cause hydrolysis of the β-lactam ring of penicillins and cephalosporins to form an inactive product. Over 300 different β-lactamase enzymes have been described;
- *Aminoglycoside-modifying enzymes*: inactivate aminoglycosides by the addition of chemical groups (phosphate, acetyl or adenylyl groups).

Interference with drug transport

- Resistance to some antimicrobials involves interference with the transport of these drugs into the bacterial cell, e.g. exclusion of glycopeptides by Gram-negative bacteria or failure to transport fusidic acid or mupirocin into the cells.

Metabolic bypass

- Bacteria may become resistant by providing a replacement for the metabolic step inhibited by an antimicrobial.
- For example, bacteria resistant to trimethoprim synthesise a trimethoprim-insensitive dihydrofolate reductase, which allows the microorganism to bypass the action of the antimicrobial. Sulphonamide resistance is mediated by a similar mechanism.

Efflux:

- Drug efflux occurs in a wide range of Gram-positive and Gram-negative bacteria.
- It is caused by increased expression of chromosomally encoded proteins, whose normal function may be to remove toxic metabolites from the cells.
- Efflux tends to result in low level resistance, but may occur with other mechanisms to produce high-level, clinically relevant resistance.
- Most classes of antimicrobial can be removed by efflux pumps including β-lactams, quinolones, tetracyclines, macrolides and aminoglycosides.

Target site protection

- Access of an antimicrobial to its target may be blocked by production of protective bacterial proteins. This mechanism contributes to resistance to tetracyclines and fluoroquinolones.

The genetics of bacterial resistance to antimicrobials

Resistance of bacteria to antimicrobials is based on genetic changes, which allow the microorganism to avoid the action of the antimicrobial agent. These genetic changes can occur *de novo* as a result of mutation or can occur via acquisition of new genetic material (antimicrobial resistance genes) from another microorganism.

Mutations occur at a low frequency during every round of cell division and chromosome replication. If a mutation happens to occur in the gene for an antimicrobial target, then this will favour survival and spread of the mutant in the presence of the antimicrobial (so called 'selection pressure'). This type of resistance is particularly common with rifampicin, due to mutations in the target RNA polymerase gene and is the reason why rifampicin should not be used as monotherapy.

Antimicrobial-resistant genes may be acquired via a number of different vectors:

- *Plasmids* are extra-chromosomal pieces of DNA containing genes that confer on the bacteria a number of different properties. These genes are often non-essential, but allow the microorganism to survive under a variety of different conditions, giving the microorganism a survival advantage. Resistance to antimicrobials is one of a number of properties that may be conferred on bacteria by plasmids.
- *Transposons* are small genetic elements consisting of individual or small groups of genes. These genetic elements have no ability to replicate, but can move from one replicating piece of DNA to another, e.g. from the bacterial chromosome to a plasmid, and vice versa. Some transposons also behave like plasmids. Transposons play an important part in the evolution of bacterial resistance.
- *Bacteriophages* are viruses that infect bacteria and may act as a vector in carrying bacterial genes from one bacterial cell to another.
- *Integrons* consist of blocks of several antimicrobial resistance genes; they usually include sulphonamide and aminoglycoside-resistance genes. New resistance genes may readily be added to an integron.

The existence of mechanisms for transferring genetic information between bacteria of the same and of different species ('horizontal transmission') by plasmids, transposons and bacteriophages, potentiates rapid spread of resistance genes.

Epidemiology of antimicrobial resistance

The principle underlying the emergence and spread of antimicrobial resistance among bacteria is that the prevalence of resistance is directly proportional to the amount of antimicrobial used. This is illustrated by the increased antimicrobial resistance found in countries with unrestricted use of antimicrobials, in hospitals compared with the community, and in intensive care units compared with general wards. Problem areas in antimicrobial prescribing include:

- the use of antimicrobials without prescription;
- the uncontrolled use of antimicrobials as growth promoters in livestock;
- poor prescribing habits;
- the absence of antimicrobial policies, particularly in hospitals.

Adverse reactions and antimicrobials (Table 20.2)

Antimicrobials may be associated with side effects common to all drugs, including allergic reactions and toxicity to various organs (e.g. hepatotoxicity, nephrotoxicity).

Specific complications associated with antimicrobials relate to their depressive effect on normal commensal flora, e.g. oral candidiasis and *Clostridium difficile* infection.

Laboratory aspects of antimicrobial therapy

Assessment of bacterial sensitivity

A number of techniques are available to assess susceptibility of bacteria to antimicrobials *in vitro*:

- *Disc diffusion tests*: antimicrobial-containing filter paper discs are placed on agar plates inoculated with the bacteria to be tested. After incubation, fully susceptible bacteria will show a large zone of growth inhibition around the disc; less sensitive (intermediate sensitive) isolates will show a smaller inhibition zone and resistant bacteria grow up to the disc edge (Figure 20.1). Results are recorded as S (sensitive), I (intermediate sensitive) or R (resistant).
- *Minimum inhibitory concentration (MIC) assays*: these give a more detailed assessment of bacterial susceptibility. Suspensions of the test bacteria are incubated overnight with doubling dilutions of the antimicrobial; the lowest concentration that inhibits growth is the MIC. Alternatively, plastic strips containing a calibrated concentration gradient of antimicrobial (e.g. E-test strips) are applied to inoculated plates.

Table 20.2 Adverse reactions of some antimicrobials

Antimicrobial	Adverse reaction
Penicillins	Allergic reactions
Cephalosporins	Allergic reactions
Carbapenems	Allergic reactions
Aminoglycosides	Nephrotoxicity
	Ototoxicity
Vancomycin	Nephrotoxicity
	Ototoxicity
Sulphonamides	Folate deficiency
	Marrow depression
	Stephens–Johnson syndrome
Rifampicin	Hepatotoxicity
Isoniazid	Hepatotoxicity
Fucidin	Hepatotoxicity
Chloramphenicol	Aplastic anaemia

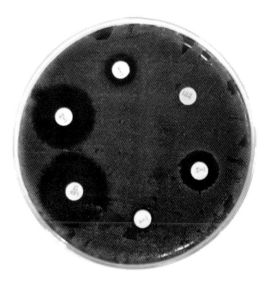

Figure 20.1 Disc diffusion sensitivity test.

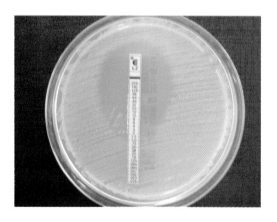

Figure 20.2 E-test to determine MIC of linezolid against an enterococcal isolate.

The MIC can be determined by direct inspection of the pattern of growth inhibition around the calibrated strip (Figure 20.2).

- *Minimum bactericidal concentration (MBC) assay*: this is similar to the MIC but the end-point is bacterial killing rather than growth inhibition; rarely used in diagnostic laboratories.
- *Agar dilution susceptibility tests*: an antimicrobial is incorporated into the medium in an agar plate at a set concentration. The test microorganism is applied to the plate in a standardised amount. Whether or not the microorganism grows will determine whether it is categorised as sensitive or resistant. Using plates containing a series of concentrations the MIC may be determined.
- *Growth rate-based susceptibility tests*: the test microorganism is placed in a container with a set concentration of antimicrobial. The rate of growth of the microorganism is measured. Slow-growing microorganisms are sensitive to the antimicrobial; faster-growing ones are resistant.

Therapeutic drug monitoring

Measurement of levels in the blood is routinely carried out for a small number of antimicrobials. This is required to:

- avoid levels associated with toxicity, e.g. amino-glycosides (including amikacin, gentamicin, tobramycin);
- ensure therapeutic levels are achieved, e.g. glycopeptides (including vancomycin).

The results are used to adjust subsequent dosing of the patient. Patients with renal or hepatic insufficiency may require monitoring of other antimicrobials.

Antibacterial agents

Antibacterials can be classified according to their site of action and their molecular structure.

Inhibitors of cell-wall synthesis

The cell wall of bacteria is essential for their growth and survival. Antimicrobial agents that block the synthesis of the bacterial cell wall are the β-lactams and glycopeptides. These agents have selective activity against bacteria, because mammalian cells have no cell wall.

β-lactam antimicrobials

Structure

This is a large group of compounds, all containing a β-lactam ring (Figure 20.3). The structure of the rings attached to the β-lactam ring determines the class of antimicrobial. Cephalosporins have a six-membered ring, whereas penicillins and carbapenems have five-membered rings, and monobactams have no additional ring. Many modifications have been made to the penicillins and cephalosporins by variation of side chains attached to the rings. These changes have significant effects upon the activity and pharmacokinetic properties.

Other β-lactams include clavulanic acid, sulbactam and tazobactam. These agents do not have useful antimicrobial activity, but they inhibit β-lactamases. They are therefore used in combination with antimicrobial β-lactams to protect against inactivation by these enzymes.

Mechanism of action

These antimicrobials interfere with the assembly of the cell-wall polymer peptidoglycan by inhibiting the transpeptidase enzymes that cross-link the linear sugar chains of the polymer. This weakens the cell wall and results in rupture (lysis) of the microorganism (Figure 20.4).

Penicillins

The penicillins comprise a large group of mainly semi-synthetic compounds based on

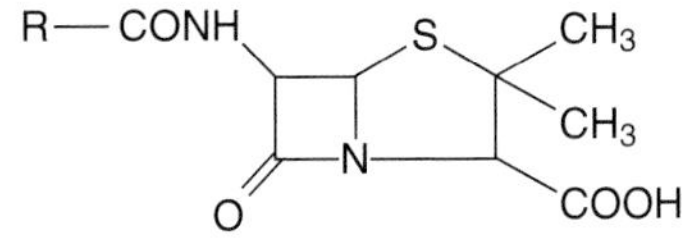

(A) Semisynthetic penicillins

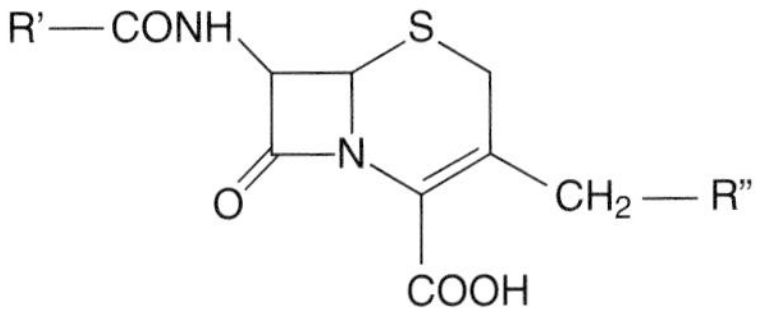

R— CONH

CH₃
CH₃
COOH

(B) Semisynthetic cephalosporins

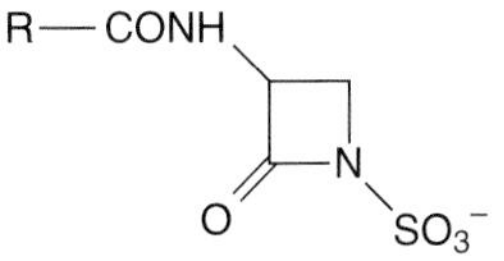

R'— CONH

CH₂ — R"

COOH

(C) Aztreonam

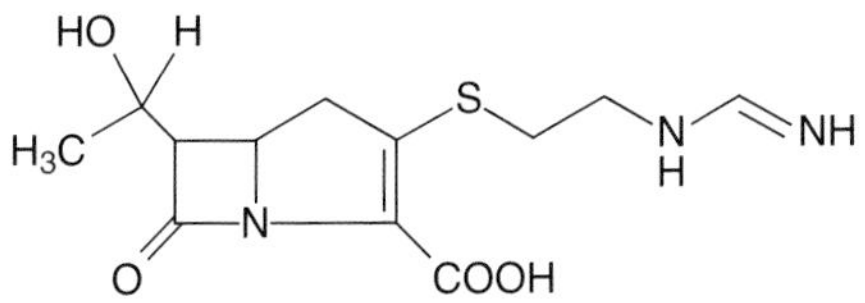

R— CONH

SO₃⁻

(D) Imipenem (+ cilastatin)

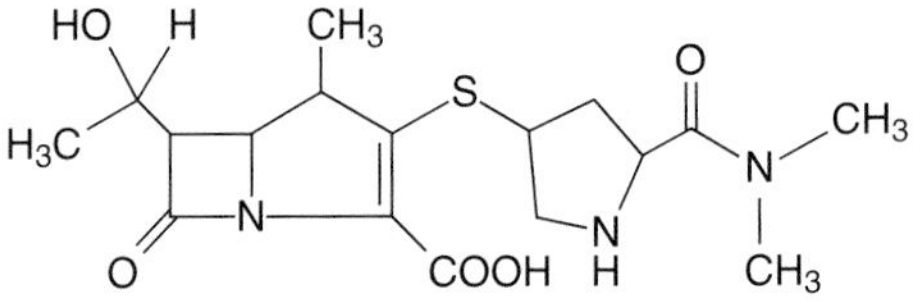

HO H
H₃C

COOH

(E) Meropenem

HO H CH₃
H₃C

COOH H CH₃

Figure 20.3 Structure of β-lactam antimicrobials: penicillins (A); cephalosporins (B); monobactams aztreonam (C); carbapenems, imipenem (D); and meropenem (E).

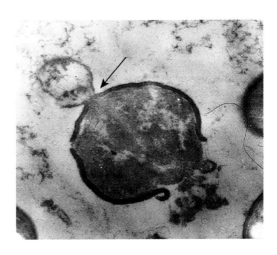

Figure 20.4 Electronmicrograph illustrating the effect of penicillin breaking the cell wall of a susceptible bacterium (arrowed).

benzylpenicillin. They can be divided into the following groups:

1 *Narrow spectrum*: benzylpenicillin, phenoxymethylpenicillin, e.g. active against streptococci;
2 *Moderate spectrum*: amoxicillin, e.g. active against a range of Gram-positive and Gram-negative bacteria;
3 *Penicillins resistant to staphylococcal β-lactamase*, e.g. flucloxacillin;
4 *Extended spectrum penicillins*: with activity against streptococci and many coliforms, e.g. ticarcillin;
5 *Penicillins with activity against Pseudomonas aeruginosa*, e.g. piperacillin.

Toxicity

Hypersensitivity reactions (e.g. immediate-type (IgE mediated)) allergy and delayed-type hypersensitivity.

Antibacterial resistance

- β-*lactamase production*: these bacterial enzymes hydrolyse the β-lactam ring; over 300 different types have been described; some β-lactams are largely unaffected by β-lactamases (e.g. flucloxacillin).
- *Alteration in target site*: e.g. meticillin-resistant *Staphylococcus aureus* (MRSA) produces a transpeptidase with low affinity for β-lactams and therefore continues to function in the

presence of β-lactam antimicrobials (including flucloxacillin).

Examples of penicillins

Benzylpenicillin

- *Pharmacokinetics*: unstable in acid and destroyed in the stomach; can be given intravenously (i.v.) or intramuscularly (i.m.). Widely distributed in the body. Excretion is predominantly renal;
- *Antimicrobial spectrum of activity*: effective mainly on Gram-positive microorganisms (e.g. streptococci) and Gram-negative cocci (*Neisseria meningitis*), some anaerobes and *Treponema pallidum*;
- *Clinical applications*: streptococcal infections, including pneumococcal pneumonia, infective endocarditis, cellulitis, meningococcal meningitis, syphilis and some more unusual infections such as actinomycosis.

Flucloxacillin

- *Pharmacokinetics*: this is a semi-synthetic penicillin. It is well absorbed orally. Part metabolised in the liver, part excreted in urine;
- *Antimicrobial spectrum of activity*: flucloxacillin is active against most β-lactamase-positive and Gram-negative strains of *Staphylococcus aureus* and *Streptococcus pyogenes*, but is not active against meticillin-resistant *Staphylococcus aureus* (MRSA).
- *Clinical applications*: *Staphylococcus aureus* infections, including cellulitis, pneumonia, endocarditis, septic arthritis and osteomyelitis.

Ampicillin and amoxicillin

- *Pharmacokinetics*: semi-synthetic penicillins; acid stable and well absorbed orally. Excretion is predominantly renal. Amoxicillin is derived from a minor chemical change in ampicillin, which improves oral absorption.
- *Antimicrobial spectrum of activity*: ampicillin and amoxicillin have almost identical antimicrobial activity, similar to benzylpenicillin, but more active against *Enterococcus faecalis*, *Haemophilus influenzae* and some Gram-negative aerobic bacilli; activity against many β-lactamase-producing bacteria can be enhanced by the co-administration of β-lactamase inhibitors, such as clavulanic acid.
- *Clinical applications*: urinary infections caused by susceptible coliforms; respiratory tract infections caused by *H. influenzae*; *Listeria monocytogenes* infections (e.g. meningitis); infections with enterococci (e.g. endocarditis).

Piperacillin with tazobactam

- *Pharmacokinetics*: a semi-synthetic penicillin, piperacillin is not absorbed orally. The principal route of excretion is via the kidneys. It is used with tazobactam, a β-lactamase inhibitor with matching pharmacokinetics.
- *Antimicrobial spectrum of activity*: piperacillin is moderately active against many Gram-positive microorganisms, Neisseria spp. and *H. influenzae*. It has wider activity than ampicillin against coliforms and is active against *Pseudomonas aeruginosa*. It is usually used in combination with the β-lactamase inhibitor tazobactam, to give a broad spectrum antimicrobial.
- *Clinical application*: severe Gram-negative aerobic bacillary infections (e.g. bloodstream infection, peritonitis, neutropenic sepsis) caused by coliforms and *P. aeruginosa*.

Cephalosporins

The cephalosporins are classified as:

1 *First-generation*: early compounds with good activity against *Staph. aureus* and some Gram-negative species, including *Haemophilus* spp. and coliforms (e.g. cephaloridine and cephalexin);
2 *Second-generation*: resistant to some β-lactamases, enhanced Gram-negative activity (e.g. cefaclor and cefuroxime);
3 *Third-generation*: enhanced anti-Gram-negative activity, usually at the expense of Gram-positive activity (e.g. cefotaxime and ceftazidime);
4 *Fourth-generation*: enhanced Gram-positive activity compared to third-generation cephalosporins with broad anti-Gram-negative activity maintained (e.g. cefepime and cefpirome).

Toxicity/side effects

Hypersensitivity reactions (as for penicillins). Patients with a penicillin allergy are more likely to react to a first-generation cephalosporin but cross reactivity with other cephalosporins is rare.

Resistance

Similar to the penicillins.

Examples of cephalosporins

Cefuroxime

- *Pharmacokinetics*: available in oral and parenteral forms. Wide distribution in the body with renal excretion;
- *Antimicrobial spectrum of activity*: *Staphylococcus aureus*, most streptococci, coliforms, (note that MRSA, *P. aeruginosa*, enterococci and anaerobes are resistant);
- *Clinical applications*: urinary tract infections, soft tissue and chest infections.

Ceftazidime

- *Pharmacokinetics*: not absorbed orally, given i.v. Distributed into many body tissues and fluids. Excretion is exclusively renal;
- *Antimicrobial spectrum of activity*: less activity against Gram-positive bacteria, but wide activity against Gram-negative aerobic bacteria including *P. aeruginosa*;
- *Clinical application*: severe Gram-negative aerobic bacillary infections (e.g. hospital acquired pneumonia, bloodstream infection) caused by coliforms and *P. aeruginosa*.

Cefotaxime

- *Pharmacokinetics*: not absorbed orally, given i.v. Good CSF and brain penetration;
- *Antimicrobial spectrum of activity*: broad spectrum of activity including *P. aeruginosa*;
- *Clinical application*: severe Gram-negative aerobic bacillary infections (e.g. hospital acquired pneumonia, bloodstream infection) caused by coliforms and *P. aeruginosa*. Use in meningitis and other CNS infections.

Carbapenems

These agents have potent, broad spectrum activity and are generally used for the treatment of severe infections or for infection caused by multiply-resistant bacteria.

Toxicity/side effects

Hypersensitivity reactions (as for penicillins). Significant cross-reactivity with penicillin allergy.

Resistance

As a result of hydrolysis by carbapenemases (β-lactamases specific for carbapenems) or reduced uptake by cell (this may be acquired during treatment).

Examples of carbapenems

Imipenem with cilastatin, and meropenem

- *Pharmacokinetics*: must be given i.v. Renal excretion. Cilastatin is combined with imipenem to inhibit renal dehydropeptidase and improve imipenem blood levels. Imipenem/cilastatin is more likely to provoke convulsions than meropenem. Meropenem is thus favoured for treating central nervous system infections.
- *Antimicrobial spectrum of activity*: active against *Enterobacteriaceae* (including those producing extended-spectrum beta-lactamase), Gram-positive bacteria (e.g. *Staphylococcus aureus* and streptococci), anaerobes and many *Pseudomonas* spp. and *Acinetobacter* spp. *Stenotrophomonas maltophilia* is resistant.
- *Clinical application*: empiric treatment of severe hospital acquired infections and neutropenic sepsis. Directed therapy for infections caused by Gram-negative pathogens resistant to other antimicrobials.

Ertapenem

- *Pharmacokinetics*: once daily iv administration;
- *Antimicrobial spectrum of activity*: active against *Enterobacteriaceae* (including those producing extended-spectrum β-lactamase), Gram-positive bacteria (e.g. *Staphylococcus aureus* and streptococci), anaerobes but not active against *Pseudomonas aeruginosa*.
- *Clinical application*: severe Gram-negative bacillary infections, (e.g. peritonitis) if *Pseudomonas* spp. or *Acinetobacter* spp. are not likely to be present. Once daily dosing allows treatment in the community, e.g. for urinary tract infections caused by multi-resistant *Enterobacteriaceae*.

Doripenem

- *Pharmacokinetics*: i.v. administration every 8 hours;
- *Spectrum*: broad spectrum, including *Pseudomonas aeruginosa* and *Acinetobacter* spp. Stable to many β-lactamases, including ESBLs;
- *Clinical application*: complicated intra-abdominal and complicated urinary tract infections, nosocomial pneumonia.

Monobactams

Activity is restricted to certain Gram-negative bacteria; these agents are resistant to many β-lactamases.

Toxicity/side effects

Hypersensitivity reactions are uncommon, no significant cross-reactivity in patients with immediate-type penicillin allergy.

Aztreonam

- *Pharmacokinetics*: must be given i.v.;
- *Antimicrobial spectrum of activity*: good activity against Gram-negative bacteria, including *Pseudomonas aeruginosa*; no activity against Gram-positive bacteria;
- *Clinical application*: used for Gram-negative and *Pseudomonas aeruginosa* infections in patients who are penicillin allergic.

Glycopeptides

Examples

Vancomycin, teicoplanin.

Mechanism of action

Block cell wall synthesis by binding to the end of the peptide chains of the peptidoglycan precursors; this prevents their incorporation into the cell wall by the transglycosylase enzyme. This results in slow cell lysis and death.

Antimicrobial spectrum of activity

Glycopeptides are bactericidal against Gram-positive bacteria, including staphylococci. They have no activity against Gram-negative bacteria.

Toxicity

Vancomycin occasionally causes nephrotoxicity and rarely causes ototoxicity. Rapid infusion can cause an erythematous rash ('red man syndrome').

Pharmacokinetics

Not absorbed from the gastrointestinal tract and must be administered i.v. for systemic infections. Widely distributed, but poor penetration into cerebrospinal fluid (CSF) and relatively poor penetration into lungs. Renally excreted.

Resistance

This is well-recognised with vancomycin resistant enterococci (VRE). *Staphylococcus aureus* with reduced (intermediate) sensitivity (VISA) are increasingly reported, but true resistance to vancomycin (VRSA) is currently very rare.

Clinical applications

Many infections caused by Gram-positive bacteria (e.g. cellulitis, wound infections) in patients with β-lactam allergy or resistant pathogens. Used for severe staphylococcal infections (especially MRSA), including endocarditis and infections of prosthetic devices caused by coagulase-negative staphylococci. Also used as oral treatment of severe *Clostridium difficile* infection. Serum levels need monitoring to ensure therapeutic levels.

Antibacterial agents acting on cell membranes

Only a few agents target the microbial membrane. These include polymyxins and lipopeptides.

Polymyxins (e.g. colistin) are similar to detergents, they disrupt the outer and cell membranes of some Gram-negative bacteria, resulting in loss of cytoplasmic content. They are nephrotoxic and usually used as topical agents, e.g. in gut sterilisation regimens. Colistin is used to treat *Pseudomonas aeruginosa* lung infections in cystic fibrosis and occasionally used to treat multi-resistant Gram-negative bacilli, e.g. *Acinetobacter* spp.

Lipopeptides (e.g. daptomycin) disrupt the cytoplasmic membrane of Gram-positive bacteria (including staphylococci), resulting in leakage of cell contents. Daptomycin has been developed relatively recently to combat increasingly resistant Gram-positive bacteria, e.g. MRSA. It is used clinically for skin and soft tissue infections and *S. aureus* infections, including bloodstream infection and endocarditis.

Inhibitors of protein synthesis

This group includes the aminoglycosides, tetracyclines, macrolides, chloramphenicol, lincosamides, oxazolidinones, fusidic acid, mupirocin and pleuromutilins, which target differences between human and bacterial protein synthesis:

- *Aminoglycosides*: e.g. gentamicin and tobramycin, bind to the 30S ribosomal subunit and interfere with their proof reading function; this results in misreading of the mRNA and production of toxic proteins through incorporation of the wrong amino acids;
- *Tetracyclines*: bind to the 30S subunit, preventing binding of aminoacyl-transfer RNA to the acceptor site in the ribosome, thereby inhibiting amino acid chain elongation;
- *Macrolides*: e.g. erythromycin, bind to the 50S subunit of ribosomal RNA and inhibit the formation of initiation complexes;
- *Chloramphenicol*: binds to the 50S subunit and interferes with the linkage of amino acids in the peptide chain formation (peptidyl transferase reaction);
- *Lincosamides*: also bind to the 50S subunit and interferes with the linkage of amino acids in the peptide chain formation;
- *Oxazolidinones*: block the initiation stage of protein synthesis in which the 30S ribosomal subunit binds to mRNA;
- *Fusidic acid*: inhibits the function of elongation factor G, a factor that generates energy for the ribosome by hydrolysis of GTP;
- *Mupirocin*: inhibits the coupling of isoleucine (1 of the 20 different amino acids found in proteins) to its tRNA;
- *Pleuromutilins*: (retapamulin) block interaction of peptidyltransferase on 50S subunit with aminoacyl-transfer RNA.

Aminoglycosides

Examples

Amikacin, gentamicin, netilmicin, streptomycin, tobramycin.

Antimicrobial spectrum of activity

Active against staphylococci and Gram-negative aerobic bacilli including *Pseudomonas* spp; they have no activity against anaerobes. They are bactericidal and enhance the antibacterial affects of some antimicrobials (e.g. β-lactams and vancomycin) against staphylococci, streptococci and enterococci.

Toxicity/side effects

Hypersensitivity, ototoxicity and nephrotoxicity.

Pharmacokinetics

Poorly absorbed from the gut; water soluble, so poor penetration into fatty tissue; excretion is almost entirely renal. Serum levels require monitoring with careful dosage adjustment particularly in renal failure.

Resistance

Mechanisms include changes in ribosomal binding of the drug, decreased permeability, increased efflux and, most importantly, inactivation by aminoglycoside-modifying enzymes.

Clinical applications

Severe infection caused by coliforms and other Gram-negative aerobic bacilli. Also used in combination with cell-wall acting antimicrobials for streptococcal and enterococcal endocarditis.

Tetracyclines

Examples

Tetracycline, doxycycline.

Antimicrobial spectrum of activity

Broad spectrum of activity against many Gram-positive and some Gram-negative bacteria; and also *Chlamydia trachomatis*, *Chlamydophila* spp., *Mycoplasma* spp and *Rickettsia* spp. All tetracyclines have very similar spectra of activity.

Toxicity/side effects

Gastrointestinal intolerance; deposition in developing bones and teeth precludes use in young children and in pregnancy; hypersensitivity occasionally, with skin rashes.

Pharmacokinetics

Can be given orally or i.v. Penetrate well into body fluids and tissues as a result of lipid solubility. Excretion is via the kidney and bile duct. Doxycycline may be given once a day.

Resistance

Efflux from cell; less commonly by protection of target from the tetracycline.

Clinical application

Important in treatment of infections caused by *Mycoplasma* spp., *Rickettsia* spp. *Coxiella burnetii* and *Chlamydia trachomatis*.

Glycylcyclines

Only one representative of this group is in clinical use: tigecycline. Tigecycline is a new antimicrobial derived from tetracycline and was developed to combat the increase in multi-resistant bacteria. Tigecycline has broad activity against many Gram-positive and Gram-negative bacteria including multi-resistant, non-fermenters such as *Acinetobacter* spp., but is not active against *Pseudomonas aeruginosa*

Macrolides and lincosamides

Macrolides

Examples

Clarithromycin, azithromycin and erythromycin.

Antimicrobial spectrum of activity

Gram-positive microorganisms; also *Haemophilus*, *Bordetella* and *Neisseria* spp. and some anaerobes. Many coliforms are resistant. Active against *Chlamydia* trachomatis, *Chlamydophila* spp., *Rickettsia* spp. and mycoplasmas.

Toxicity/side effects

Gastrointestinal upsets, rashes, hepatic damage (rare).

Pharmacokinetics

Absorbed following oral administration; also given i.v. They are well distributed and excretion is mainly in the bile.

Resistance

This is by alteration of the RNA target, which results in cross-resistance with clindamycin, or drug efflux (with no cross-resistance to clindamycin).

Clinical applications

Streptococcal and staphylococcal soft tissue infections; respiratory infections including those caused by *Mycoplasma pneumoniae*, *Legionella* spp. and *Chlamydophila pneumoniae*; *Campylobacter* enteritis.

Lincosamides

Examples

Lincomycin (not in clinical use) and clindamycin.

Antimicrobial spectrum of activity

Similar to macrolides, but more active against anaerobes.

Toxicity

Associated with pseudomembranous colitis, but probably no more than many other antimicrobials.

Pharmacokinetics

Usually given orally, but can be given i.v. or i.m. Penetrates well into the bone; metabolised in the liver.

Resistance

See macrolides.

Clinical applications

Clindamycin is primarily used to treat cellulitis and osteomyelitis caused by susceptible microorganisms, as an alternative to flucloxacillin.

Oxazolidinones

Example

Linezolid.

Antimicrobial spectrum of activity

Active against a wide range of Gram-positive bacteria, including MRSA and glycopeptide-resistant enterococci and some anaerobes. Not active against Gram-negative bacteria.

Toxicity

Following prolonged use (>2 weeks) may cause thrombocytopenia and anaemia (check blood counts). Can interact with monoamine oxidase inhibitors. Rarely causes optic neuropathy.

Pharmacokinetics

Excellent oral absorption; oral dose is equivalent to intravenous. Can be used in renal failure. Good penetration of skin and soft tissues, bones, joints and the central nervous system (CNS).

Resistance

Found rarely in *Staphylococcus aureus* and enterococci. Usually the result of ribosomal mutations. May be acquired during treatment.

Clinical applications

Treatment of infections caused by MRSA and glycopeptide-resistant enterococci, including skin and soft tissue infections; ventilator-associated pneumonia; bone and joint, and CNS infections.

Chloramphenicol

Antimicrobial spectrum of activity

Effective against a wide range of microorganisms, including Gram-negative and Gram-positive bacteria, chlamydiae, mycoplasma and rickettsiae.

Toxicity and side effects

Chloramphenicol has a dose-related, but reversible, depressant effect on bone marrow; rarely, irreversible, potentially fatal, marrow aplasia. Toxicity in neonates causes grey baby syndrome.

Pharmacokinetics

Rapidly absorbed after oral administration, with good penetration into many tissues, including the CSF and brain. Metabolised in the liver to inactive metabolites, which are excreted via the kidney.

Resistance

This occurs as a result of inactivation by an inducible acetylase enzyme; reduced permeability.

Clinical applications

Used infrequently in the UK because of concerns about toxicity. Can be used for treatment of meningitis and brain abscesses (e.g. in penicillin allergic patients); used topically for eye infections.

Fucidin (fusidic acid)

Antimicrobial spectrum of activity

Active against staphylococci.

Toxicity and side effects

Causes hepatic damage.

Pharmacokinetics

Well-absorbed, good penetration into bone and joints.

Resistance

Develops rapidly if used as monotherapy.

Clinical applications

Used in combination with flucloxacillin for serious staphylococcal infections (e.g. osteomyelitis, endocarditis).

Mupirocin

Antimicrobial spectrum of activity

Active against staphylococci and streptococci.

Toxicity and side effects

Causes hepatic damage.

Pharmacokinetics

Topical only.

Resistance

Develops rapidly if used continuously.

Clinical applications

Topical treatment of bacterial skin infections and removal of nasal carriage of MRSA.

Pleuromutilins (retapamulin)

Antimicrobial spectrum of activity

Active against staphylococci and streptococci.

Pharmacokinetics

Topical only.

Clinical applications

Topical treatment of impetigo (*Staphylococcus aureus* and *Streptococcus pyogenes*).

Inhibition of nucleic acid synthesis and function

Several classes of antimicrobial agents act on microbial nucleic acid, including the quinolones, sulphonamides, diaminopyrimidines, rifampicin and nitroimidazoles.

Quinolones

Examples

Nalidixic acid and fluoroquinolones, e.g. ciprofloxacin, ofloxacin, norfloxacin, levofloxacin and moxifloxacin.

Mechanism of action

Inhibit the action of bacterial DNA gyrases (topoisomerases), which are important in 'supercoiling' (folding and unfolding of DNA during chromosome replication).

Nalidixic acid

Antimicrobial spectrum of activity

Bacteriostatic against a wide range of *Enterobacteriaceae*; no activity against *Pseudomonas aeruginosa* or Gram-positive microorganisms.

Toxicity and side effects

Gastrointestinal and neurological disturbances.

Pharmacokinetics

Rapidly absorbed after oral administration and almost entirely excreted in the urine.

Resistance

Changes in DNA gyrases result in reduced affinity for nalidixic acid; efflux pumps; less commonly may be caused by target protection. Resistance may be acquired during treatment as a result of chromosomal mutation.

Clinical application

Uncomplicated urinary tract infections.

Fluoroquinolones

Antimicrobial activity

Fluoroquinolones with a Gram-negative spectrum, e.g. ciprofloxacin, have a wider spectrum of activity than nalidixic acid; includes *Pseudomonas* spp, Enterobacteriaceae, legionellae, chlamydiae, mycoplasmas and rickettsiae; poor activity against pneumococci. Fluoroquinolones with better Gram-positive activity (moxifloxacin, levofloxacin) have activity against pneumococci. None of the fluroquinolones have any useful activity against streptococci, enterococci or anaerobes.

Toxicity and side effects

Gastrointestinal disturbances, photosensitivity, rashes, neurological disturbances, including seizures (rare) and ruptured Achilles' tendon. Possible effect on growing cartilage relatively contraindicates use of fluoroquinolones in children.

Pharmacokinetics

Generally good absorption after oral administration; penetrate well into body tissues and fluids. Eliminated by renal excretion and liver metabolism, with some excretion in bile.

Resistance

Has developed extensively through overuse; mechanisms involve mutation in the target DNA gyrase and active removal from the cells (efflux).

Clinical applications

For fluoroquinolones with Gram-negative spectrum: urinary tract infections, gonorrhoea, respiratory and other infections caused by Gram-negative aerobic bacilli, including *Pseudomonas aeruginosa*; also effective for enteritis caused by *Shigella* spp. and *Salmonella* spp.; for prophylaxis in contacts of meningococcal disease. For fluoroquinolones with more Gram-positive spectrum: community-acquired pneumonia, exacerbation of chronic obstructive pulmonary disorder (COPD), sinusitis, otitis media.

Sulphonamides

Example

Sulfamethoxazole.

Mechanism of action

Inhibits folic acid synthesis in bacteria as a competitive antagonist of *p*-aminobenzoic acid, resulting in inhibition of purine and thymidine synthesis (Figure 20.5). Note: trimethoprim also acts on the folic acid synthesis in the next step in the metabolic pathway.

Pharmacokinetics

Well absorbed after oral administration. Distributed throughout the body and excreted mainly in the urine.

Antimicrobial spectrum of activity

Broad spectrum of activity, including streptococci, neisseriae, *H. influenzae.*

Toxicity

Hypersensitivity reactions, causing renal damage, rash; rarely Stevens-Johnson syndrome (a serious

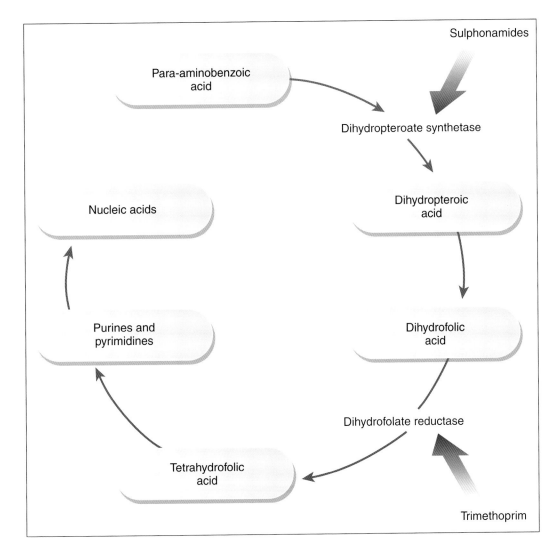

Figure 20.5 Action of sulphonamides and trimethoprim.

form of erythema multiforme); bone marrow failure.

Resistance

Many Enterobacteriaceae are now resistant, as a result of production of an altered dihydropteroate synthetase with decreased affinity for sulphonamide.

Clinical applications

Limited by resistance and toxicity, but include treatment of *Nocardia* infections and also occasionally used in combination with trimethoprim ('co-trimoxazole') for treatment of non-severe urinary tract, respiratory tract or soft tissue infections caused by pathogens resistant to commonly used antibacterials.

Diaminopyrimidines

Example

Trimethoprim.

Mechanism of action

Prevents synthesis of tetrahydrofolic acid by inhibiting dihydrofolate reductase (Figure 20.5).

Antimicrobial spectrum of activity

Broad spectrum of activity against many Gram-positive and Gram-negative bacteria. *Pseudomonas* spp. are resistant.

Toxicity

Folate deficiency.

Pharmacokinetics

Rapidly absorbed after oral administration. Excretion is via urine.

Resistance

Mainly as a result of modification or production of multiple copies of the target enzyme, dihydrofolate reductase.

Clinical applications

Urinary tract infections.

Co-trimoxazole (trimethoprim combined with sulfamethoxazole)

This was prescribed commonly in general practice for the treatment of urinary tract and respiratory infections; however, it is now recognised that trimethoprim alone is probably just as effective and does not have the toxicity problems associated with sulphonamides.

Rifamycins

Example

Rifampicin.

Mechanism of action

Binds to RNA polymerase and blocks synthesis of mRNA.

Antimicrobial spectrum of activity

Active against many staphylococci, streptococci, *H. influenzae*, neisseriae, legionellae, mycobacteria and many anaerobes. Enterobacteriaceae and *P. aeruginosa* are resistant.

Toxicity

Adverse reactions include skin rashes and transient liver function abnormalities; a rare cause of hepatic failure. Potent inducer of hepatic enzymes, reducing the effect of warfarin and oral contraceptives.

Pharmacokinetics

Well absorbed after oral administration; widely distributed in the body, including CSF. Metabolised in the liver and elimination primarily by biliary secretion.

Resistance

Resistant mutants emerge during therapy, when used as a single agent; resistance is the result of the change in a single amino acid of the RNA polymerase target site. Often used in combination with other agents, to prevent the development of resistance.

Clinical applications

Tuberculosis (as part of combination therapy); in combination with other antimicrobials for endocarditis and osteomyelitis; in combinations for some MRSA infections; as prophylaxis for close contacts of meningococcal and *H. influenzae* meningitis.

Nitroimidazoles

Example

Metronidazole.

Mechanism of action

Metabolised by nitroreductases to active intermediates, which cause DNA breakage.

Antimicrobial spectrum of activity

It is active against *Bacteroides* spp., *Clostridium* spp. and other anaerobes. (Note: also active against *Giardia lamblia*, *Trichomonas vaginalis* and other parasites.)

Toxicity

Nausea, metallic taste; rarely peripheral neuropathy.

Pharmacokinetics

Well absorbed orally or *per rectum* and distributed into most tissues; metabolised in the liver and metabolites excreted in the urine.

Resistance

Rare, but may occur as a result of reduced uptake or decreased nitroreductase activity.

Clinical applications

Treatment of anaerobic infections.

Other antimicrobials

Nitrofurantoin

This agent is only used in uncomplicated urinary tract infections, because no significant blood levels are achieved.

Antimycobacterial agents

Rifampicin and the specific antimycobacterial agents, isoniazid, pyrazinamide and ethambutol are used in treatment of tuberculosis.

21

Antifungal agents

Elizabeth Johnson
Health Protection Agency Mycology Reference Laboratory, Bristol, UK

As fungi are eukaryotic like their human hosts, there are fewer potential targets for antifungal agents but certain groups of agents do have the required selective toxicity. Potential targets in the fungal cell are ergosterol in the fungal cell membrane, which fungal cells contain in place of cholesterol in human cell membranes and components of the fungal cell wall, which human cells lack. The principal agents used in clinical practice are the azoles, the echinocandins, flucytosine, griseofulvin, terbinafine and the polyenes.

Azoles

- *Mechanism of action*: azoles alter the fungal cell membrane by blocking biosynthesis of ergosterol, resulting in build-up of toxic intermediary metabolites, leakage of cell contents and reduced function of membrane-bound enzymes.
- *Toxicity*: they may cause transient abnormalities of liver function; severe hepatotoxicity is a rare complication of ketoconazole therapy.

Fluconazole

- *Antifungal activity*: active against *Candida* species (some species such as *C. krusei* are resistant or have reduced susceptibility, such as

C. glabrata), *Cryptococcus* species and *Histoplasma capsulatum*, dermatophytes; ineffective against most other moulds, including *Aspergillus* and *Mucorales*.
- *Pharmacokinetics*: oral and intravenous preparations are available; good penetration into various body sites, including CSF and the eye. Fluconazole is excreted unchanged in urine. Adverse effects uncommon.
- *Clinical applications*: mucocutaneous and invasive candidiasis; cryptococcal infections, antifungal prophylaxis in immunocompromised patients (e.g. AIDS patients and transplant recipients).

Itraconazole

- *Antifungal activity*: active against *Candida* spp., *Histoplasma capsulatum*, *Aspergillus* spp., *Scedosporium* spp., some mucorales and dermatophytes;
- *Pharmacokinetics*: oral and intravenous preparations are available. It is highly protein bound and degraded into an active metabolite hydroxy-itraconazole and a large number of inactive metabolites and excreted in bile. Accumulates in keratinised tissue, so good for treatment of onychomycosis;
- *Clinical applications*: dermatophytoses, mucocutaneous and invasive candidiasis, aspergillosis, histoplasmosis, blastomycosis , prophylaxis.

Medical Microbiology and Infection Lecture Notes, Fifth Edition. Edited by Tom Elliott, Anna Casey, Peter Lambert and Jonathan Sandoe.
© 2011 Blackwell Publishing Ltd. Published 2011 by Blackwell Publishing Ltd.

Ketoconazole

Available as oral or topical forms and used principally as topical therapy for dermatophyte infections and cutaneous candidiasis.

Miconazole

Available as topical, oral and parenteral forms; used principally as topical therapy for dermatophyte infections and mucosal or cutaneous candidiasis.

Voriconazole

- *Antifungal therapy:* active against a wide range of moulds and yeasts, including *Aspergillus* spp., *Fusarium* spp., some *Scedosporium* spp., *Candida* spp. and many other yeast genera. The spectrum excludes members of the mucorales.
- *Pharmacokinetics:* oral and intravenous preparations available. Cleared mainly by hepatic metabolism; has several notable drug interactions (e.g. warfarin, ciclosporins); generally well tolerated; can cause visual disturbances, hepatotoxicity.
- *Clinical applications:* invasive aspergillosis, other invasive mould infections, invasive yeast infections.

Posaconazole

- *Antifungal therapy:* active against a wide range of moulds and yeasts, including the mucorales;
- *Pharmacokinetics:* oral preparation only, few side effects and a limited number of drug interactions;
- *Clinical applications:* salvage invasive aspergillosis, other mould infections, including mucraceous moulds, prophylaxis.

Flucytosine (5-fluorocytosine)

- Synthetic fluorinated pyrimidine;
- *Mechanism of action:* deaminated in fungal cells to 5-fluorouracil, which is incorporated into RNA in place of uracil, resulting in abnormal protein synthesis and inhibition of DNA synthesis. Resistance may arise during treatment;
- *Pharmacokinetics:* intravenous and oral forms available; good tissue and cerebrospinal fluid (CSF) penetration; excreted via the urine;

- *Antimicrobial spectrum of activity:* effective against most yeasts, including *Candida* (some innate resistance in *C. krusei* and *C. tropicalis*) and *Cryptococcus neoformans*. Resistance may occur during treatment, so used in combination therapy;
- *Toxicity:* hepatotoxicity and marrow aplasia; need to monitor serum levels;
- *Clinical applications:* combined with amphotericin B in the treatment of cryptococcal meningitis and some forms of systemic candidiasis.

Griseofulvin

- *Mechanism of action:* inhibition of nucleic acid synthesis and damage to cell wall by inhibiting chitin synthesis; resistance is rare;
- *Pharmacokinetics:* available in oral preparation only; well absorbed and concentrates in keratin, so useful in the treatment of dermatophytosis. Griseofulvin is metabolised in the liver and metabolites are excreted in the urine;
- *Antimicrobial spectrum of activity:* restricted to dermatophytes;
- *Toxicity and side effects:* generally well tolerated; headaches and urticarial rashes may occur;
- *Clinical applications:* dermatophytoses.

Terbinafine

- *Mechanism of action:* inhibition of ergosterol biosynthesis;
- *Pharmacokinetics:* available as an oral preparation or cream for topical administration;
- *Antimicrobial spectrum:* for the treatment of dermatophytosis, including scalp and nail infection. Some activity against other moulds;
- *Toxicity and side effects:* may cause hepatotoxicity;
- *Clinical applications:* dermatophytoses.

Amphotericin B

- *Mechanism of action:* damages the fungal cell membrane by binding to sterols; this results in leakage of cellular components and cell death.
- *Pharmacokinetics:*
  - topical preparations (lozenges/mouth washes) for oral candidiasis;
  - parenteral preparation for intravenous administration; highly protein bound with low

penetration into many body sites, including CSF; metabolised in the liver.
- *Antimicrobial activity:* broad spectrum of activity, including *Aspergillus, Candida, Blastomyces* and *Coccidioides,* spp., *Cryptococcus neoformans, Histoplasma capsulatum* and mucoraceous moulds. Resistance is rare.
- *Toxicity:*
  - anaphylactic reactions occur in some patients (a small test dose should be given before starting therapeutic doses); fever and chills are common.
  - renal tubular damage is a serious problem; renal function should be monitored regularly; doses should be increased slowly.
  - lipid amphotericin preparations (amphotericin complexed to microscopic lipid micelles or strings) have been developed that allow higher doses of amphotericin to be used with reduced toxicity.
- *Clinical applications:* amphotericin remains an effective therapy for systemic mycoses, including disseminated candidiasis, cryptococcosis, aspergillosis and mucormycoses.

Nystatin

- *Mechanism of action:* interferes with the permeability of the cell membrane of sensitive fungi by binding to sterols;
- *Antifungal activity:* mainly against Candida spp.;
- *Pharmakinetics:* poorly absorbed via gastrointestinal tract; not absorbed via skin or mucous membrane when applied topically;
- *Clinical application:* used for treatment of oral, cutaneous and mucosal candidiasis.

Echinocandin antifungal agents

- *Mechanism of action:* inhibit synthesis of cell wall, resulting in cell lysis and death of *Candida* spp., destroys the growing tips of *Aspergillus* spp.;
- Includes anidulafungin, caspofungin and micafungin;
- *Antifungal activity:* active against *Candida* and *Aspergillus* spp.; not active against *Cryptococcus neoformans,* other basidiomycete yeasts, some other moulds including mucorales species;
- *Pharmakinetics:* intravenous use only. Caspofungin and micafungin are metabolized by spontaneous degradation and in liver, anidulafungin by spontaneous degradation only. Drug interactions with caspofungin and micafungin include cyclosporin, rifampicin; anidulafungin, no significant drug interactions; all echinocandins side effects infrequent; not hepatotoxic or nephrotoxic;
- *Clinical application:* all echinocandins treatment of invasive candidiasis, caspofungin salvage aspergillosis. Caspofungin license includes empirical treatment of neutropenic fever; micafungin license includes prophylaxis and treatment of neonates.

Antiviral agents

Eleni Nastouli
University College London Hospitals NHS Trust and Great Ormond Street Hospital for Children NHS Trust, London, UK

A number of antiviral agents are licensed for treatment and new drugs are being developed. Antivirals are mainly used for the treatment of human immunodeficiency virus (HIV), hepatitis B and C, herpesviruses (herpes simplex virus (HSV), varicella-zoster virus (VZV), cytomegalovirus (CMV), human herpesviruses (HHV-6 and-7)), influenza virus and respiratory syncytial virus (RSV).

Mechanisms of action

Antiviral agents can:

1 inactivate intact viruses (viricidal) including: ether, detergents, ultraviolet (UV) light, but these are not used for treating patients;
2 inhibit viral replication (antivirals);
3 modify host responses (immunomodulators).

Antivirals inhibit:

- virus attachment to cell receptors;
- virus uncoating;
- viral genome transcription and replication;
- virus maturation;
- virion assembly and release.

Immunomodulators enhance host-immune responses.

Drug resistance

Resistance results from point mutations within the viral genome, and testing for resistance is an essential part of the clinical management of patients treated with antivirals. It is mainly encountered when treating immunocompromised patients. Transmission of drug resistant viruses is well documented, particularly for HIV.

Anti-HIV compounds

Current treatment guidelines for HIV infection suggest the use of three active drugs from at least two classes, i.e. two nucleoside reverse transcriptase inhibitors (NRTI) and a non-nucleoside reverse transcriptase inhibitor (NNRTI) or two NNRTI and a protease inhibitor (PI).

Nucleoside analogue reverse transcriptase inhibitors (NRTI)

Examples include: zidovudine (AZT), didanosine (ddI), zalcitabine (ddC), stavudine (d4T), lamivudine (3TC), abacavir (ABC) and emtricitabine (FTC).

Medical Microbiology and Infection Lecture Notes, Fifth Edition. Edited by Tom Elliott, Anna Casey, Peter Lambert and Jonathan Sandoe.

Table 22.1 Nucleoside analogue reverse transcriptase inhibitors

Naturally occurring nucleoside	Drug analogue
Thymidine	AZT, d4T
Cytidine	ddC, 3TC, FTC
Adenosine	ddI
Guanosine	ABC

Structure

Analogues of naturally occurring nucleosides (Table 22.1)

Mechanism of action

Activated by phosphorylation by cellular enzymes to the triphosphate form. Inhibition of viral RNA-dependent DNA polymerase (reverse transcriptase, RT) and chain termination of the viral RT reaction.

Activity

HIV-1 and -2, hepatitis B (3TC and FTC only).

Clinical applications

HIV treatment and post-exposure prophylaxis.

Route of administration

Orally.

Toxicity-side effects

- Lactic acidosis, steatosis, lipoatrophy (effects of mitochondrial toxicity);
- Abacavir can cause hypersensitivity reactions in HLA-B*5701 positive individuals, therefore HLA testing is indicated prior to treatment;
- AZT: granulocytopenia and/or anaemia;
- d4T, ddI: peripheral neuropathy, pancreatitis.

Nucleotide analogue reverse transcriptase inhibitor (NtRTI)

i.e. tenofovir.

Structure

Acyclic phosphonate analogue of adenosine monophosphate.

Mechanism of action

Activated by phosphorylation by cellular enzymes to the diphosphate form and then as above.

Activity

HIV-1 and -2, hepatitis B.

Clinical applications

HIV infection.

Route of administration

Orally.

Toxicity-side effects

Renal tubular dysfunction, bone demineralisation.

Non-nucleoside reverse transcriptase inhibitors (NNRTI)

Examples include nevirapine, efavirenz and etravirine (the newest in the class, active against viruses resistant to other NNRTI).

Mechanism of action

Non-competitive inhibitors of RT. They bind to a hydrophobic pocket on RT, separate from the active site.

Activity

HIV-1. Not active against HIV-2.

Clinical applications

HIV infection.

Route of administration

Orally.

Toxicity-side effects

- *Nevirapine*: rash, hepatitis, Stevens-Johnson syndrome, usually first 12 weeks;
- *Efavirenz*: mood changes, vivid dreams, common but usually short lived;

- *Etravirine*: Stevens-Johnson syndrome, toxic epidermal necrolysis, erythema multiforme, organ dysfunction, such as hepatic failure.

Protease inhibitors

Examples include saquinavir, ritonavir, indinavir, nelfinavir, amprenavir, lopinavir, atazanavir, tipranavir and darunavir.

Structure

Oligopeptide analogues of the natural substrate of viral protease.

Mechanism of action

Binding to the protease active site and inhibition.

Activity

HIV-1 and -2.

Clinical applications

HIV infection.

Route of administration

Orally.

Toxicity-side effects

Lipodystrophy, hyperlipidaemia, diabetes mellitus, important interactions with a range of other drugs.
  Atazanavir can cause jaundice and elevated total bilirubin.

Viral entry inhibitors (fusion inhibitors)

Enfuvirtide (T20)

Structure

A peptide made up of 36 amino acids corresponding to amino acid residues of the viral glycoprotein precursor gp160 and gp41.

Mechanism of action

Inhibition of virus-cell fusion, mimicking a homologous region in gp41.

Activity

HIV-1.

Clinical applications

HIV infection.

Route of administration

Subcutaneous injection.

Toxicity-side effects

Local injection site reactions common.

Maraviroc

Structure

A cyclohexane carboxamide.

Mechanism of action

An antagonist of human chemokine receptor CCR5, a coreceptor used by the virus for cell entry. Co-receptor tropism of the virus infecting the patient needs to be determined with a specific assay. This is because HIV-1 can also use CXCR4, usually in advanced infection. Maraviroc is not effective against CXCR4-tropic, dual- or mixed-tropic virus.

Activity

HIV-1.

Clinical applications

Treatment experienced HIV infected patients – not currently recommended as first-line therapy.

Route of administration

Orally.

Integrase inhibitors

Examples: raltegravir.

Structure

A pyrimidine carboxamide potassium salt.

Mechanism of action

Inhibition of viral integrase, the enzyme integrating viral linear DNA to the host cell genome.

Inhibition of provirus formation, a critical step in viral life cycle.

Activity

HIV-1.

Clinical applications

HIV infection.

Route of administration

Orally.

Drug combinations

Formulations of fixed dose drug combinations in one tablet, i.e. NRTI (AZT-3TC, tenofovir-FTC, abacavir-3TC, abacavir-3TC-AZT) and multi-class combinations (tenofovir-FTC-efavirenz).

Resistance in HIV infection

This develops gradually, resulting in high-level resistance. Usually relates to ongoing viral replication due to suboptimal adherence. Resistant mutants can be transmitted. NNRTI compared to PI exhibit lower genetic barrier to resistance, i.e. the virus has an easier route to high level resistance, in some cases requiring only one point mutation.

Anti-hepatitis B compounds

Nucleoside analogue reverse transcriptase inhibitors (NRTI)

Lamivudine (3TC) and Emtricitabine (FTC)

See above, as for anti-HIV compounds.

Entecavir

Structure

A guanosine nucleoside analogue.

Mechanism of action

Phosphorylation by cellular enzymes to the tri-phosphate form. A chain terminator in the RT reaction.

Activity

Hepatitis B, HIV.

Clinical applications

Hepatitis B. Inadequate activity for use against HIV.

Route of administration

Orally.

Nucleotide analogue reverse transcriptase inhibitor (NtRTI)

Adefovir

Structure

Acyclic phosphonate analogue of adenosine monophosphate.

Mechanism of action

Phosphorylation by cellular enzymes to the di-phosphate form. Inhibition of RT and chain termination in the RT reaction.

Activity

Hepatitis B, HIV and other retroviruses and to lesser extent also herpes viruses.

Clinical applications

HBV infection, particularly for the treatment of lamivudine-resistant HBV infections. Inadequate activity for clinical treatment of HIV infection

Route of administration

Orally.

Tenofovir

As above in anti-HIV compounds.

Resistance in hepatitis B

Lamivudine exhibits low, adefovir intermediate, and tenofovir/entecavir higher genetic barrier to resistance. Therefore, both the latter are the pre-ferred first-line options. Patients with hepatitis B and HIV requiring treatment should receive fully active antiretroviral treatment, including an agent active against hepatitis B, i.e. tenofovir. Entecavir should not be used for HBV infection in HIV/HBV co-infected patients, without full treatment of HIV.

Anti-hepatitis C compounds

Interferon-α and pegylated interferon-α

Interferons are host cell proteins synthesised by eukaryotic cells that can inhibit growth of viruses. There are three major classes: α, β and γ.

Mechanism of action

Complex direct antiviral effects and enhancement of immune responses.

Activity

Mainly hepatitis B and C and papillomaviruses. Pegylated interferon is interferon-α attached to polyethylene glycol, slowing down the elimination rate and enabling less frequent dosing.

Clinical applications

Chronic hepatitis C; other possible applications include papillomavirus infections.

Route of administration

Subcutaneuos injection.

Toxicity-side effects

May cause or aggravate neuropsychiatric, autoim-mune, ischaemic, infectious disorders.

Ribavirin

Structure

A synthetic triazole guanosine analogue.

Mechanism of action

Interference with viral mRNA production.

Activity

Inhibits a wide range of RNA and DNA viruses, in particular paramyxoviruses (RSV), arenaviruses (Lassa, Junin) and adenoviruses.

Resistance

Not recognised, since activity is thought to be mediated through cellular processes

Clinical applications

Orally, in combination with interferon-α for the treatment of hepatitis C and as an aerosol for the treatment of RSV infections in high-risk patients.

Route of administration

Orally.

Toxicity-side effects

Haemolytic anaemia. Teratogenicity.

STAT-C

Specifically Targeted Antiviral Treatment for hep-atitis C (STAT-C) includes drugs that directly in-hibit viral replication (protease and polymerase inhibitors) in combination with interferon-α and ribavirin. Currently in phase 3 clinical trials.

Anti-herpesvirus compounds

Aciclovir and valaciclovir

Structure

A deoxyguanosine analogue. Valaciclovir is the L-valine ester of aciclovir; a pro-drug of aciclovir with better absorption.

Mechanism of action

Activation by viral thymidine phosphokinases and cellular kinases to the triphosphate form. Inhibition of viral DNA polymerases and chain termination.

Activity

HSV-1 and -2 and VZV.

Resistance

Several mechanisms exist, including deletion/al-teration of viral thymidine kinase and altered DNA polymerase. Mainly in immunocompromised patients.

Clinical applications

Mucosal, cutaneous and systemic HSV-1 and -2 infections, i.e. keratitis, encephalitis, genital herpes, neonatal herpes and for VZV infections including chickenpox and shingles.

Route of administration

Aciclovir (orally and intravenous IV infusion), valaciclovir (orally).

Penciclovir and famciclovir

Structure

Penciclovir is a deoxyguanosine analogue. Famciclovir is the diacetyl ester of penciclovir, a pro-drug of penciclovir with increased bioavailability.

Mechanism of action

Similar to aciclovir. Inhibition of viral DNA synthesis.

Activity

HSV-1 and -2 and VZV.

Resistance

Mainly in immunocompromised patients. Cross resistance with aciclovir resistance.

Clinical applications

HSV-1 and -2 and VZV infections.

Route of administration

Orally.

Ganciclovir and valganciclovir

Structure

Deoxyguanosine analogues. Valganciclovir is the L-valine ester of ganciclovir, a pro-drug with higher tissue concentration.

Mechanism of action

Activation by viral HSV thymidine phosphokinases, CMV protein kinases and cellular kinases to the triphosphate form. Inhibition of viral DNA polymerases and chain termination.

Toxicity and side effects

Myelosuppression: neutropenia (up to 40% of patients); thrombocytopenia (up to 20%); reversible on cessation.

Activity

CMV, HHV-6 and -7, HSV-1 and -2.

Resistance

Mainly in immunocompromised patients.

Clinical applications

CMV infections, particularly in immunocompromised patients; prevention of CMV disease after organ transplantation.

Route of administration

Ganciclovir (I.V.), valganciclovir (orally).

Foscarnet

Structure

An inorganic pyrophosphate analogue. It inhibits herpesviruses and most ganciclovir-resistant CMV and aciclovir-resistant HSV and VZV mutants.

Mechanism of action

Interference with the binding of pyrophosphate to its binding site and direct inhibition of the viral DNA polymerase.

Toxicity and side effects

Nephrotoxicity; hypo- and hypercalcaemia and hypokalaemia.

Activity

HSV-1 and -2, VZV, CMV and HHV-6 and -7.

Resistance

Mainly in immunocompromised patients.

Clinical applications

CMV infections, aciclovir-resistant HSV and VZV infections.

Route of administration

I.V.

Cidofovir

Structure

A deoxycytosine analogue.

Mechanism of action

Phosphorylation by cellular enzymes to the diphosphate form. Inhibition of viral DNA polymerase and chain termination.

Toxicity

Nephrotoxic.

Activity

HSV-1 and -2, VZV, CMV, HHV-6 and -7, papilloma-, polyoma-, adeno- and poxviruses.

Resistance

Mainly in immunocompromised patients.

Clinical applications

CMV, HHV-6 and -7 infections, aciclovir-resistant HSV and VZV infections, laryngeal and cutaneous papillomatous lesions, adenovirus infections.

Route of administration

I.V.

Anti-influenza compounds

Amantadine/rimantadine

Structure

Tricyclic amines.

Mechanism of action

Inhibition of uncoating of viral RNA.

Activity

Influenza A.

Resistance

Readily selected; up to 30% of treated patients develop resistance.

Clinical applications

Treatment and prevention of influenza A virus infection.

Route of administration

Orally.

Neuraminidase inhibitors (Zanamivir, Oseltamivir, Peramivir)

Structure

N-Acetylneuraminic acid (sialic acid) analogues.

Mechanism of action

Inhibition of viral neuraminidase, prevention of release of progeny virus particles from infected cells.

Activity

Influenza A and B.

Resistance

Rare unless immunocomprmised.

Clinical application

Treatment and prevention of influenza A and B infections.

Route of administration

Zanamivir by inhalation and I.V., oseltamivir orally. Peramivir can be given I.V.

Toxicity-side effects

Zanamivir can cause paradoxic bronchospasm.

Part 3

Infection

Diagnostic laboratory methods

Tony Worthington
Aston University, Birmingham, UK

This chapter summarises the common diagnostic techniques and procedures undertaken by the Clinical Microbiology Laboratory. The role of the laboratory in the diagnosis of infections can be considered in six major steps. A diagnostic template outlining the sequence of events is given in Figure 23.1.

Clinical request form

A detailed request form that accompanies a clinical sample is pivotal in ensuring the appropriate diagnostic procedures are undertaken; information should include: patient details, clinical diagnosis, onset of symptoms, sample type, time of collection, treatment history and concurrent antimicrobial therapy and any health and safety issues. Supporting clinical information, including travel history and contact with infected individuals, is also important.

Sample collection

Samples for microbiological investigation require careful collection, without contamination from external sources (e.g. healthcare worker collecting sample/clinical environment) or the patient's own flora. Table 23.1 demonstrates body sites that have a normal microbiological flora and those areas that are sterile. When taking clinical samples, it is important to: use sterile, leak-proof containers; label the specimen correctly; take care whilst obtaining samples through an area containing a normal flora, e.g. venepuncture through skin to obtain blood culture (Figure 23.2); in this instance the skin should be decontaminated with an appropriate antiseptic prior to collecting blood. If possible, specimens for microbiological culture should be taken prior to commencement of antibiotic therapy, to avoid false-negative results.

Medical Microbiology and Infection Lecture Notes, Fifth Edition. Edited by Tom Elliott, Anna Casey,
Peter Lambert and Jonathan Sandoe.
© 2011 Blackwell Publishing Ltd. Published 2011 by Blackwell Publishing Ltd.

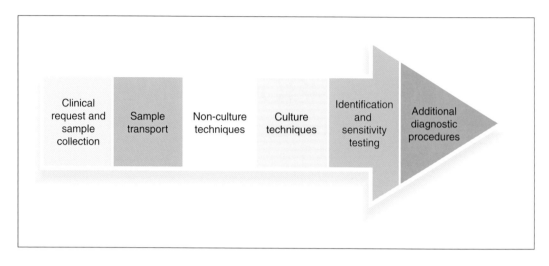

Figure 23.1 Diagnostic template.

Transport of clinical samples

Rapid transport of samples to the microbiology laboratory is essential, as many fastidious microorganisms, such as *Neisseria gonorrhoeae* and *Haemophilus influenzae*, die during transit. Furthermore overgrowth by contaminating normal flora obscuring the pathogen may also occur. To minimise these complications, the microbiology department may adopt several strategies: use of transport media (Table 23.2); refrigeration of sample at 4 °C when a short delay in processing is anticipated, freezing at − 70 °C or below in the presence of a stabilising fluid, e.g. glycerol or serum.

Non-culture techniques

Following receipt of the sample, the microbiology laboratory may utilise non-culture techniques to provide rapid clinical information, which may benefit patient management. There are several situations where non-culture techniques are of importance:

• Microorganism cannot be readily cultured *in vitro*;

Table 23.1 Sterile and non-sterile sites of the human body

Normally sterile sites of the body	Sites having a normal flora
Blood	Upper respiratory tract: oral ('viridians') streptococci, *Candida albicans*, anaerobes
Bone marrow	
Subcutaneous tissue/muscle/bone	Skin: coagulase-negative staphylococci, diphtheroids
Cerebrospinal fluid/brain	Gastrointestinal tract: Coliforms, e.g. *Escherichia coli*, anaerobes, enterococci ('faecal flora')
Lower respiratory tract	
Heart	Vagina: lactobacilli, anaerobes
Bladder/kidneys/prostate/uterus	Urethra: skin microorganisms and faecal flora
Liver/pancreas/adrenals/gall bladder	

- Microorganism is slow-growing;
- Rapid laboratory diagnosis significantly influences clinical management of the patient.

Non-culture techniques include direct microscopy, immunological methods, serology, and nucleic acid amplification techniques (NAAT).

Direct microscopy

Many clinical samples may be visualised by direct microscopy; unstained wet mounts, stained preparations (e.g. Gram, Ziehl-Neelsen, auramine, acridine orange) or fluorescent antibody stains can be examined.

Unstained wet mounts

Commonly used to identify the presence of motile *Trichomonas vaginalis* in fresh high vaginal specimens (HVS) and cysts/ova/larvae of gastrointestinal parasites in faecal samples, e.g. *Ascaris lumbricoides, Giardia lamblia, Entamoeba histolytica, Strongyloides stercoralis*. This may also be of value in the diagnosis of some fungal infections, e.g. dermatophyte infection through detection of fungal filaments in clinical samples.

Stained preparations

Gram stain

Most widely used stain; classifies bacteria into Gram-positive cocci/bacilli, Gram-negative cocci/bacilli and establishes the presence of

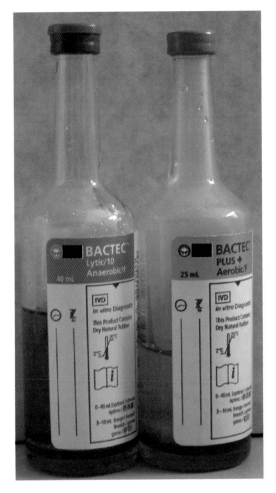

Figure 23.2 Aerobic and anaerobic blood culture bottles.

Table 23.2 Common transport media

Microorganism type	Medium	Comments
Bacteria	Stuart's transport medium	Contains charcoal to inactivate toxic by-products of bacterial growth
	1.8% (w/v) boric acid	Prevents bacterial multiplication in urine
Viruses	Viral transport medium (VTM)	Buffered salt solution containing serum and also antimicrobials to inhibit bacterial and fungal growth
Chlamydiae	Chlamydial transport medium	Similar to VTM but without antimicrobials detrimental to Chlamydiae
Parasites	Merthiolate-iodine-formalin	Preserves ova and cysts and kills bacteria. Unsuitable for protozoal trophozoites

inflammatory cells (e.g. polymorphonucleocytes) (box 23.1). Also facilitates the diagnosis of many fungal infections, e.g. budding cells and pseudo-mycelium of *Candida albicans*. Particularly useful in diagnosing infections from sterile sites, e.g. Gram-negative diplococci (*Neisseria meningitidis*) in cerebrospinal fluid (CSF) or when microorganisms have a characteristic morphology, e.g. *Streptococcus pneumoniae* in sputum samples.

BOX 23.1 Gram stain method

1 Spread specimen thinly on glass microscope slide and heat fix;
2 Stain with crystal violet (purple);
3 Add Lugols iodine (this fixes the dye in Gram-positive bacteria only);
4 Decolourise with acetone or alcohol (only Gram-negative bacteria are decolourised; Gram-positive remain purple);
5 Counter stain; carbol fuchsin (stains Gram-negative bacteria pink; Gram-positive bacteria remain purple).

Ziehl-Neelsen (ZN) stain

ZN stains can be performed on many clinical samples, principally to identify mycobacterial infection when suspected (box 23.2).

BOX 23.2 Ziehl–Neelsen stain

1 Spread specimen thinly on glass microscope slide and heat fix;
2 Stain with HOT carbol–fuchsin dye (all bacteria are stained pink);
3 Decolourise with 20% sulphuric acid (mycobacteria retain dye and are therefore 'acid-fast');
4 Counter stain with methylene blue or malachite green to reveal non-mycobacterial microorganisms. Mycobacteria are stained pink, non-mycobacteria are blue or green.

Fluorescent stains

Auramine: most widely used for detection of *Mycobacterium tuberculosis* in clinical specimens and *Cryptosporidium parvum* in faecal samples.

Acridine orange: commonly used to detect *Trichomonas vaginalis* in HVS.

Fluorescent antibody stains

Monoclonal or polyclonal antibodies are complexed with fluorescent molecules for diagnosis of several infections (Figure 23.3) including *Pneumocystis jirovecii* pneumonia, syphilis and *Legionella pneumophila* pneumonia.

Electron microscopy (EM)

EM is used to visualise and rapidly identify viruses in some clinical samples, e.g. rotavirus/norovirus in faecal samples or herpes simplex and varicella zoster in blister fluids.

Immunological methods

Immunological methods may be used for the detection of bacterial antigen in clinical samples, identification of specific bacterial antigen post-culture or serological detection of antibody/antigen in the patient's serum. The antibody-antigen reaction must be made visible and can be achieved by various techniques.

Antigen detection in clinical samples (Table 23.3)

Some microbial antigens may be detected in clinical samples using commercially available kits to provide a rapid diagnosis of infection, e.g. *Cryptococcus neoformans* capsular antigen in CSF samples, using latex beads coated with specific antibody; *Streptococcus pneumoniae* antigen in urine samples using specific antibody to *S. pneumonia* bound to a nitrocellulose base; *Clostridium difficile* toxin in faecal samples; fluorescent antibody stains (see above). Specific antibodies may also be labelled with enzymes (enzyme-linked immunosorbent assay (ELISA)) which, after binding, can be visualised by the addition of a substrate that is converted to a coloured product, e.g. for the detection of rotavirus in faeces.

Serology (estimation of serum antibody levels)

Detection of antibody by labelled antibody techniques requires an additional step. These assays

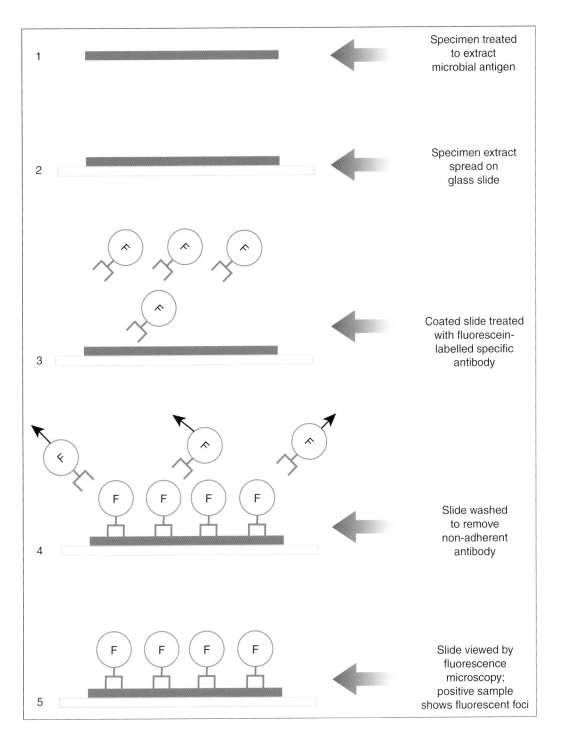

Figure 23.3 Direct detection of microorganisms or their antigens by fluorescein-labelled antibodies.

Table 23.3 Direct detection of bacterial antigens in clinical samples

Clinical specimen	Microorganism/antigen	Technique
Respiratory samples	Influenza/Parainfluenza virus	Immunofluorescence
	Respiratory syncytial virus (RSV)	
	Adenovirus	
	Legionella pneumophila	
	Pneumocystis jirovecii;	
Urogenital specimens	Chlamydia trachomatis	ELISA, Immunofluorescence
	Streptococcus pneumoniae	Enzyme immunoassay (EIA)
Cerebrospinal fluid	Haemophilus influenzae	Co-agglutination
	Neisseria meningitidis	
	Streptococcus pneumoniae	
Faeces	Rotavirus	ELISA/EIA
	C. difficile toxin	

are often carried out in 96-well microtitre trays. Individual wells are precoated with known microbial antigen and the patient's serum added. The well is washed to remove unbound antibody and the remaining bound antibody is detected by adding antibody to human immunoglobulin-labeled with fluorescein or enzyme (ELISA, Figure 23.4).

Antibodies of the various human classes, IgG, IgM or IgA can be detected individually. Another method for capturing specific IgG and IgM antibodies is to coat wells with anti-human immunoglobulins. The patient's serum is added to the wells and bound antibodies are detected by the addition of specific antigens, followed by a labelled antibody (Figure 23.4). Serological diagnosis is important for detecting infections caused by pathogens that are difficult to culture by standard laboratory methods, e.g. *Mycoplasma pneumoniae, Chlamydophila psittaci, Treponema pallidum, Coxiella burnetii,* hepatitis A, B and C (HAV, HBV, HCV) and HIV. Active infection is diagnosed by either detection of specific IgM or a four-fold increase in IgG antibodies in paired sera (acute and convalescent samples) taken 10–14 days apart. Immune status testing (e.g. hepatitis B immunisation) is performed by detection of IgG antibodies. Many serological assays are now automated or semi-automated in modern diagnostic laboratories.

Co-agglutination reactions

Specific antibody or antigen fixed to a carrier, e.g. latex beads. Positive results are indicated by visible agglutination. May be used for identifying group-specific carbohydrate antigen of β-haemolytic streptococci (Lancefield grouping), detection of bacterial antigen in CSF for diagnosing meningitis, e.g. *Neisseria meningitidis,* and for confirming culture isolates of *Staphylococcus aureus*/MRSA (Figure 23.5).

Nucleic Acid Amplification Tests (NAAT)

Molecular biology techniques for the detection and amplification of microbial nucleic acids in specimens are now widely used for diagnosis of a large number of infections. NAAT are useful for microorganisms that are difficult or slow to culture (e.g. mycobacteria, Hepatitis B/C, HIV) or where rapid results are necessary, e.g sexually transmitted infection due to *Chlamydia trachomatis* or *Neisseria gonorrhoeae,* or for MRSA screening. NAAT have greater sensitivity than many serological methods. Many NAAT are now available as commercial kits and in automated systems.

Available techniques include:

- *Polymerase chain reaction (PCR)*: uses thermostable DNA polymerase enzyme to extend

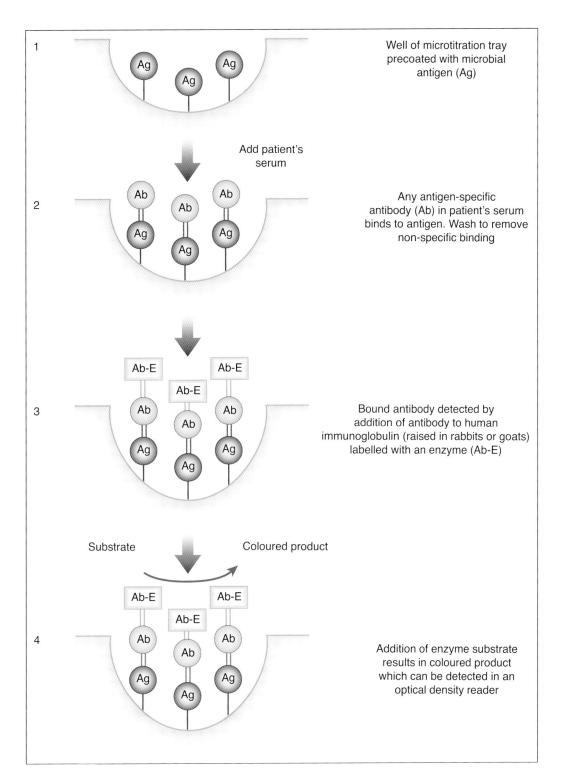

1 Well of microtitration tray precoated with microbial antigen (Ag)

Add patient's serum

2 Any antigen-specific antibody (Ab) in patient's serum binds to antigen. Wash to remove non-specific binding

3 Bound antibody detected by addition of antibody to human immunoglobulin (raised in rabbits or goats) labelled with an enzyme (Ab-E)

Substrate → Coloured product

4 Addition of enzyme substrate results in coloured product which can be detected in an optical density reader

Figure 23.4 Detection of antibodies by ELISA.

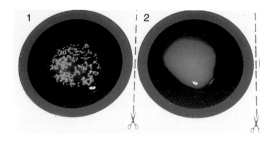

Figure 23.5 Latex agglutination test for *Staphylococcus aureus*: (1) positive agglutination; (2) no agglutination.

oligonucleotide primers complementary to the target nucleic acid in consecutive cycles of denaturing, annealing and extension. This results in amplification of target DNA (Figure 23.6). The technique can be used as a *multiplex PCR* to detect several targets within a specimen in one PCR reaction. *Real-time PCR* allows the reaction to be undertaken within a closed system, using very rapid temperature cycling times and results in completion of a PCR reaction and detection of the product within minutes.

- *Ligase chain reaction* (*LCR*): involves hybridisation of two oligonucleotide probes at adjacent positions on a strand of target DNA, which are subsequently joined by a thermostable ligase enzyme.
- *Nucleic acid sequence-based amplification* (*NASBA*): uses RNA as a target and utilises three enzymes simultaneously: reverse transcriptase, RNAase H and DNA-dependent RNA polymerase.

- *Strand displacement amplification* (*SDA*): utilises oligonucleotide primers containing a restriction enzyme site, DNA polymerase and a restriction enzyme at a constant temperature, to produce exponential amplification of the target.

Culture techniques

Most medically important bacteria and fungi can be cultured on laboratory agar or in enrichment broths. Recovery of pathogenic microorganisms by culture remains the definitive method of confirming a diagnosis of infection. Various types of microbiological media exist:

- *Basic agar*: e.g. nutrient agar: recovers the majority of medically important bacteria;
- *Enriched agar*: e.g. horse blood/chocolate agar: recovers clinically important bacteria including fastidious microorganisms, e.g. *Neisseria gonorrhoeae*, *Haemophilus influenzae*;
- *Selective agar*: contains antimicrobial agents to suppress growth of normal flora from sites that are normally colonised, allowing recovery of specific pathogens from a mixture of bacteria (Table 23.1), e.g. cefoxitin cycloserin fructose agar (CCFA) for recovery of *Clostridium difficile* from faeces;
- *Differential agar*: contains an indicator (usually a dye) to allow differentiation of bacteria, e.g. cysteine lactose electrolyte deficient (CLED) agar, which differentiates lactose fermenting microorganisms from non-lactose fermenters by formation of yellow colonies;

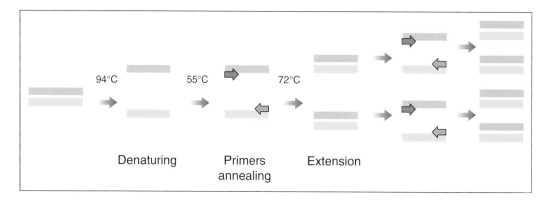

Figure 23.6 Nucleic acid amplification by PCR.

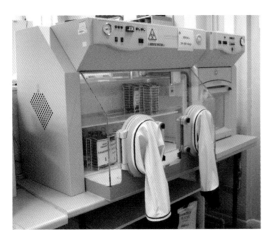

Figure 23.7 Anaerobic cabinet used for growing anaerobic bacteria.

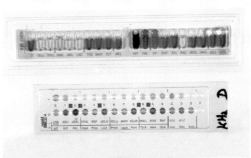

Figure 23.8 Commercial biochemical-based identification system (API).

- *Enrichment broth*: nutritious broth, which allows recovery and enrichment of small numbers of microorganisms within a clinical sample, e.g. brain heart infusion (BHI), cooked meat broth;
- *Selective enrichment broth*: enrichment broth containing antimicrobial agents allowing recovery and enrichment of specific pathogens from non-sterile sites, e.g. sodium selenite broth for selective enrichment *of Salmonella* from faeces.

Following inoculation, microbiological media are incubated under specific atmospheric conditions to allow growth of microorganisms, e.g. at 37 °C under anaerobic (Figure 23.7) or aerobic conditions usually for 24–48 hrs.

Bacterial identification

To ensure correct and appropriate treatment of infection, is it essential to accurately identify pathogens recovered from samples. Identification techniques include:

- *Growth characteristics*, e.g. strictly aerobic/anaerobic, facultative anaerobe; speed of growth;
- *Colonial characteristics*, e.g. size, shape, haemolysis, odour;
- *Microsopical appearance*, e.g. Gram positive/negative; presence of hyphae/spores; bacillus/coccus;
- *Antigenic characteristics*, e.g. group specific carbohydrates (Lancefield grouping of β-haemolytic streptococci), presence of clumping factor/

protein A (*S. aureus*), somatic/flagella antigens (identification of *Salmonella* spp.);
- *Biochemical properties*, e.g. fermentation of sugars, enzyme production (Figure 23.8);
- *Specific growth factor requirement*, e.g. X and V dependency of *Haemophilus influenzae*;
- *Gene probes*, e.g. specific gene probes to identify bacterial DNA/RNA, e.g. identification of mycobacteria;
- *Toxin production*, e.g. Nagler test for *Clostridium perfringens*, ELISA for *C. difficile* toxins.

Antibiotic Susceptibility Testing (AST)

Microorganisms of clinical significance are investigated for antibiotic susceptibility. Various AST methods are used in the laboratory and include disc diffusion susceptibility test (Figure 23.9), determination of minimum inhibitory/bactericidal concentrations (MIC/MBC), and agar dilution assay. Many modern laboratories now incorporate semi- or fully automated systems for rapid (same day) bacterial identification and susceptibility results, e.g. VITEK®2 (bioMérieux, Figure 23.10). In the UK, susceptibility testing is undertaken in line with the British Society for Antimicrobial Chemotherapy (BSAC) guidelines.

Additional diagnostic procedures

- *Further identification*: Identification to genus or species level is normally satisfactory in routine diagnostic laboratories; however, further characterisation (typing) may be necessary in

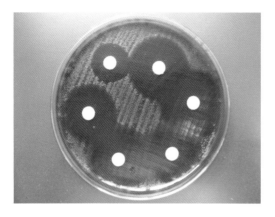

Figure 23.9 Antibiotic sensitivities of a group A streptococcus (*S. pyogenes*) by the BSAC disc diffusion susceptibility test.

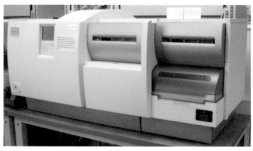

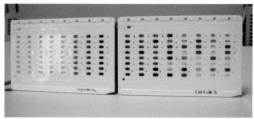

Figure 23.10 Vitek®2 machine and cards used for automated identification and antibiotic sensitivity testing.

outbreak situations to identify the relatedness of strains. Microorganisms can be further characterised by phenotypic methods, e.g. antibiogram profiling, biochemical profiling, phage typing (e.g. *S. aureus*), serotyping (e.g. *Salmonella* spp.) or by genotypic techniques, e.g. ribotyping (*C. difficile*), pulsed field gel electrophoresis (PGFE), multilocus sequence typing (MLST).

• *Further AST*: Multi–resistant microorganisms may need to be tested against an additional panel of further antibiotics prior to issuing the final report.

• *Reporting of infectious disease*: Notification of a number of specified infectious diseases, e.g. tuberculosis, meningitis and food poisoning is required under the Public Health (Infectious Diseases) 1988 Act and the Public Health (Control of Diseases) 1984 Act. In the UK, notifications are sent to the Office of National Statistics (ONS) and the Communicable Disease Surveillance Centre (CDSC).

Epidemiology and prevention of infection

Barry Cookson
Health Protection Agency, Microbiology Services, Colindale, London, UK

Community-acquired infections are those acquired in the community, rather than as a result of admission to healthcare establishments such as hospitals. Hospital-acquired (also called nosocomial) infections are defined as those infections presenting during hospitalisation (at least 2 days after admission) by a patient who was not incubating that infection upon admission. Patients may also present after their discharge with a hospital-acquired infection to their GP, or to follow-up care establishments (including outpatients) or if they are re-admitted to a hospital.

The incidence of hospital-acquired infection is between 5 and 10% of all inpatients in the UK; it can be much higher in less well resourced countries. A UK prevalence study in 2006 demonstrated that the principal sites of infection were of:

- the urinary tract (20%);
- surgical sites (15%);
- lower respiratory tract (14%);
- skin (11%);
- bloodstream (7%);
- gastro-intestinal tract (21%) (e.g. Norovirus and *Clostridium difficile*).

Increased risk of infection is related to prolonged hospitalisation, intensive care, the use of invasive prosthetic devices (e.g. intravenous catheters, urinary catheters, endotracheal tubes) and immunocompromised patients, including those with impaired local host defences (e.g. burns, trauma). The widespread use of antimicrobials in hospitals results in the selection of antimicrobial-resistant microorganisms in the hospital environment; patients in hospital who receive antimicrobials frequently become colonised with these microorganisms, some of which may subsequently cause infection.

Strategies to prevent and control infection in the community and healthcare establishments, including hospitals, require an understanding of the sources and modes of transmission of microorganisms causing these infections and the dynamics of pathogenesis.

Epidemiology of infection

Epidemiology of infection is the study of the aetiology and occurrence of infections in populations. It includes knowledge of the 'time, place and person' of those patients infected or colonised with the implicated microorganisms. Infections may be either sporadic, or occur in outbreaks, with two or more related patients, suggesting that

Medical Microbiology and Infection Lecture Notes, Fifth Edition. Edited by Tom Elliott, Anna Casey, Peter Lambert and Jonathan Sandoe.

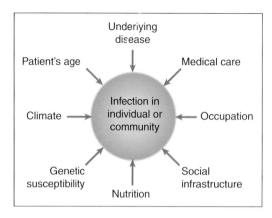

Figure 24.1 Factors affecting the epidemiology of infection.

transmission has occurred. Typing of microorganisms isolated from infected or colonised patients enables the hypotheses of spread to be confirmed or refuted. Factors affecting the epidemiology of infections are shown in Figure 24.1.

Definitions

- The *incidence rate* is the number of new cases of acute disease in a specified population over a defined period, and is expressed as a proportion of the total population studied.
- The *prevalence rate* is the total number of cases present in a defined population at a certain time point or over a certain period. Prevalence exceeds incidence. However, for healthcare associated infection studies, as length of stay in these establishments decreases, so the two become more similar.
- The *attack rate* is the proportion of the total population at risk, who became infected during an outbreak.
- Infections that remain present in a population are described as *endemic*; an increase in incidence above the endemic level is described as hyper-endemic.

The cycle of infection

This term describes the classical cycle for any infection and is used by epidemiologists when investigating possible outbreaks of infection. This is shown for hospital-acquired infection in Figure 24.2, but can be used for any infection. The reservoir comprises potential locations of the causative microorganism. The epidemiology of the outbreak may suggest several sources of infection, one of which may be supported by the typing of microorganisms isolated from an outbreak. For a source to be a focus of infection, there has to be a 'route of transmission' and a 'portal of entry' into the subjects involved. Those exposed may then become infected or merely colonised by the microorganism. In either case, these individuals add to the reservoir of the microorganism and may become additional sources for new infections or colonisations. For many infections, especially those occurring in hospitals, about three times as many patients are colonised as infected. An important point regarding control of outbreaks, especially in healthcare establishments, is that colonised and infected patients need to be identified, as either can be the source for further transmissions.

Sources of infection

Endogenous

These are infections caused by microorganisms that are part of the host's normal flora.

Exogenous

These infections are caused by microorganisms acquired from other humans, animals or the environment:

- *Humans*: infections are commonly acquired from other humans, who may be infected or carry a microorganism asymptomatically; carriers may be convalescent (i.e. recovered from the infection, but continuing to excrete the microorganism, e.g. typhoid carriage in the gall bladder); or healthy carriers who have not had an infection (e.g. a third of the population persistently carry *Staphylococcus aureus* in the nose).
- *Animals*: human infections acquired from animals are termed 'zoonoses'. Both domestic and wild animals may be sources of infection; the animal may be infected or carry the microorganism asymptomatically.

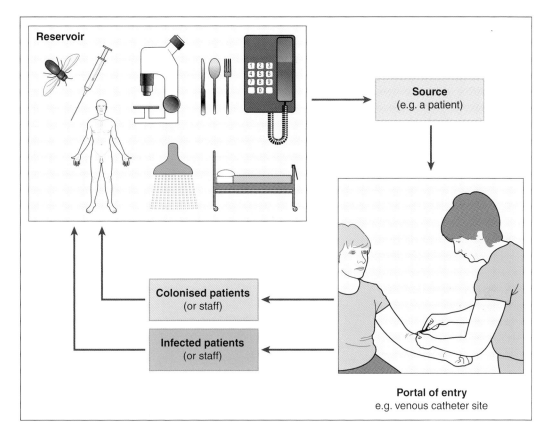

Figure 24.2 Cycle of Infection.

- *Environment*: large numbers of microorganisms are found in soil and water, but very few are associated with human infection (e.g. *Clostridium tetani*; *Aspergillus* spp, *Legionella* spp).

- *Shed squamous epithelial cells*: which may act as airborne vehicles for microorganisms (e.g. staphylococci);
- *Aerosolised spores*: (e.g. *Aspergillus fumigatus*) from contaminated air-handling plants.

Routes of spread of infection

Airborne

Airborne spread can occur via:

- *Droplets*: produced by patients with a respiratory infection (e.g. influenza virus, *Mycobacterium tuberculosis*), from ventilator nebulisers (e.g. *Pseudomonas aeruginosa*) or from air-conditioning systems (e.g. *Legionella pneumophila*);

Contact transfer (Tables 24.1 and 24.2)

Sources of microorganisms (e.g. respiratory secretions, exudates from wounds and other skin lesions, urine, faeces) may be transferred to an individual either directly or via a vector such as the hands of staff or objects ('fomites'), e.g. surgical instruments, utensils, medical equipment. Other vectors include food, water and insects (e.g. flies). Many infections can also be spread via oral-oral or sexual contact. Faecal-oral transmission is a very important mechanism of spread of infection.

Table 24.1 Examples of oral transmission of infectious agents

Vector	Infection (example)
Direct; person to person	Shigellosis
	Rotavirus infection
Food	Salmonellosis
	Campylobacter enteritis
Milk	Brucellosis
	Tuberculosis
Water	Cholera
	Typhoid

Vertical transmission (transmission from mother to foetus/baby)

This can occur either as a blood borne transmission *in utero* via the placenta e.g. rubella or via contact transmission in the birth canal during delivery (e.g. herpes simplex virus, HIV).

Direct inoculation

Another portal of entry is that of injection, e.g. needles, infusions (drugs, blood, fluids), tick or mosquito bites.

Table 24.2 Examples of transmission by direct contact or transfer

Contact	Infection
Skin	Dermatophyte infection
	Leprosy
Oral	Glandular fever
Sexual	Gonorrhoea
	Chlamydia
	HIV
	Hepatitis B
Inoculation injury from infected source	Hepatitis B, Hepatitis C and HIV
Insect transmission	Malaria from infected mosquitoes

Examples of factors affecting transmission of microorganisms

Survival in the environment

Respiratory viruses survive poorly outside the host; successful transmission requires the production of large numbers of infectious virions. However, the number of virions that are sufficient to cause infection may be small.

M. tuberculosis and *C. difficile* can survive outside the host, and infection can follow the transmission of only a few bacteria.

Neisseria gonorrhoeae dies rapidly outside the host, so transmission is dependent on direct mucous membrane contact (e.g. sexual contact).

Establishment on new host

To attach and survive on a new host, a microorganism must overcome the physical, chemical and immunological barriers that protect the host at each port of entry (e.g. skin, respiratory, gastrointestinal and urogenital tracts). Microorganisms have a variety of virulence factors that promote attachment and survival. When considering the pathogenesis of infection, an analogy can be made of the interactions between the seed (infecting microorganism), the soil (the patient or member of staff) and the climate (all aspects of the environment, e.g. antimicrobials, intravenous devices, the healthcare delivery system).

Key strategies to prevent infections

Reduce or eliminate exposure to sources of infection

Complete *elimination* of an infection worldwide is complex, but has been achieved with smallpox and is aimed for poliomyelitis and measles. Examples of strategies for reducing the source of infection are shown in Table 24.3. The decreased incidence of many infections in developed countries is associated with improved

Table 24.3 Examples of actions which reduce potential sources of infection

Source	Infection	Action
Human	Salmonellosis	Screening of food handlers for *Salmonella* carriage followed by isolation and treatment as appropriate
	Tuberculosis	Isolation; follow-up cases; contact tracing; investigation and treatment of contacts
Animal	Rabies	Quarantine; immunisation of pets
	Anthrax	Burning infected dead animals; immunisation of animals
Environment	Legionellosis	Improved design and maintenance of humidification systems and air conditioning systems including chlorination

social conditions, thereby reducing airborne, faecal-oral and direct contact transmission.

Prevent transmission of infection

Airborne

Isolation of patients with infections that spread by respiratory droplets is feasible for a limited number of conditions (e.g. preventing hospital spread of tuberculosis).

Water

Separate sewage from drinking water and provision of potable water.

Food

Food contamination is an important public health problem; many cases of food poisoning occur per annum in the UK. Preventative measures include:

- Efficient refrigeration of certain foods, e.g. milk;
- Separate storage and preparation areas for possibly contaminated foods (e.g. uncooked poultry) from cooked produce;
- Thorough cooking and reheating procedures; complete defrosting before cooking;
- Catering facilities should have staff with high standards of personal hygiene; exclude from work any staff with infections (e.g. staphylococcal skin infections, diarrhoea, *Salmonella* carriers).

Direct and contact transfer

- Good personal hygiene and isolate patients, e.g. for enteropathogenic pathogens, to prevent faeco-oral spread;
- Sexually transmitted infections can be prevented by safe sex, contact tracing and health education campaigns;
- Blood-borne virus infections (e.g. hepatitis viruses B and C, and HIV) can be prevented (e.g. safe sharps practice, provision of sterile needles for intravenous (IV) drug abusers, and screening of blood and organ donors).

Increasing host resistance

Malnutrition and parasitic infections are important factors that weaken host resistance to other infections.

Immunisation against a variety of potential diseases; including *Haemophilus influenzae*, pertussis (whooping cough), mumps, diphtheria, polio, *Streptococcus pneumoniae* (pneumococcus), *Neisseria meningitidis* and *Clostridium tetani* (tetanus).

Antimicrobial prophylaxis

Includes:

- Preoperative for certain surgical procedures, long-term for specific conditions, e.g. post splenectomy to prevent pneumococcal infection;
- Immunocompromised patients, e.g. AIDS patients to prevent *Pneumocystis* pneumonia;
- Transplant patients to prevent CMV infection;
- Short-term for travellers going to endemic areas, e.g. anti-malarials.

Healthcare-associated infections

Infection prevention and control (IPC) is an important aspect of patient care in the community, as well as in the hospital environment. Infections may result from medical interventions (e.g. a haemodialysis line infection) that are associated with medical care, but not necessarily related to a hospital admission, hence the term healthcare associated infection. Infections not present at the time of admission to a hospital can be either derived in the community (community-acquired infections) or acquired during hospitalisation (hospital-acquired infections).

The source of microorganisms causing HCAI are predominantly from the patient's own body microflora (endogenous), and may be prevented by protecting the potential portals of entry. Prevention includes good aseptic technique and the appropriate use of antimicrobial prophylaxis for certain procedures, e.g. colonic or orthopaedic operations. Infections may also be acquired from external sources. There are two main sources of these. Firstly, cross infection from other patients; these are prevented by interrupting the route of transmission. Methods include appropriate patient isolation and staff hand hygiene measures, e.g. alcohol hand rubs for unsoiled hands. Secondly, acquisition of microorganisms can be from the environment. These can be prevented by correct decontamination procedures, e.g. sterilisation of equipment in hospital sterilisation and decontamination units, or regular cleaning of the hospital environment and equipment, particularly in the patient's immediate environment.

Specific microorganisms associated with healthcare-acquired infection

Microorganisms causing HCAI may be more resistant to antimicrobial agents and include meticillin-resistant *S. aureus* (MRSA), *Pseudomonas aeruginosa* and vancomycin-resistant enterococci (VRE). These need specific preventative and control strategies, in addition to approaches outlined above.

Examples of healthcare-associated infection

Examples of sources and microorganisms associated with different healthcare-associated infections are given in Table 24.4. and are described in more detail below.

Urinary tract infection

This, in many surveys, is the most common nosocomial infection, and is often a complication of urethral catheterisation or other urinary tract operative procedures.

The source of the infecting microorganism may be endogenous or exogenous (being introduced during urological procedures or manipulation of catheter drainage systems). Prevention includes the use of sterile instruments, closed-drainage urinary catheter systems, and careful aseptic technique during urinary catheterisation and subsequent catheter care.

Table 24.4 Examples of sources and microorganisms associated with healthcare-associated infection

Type	Common pathogen	Source/spread
Urinary tract infection	Coliforms	Urinary catheterisation, patient's own flora
Post-operative wound infections	*Staphylococcus aureus*	Patients own flora, environment, hand spread, carriage by staff
Ventilation-associated respiratory tract infection	Coliforms	Hospital source or patient's own flora
Intravascular catheter related infection	Coagulase-negative staphylococci	Patient's skin flora

Table 24.5 Incidence of wound infections relative to surgery undertaken

Type of surgical wound	Example of surgery	Maximal incidence of wound infections (%)*
'Clean': does not involve gastrointestinal, respiratory or genitourinary tracts	Orthopaedic or cardiac surgery	5
'Contaminated': involves site with normal flora (apart from skin)	Operations on gall bladder, genitourinary tract	Up to 20
'Infected': operation site infected at time of surgery	Emergency surgery for burst, infected appendix	Up to 50

*There should be systems in place to ensure that rates of infection are far lower than these potential maxima.

Surgical site infection

The incidence of surgical site (wound) infection varies according to the type of surgery (Table 24.5). Causative microorganisms depend on the site and type of procedure and include:

- *S. aureus*: the most common cause after surgery;
- *Coliforms and anaerobes*: associated most commonly with operations involving the gastrointestinal tract;
- *Coagulase-negative staphylococci*: a frequent cause of device-associated infections;
- *Clostridium perfringens*: may result in gas gangrene, now rare in well resourced countries, but still remaining a problem in less well resourced (developing) countries;
- *Beta-haemolytic strepto*cocci, e.g. *Streptococcus pyogenes*: less common than staphylococcal infections, but may result in rapid local spread (cellulitis or fasciitis) and bloodstream infection.

Surgical wound infections are frequently endogenous. Exogenous acquisition may occur intra-operatively or post-operatively, either by the airborne route or by direct contact (cross-infection).

Prevention includes:

- Preoperative measures:
  - o decontamination of skin surfaces pre-operatively with antiseptics;
  - o prophylactic antimicrobials for operations with a significant risk of wound infection. The right dose of the right antimicrobial(s) have to be given at the right time pre-operatively and for the appropriate period (usually one dose);
- Intra-operative measures:
  - o modern operating theatres provide positive pressure ventilation and deliver filtered air to clean areas first (e.g operating theatre) and then to less clean areas (e.g. anaesthetic room); the ventilation systems reduce the number of microorganisms entering the theatres and, by directing the airflow away from the patient, the number of microbial-carrying particles generated around the operative site is minimised;
  - o the use of sterile instruments, careful hand-washing techniques and the wearing of sterile surgical gloves, headwear and close-woven operation gowns;
  - o good surgical technique to reduce devitalisation of tissue and haematoma formation.
- Postoperative measures:
  - o 'no-touch' techniques in the cleaning and dressing of wounds and manipulating drains;
  - o the use of specially ventilated ward areas for dressing of extensive wounds, such as burns;
  - o isolation of patients with heavily infected wounds, particularly with antimicrobial-resistant microorganisms.

Lower respiratory tract infection

This important cause of morbidity and mortality in hospitalised patients is often a complication of intubation (anaesthesia, intensive care), which by-passes the normal physical defenses of the respiratory tract (e.g. mucus trapping, ciliated epithelium).

Prevention

Many infections are endogenous and isolation of infected patients is of limited value. The use of 'closed' suction and single-use suction catheters, sterile anaesthetic circuits with inspiratory and expiratory microbial filters reduces the chance of cross-infection.

Intravascular catheter infections

The use of both peripheral and central vascular catheters (CVC) is associated with infection, ranging from insertion site infections to bloodstream infection and severe sepsis. The source of infection is primarily from the patient's own skin microflora, with microorganisms gaining access to the catheter at the time of insertion, from the skin insertion site or via connectors.

Isolation procedures

Hospitals require a policy for isolating patients with specific transmissible infections (source isolation) and for isolating certain immunocompromised patients (e.g. bone marrow transplant recipients) to prevent them acquiring infection (protective isolation):

- *Source isolation* for conditions such as chickenpox, measles, infections with MRSA and other multiple antimicrobial-resistant microorganisms, especially if airborne spread is likely (as determined by risk assessment): includes single-room accommodation with closed door and a ventilation system that provides a *negative* air pressure within the room compared to outside; disposable gloves and aprons should be worn when attending the patient, and hands should be washed before leaving the room. For enteric infections, procedures are required for safe disposal of faeces and urine.

  Where side rooms are in limited supply, patients with MRSA and other multi-resistant microorganisms, who are not likely to spread the microorganisms by the air-borne route, can be nursed together, e.g. in four-bedded bays. Some hospitals have specific infectious diseases wards or isolation wards for such patients.
- *Strict isolation* is required for highly dangerous conditions, e.g. Lassa fever, viral haemorrhagic fever: these patients require treatment in designated isolation hospitals with special facilities (so-called category IV wards).
- *Protective isolation*: to protect compromised patients (e.g. bone marrow transplant recipients) from infection. Facilities include single-room accommodation, with a ventilation system that provides a *positive* pressure within the room and highly efficient particulate (HEPA) filtered air. Gowns, aprons and masks need to be worn by all those entering the room; hands should be washed before and after entering.

The prevention and control of infection in hospitals

Each hospital should have an IPC team and IPC committee. Within the team there are various key members. These are outlined below:

- *IPC doctor*: a registered medical practitioner with experience in hospital infection; usually a Consultant Medical Microbiologist, who takes a leading role in the effective functioning of the IPC team (see below), and is involved in producing policies and preventive programmes for healthcare-associated infections;
- *IPC nurse*: is a registered nurse with additional qualifications in IPC. Serves as an adviser to the IPC team, providing specialist nursing input into the identification, prevention, monitoring and control of infection;
- *Consultant in communicable disease control (CCDC)*: involved in surveillance, prevention and control of communicable diseases and infections within the boundaries of a health authority. They have responsibility for ensuring adequate arrangements for prevention of communicable disease, IPC in the community and will liaise with the hospital IPC team;
- *IPC link staff*: IPC is the responsibility of all healthcare workers. A legal code of practice is in place, which ensures this and the Care Quality Commission inspects healthcare establishments against this code. It is recommended that all wards have designated IPC staff (e.g. link nurses), which have additional training in IPC and report to the IPC team. Duties can include the audit of hand hygiene procedures. This Code is now extended into all healthcare establishments in England;
- *Director of Infection Prevention and Control (DIPC)*: A senior manager or IPC doctor or nurse,

who is either a member of the board or reports directly to the Chief Executive with a responsibility for ensuring that there is an annual IPC programme in place, and reports regularly to the Board on how well its agreed goals are being met. The DIPC also ensures that infection policies and procedures are in place and audited regularly, and results of these audits reported back to the appropriate staff that need to be informed.

IPC team

Is responsible for the operational running of an IPC programme. The team produces policies and procedures in IPC with regular updates, and is also involved in education of staff in IPC and surveillance of infection. Provides advice on all matters relating to the prevention and spread of infection.

IPC committee

Has responsibility for the strategic planning and evaluation of matters relating to IPC. This involves senior management of the healthcare organisation. In addition, occupational health should be represented on this committee, to ensure that the risk of infection to healthcare workers is minimised. Local Health Protection Units are usually represented as well.

Surveillance

It is important in IPC that an appropriate surveillance programme is in place to identify early cases of possible sources of transmissible infections and to prevent spread of infection by ensuring that appropriate IPC measures are implemented. Surveillance can also help in determining trends, so that IPC measures can be directed towards particular problems. There are various methods of surveillance, including laboratory-based surveillance, e.g. numbers of MRSA bacteraemia or ward surveillance, e.g. numbers of cases of *Clostridium difficile* diarrhoea. The surveillance of some infections, e.g. MRSA bacteraemia, is mandatory and has to be reported to a National Database. England is unusual in also setting and reviewing targets for reductions in infections included in some of the mandatory surveillance activities. Lengths of hospital stay are now so short for some conditions (including day surgical cases) that surveillance

methods need to consider ways of detecting infections occurring after patient discharge into the community. Methods include patients carrying infection reporting cards that they give to healthcare workers, e.g. general practitioner staff, district nurses, midwives, healthcare workers in outpatients or Accident and Emergency, whom they see when suffering from such infections and recording systems when re-admitted to hospitals or other healthcare establishments.

Major outbreaks

It is important that hospitals, as well as the community, have in place systems for managing major outbreaks. Medical staff have a statutory duty to notify certain infectious diseases to the CCDC (Table 24.6), to ensure that any infections that may affect both the hospital and the community are coordinated in terms of control. If an outbreak occurs, there are several stages in the investigation, including collection of epidemiological data, screening of hospital cases and putting in place an appropriate outbreak control management plan. Most outbreaks of healthcare-associated infection include colonised and infected patients. Screening measures are designed to include all potentially exposed cases.

Table 24.6 List of some of the infectious diseases that must be notified to a CCDC

Common	Less common
Confirmed measles	Acute poliomyelitis
E. coli O157	Psittacosis
Hepatitis B	Leptospirosis
All meningitis	Relapsing fever
Typhoid and Paratyphoid fever	Yellow fever
	Anthrax
Diphtheria	Cholera
Meningococcal disease	Plague
Confirmed mumps	Tetanus
Legionnaires disease	Viral haemorrhagic fever
Confirmed rubella	Botulism
	Leprosy
	Rabies
	Typhus

Biological warfare

Plans need to be in place, both in hospitals and the community, in case of contamination with biological material, including smallpox and anthrax. Precautions include appropriate protective clothing, prophylaxis and immunisation.

Prevention of infection to healthcare workers

Healthcare workers can protect themselves from acquiring infections by several mechanisms:

- *Immunisation*: against various infections including hepatitis B;
- *Barrier protection*: healthcare workers should carry out a risk assessment when dealing with any patient, and should assume that a patient may be potentially infectious and apply universal precautions. These are precautions that should be taken for every patient contact to prevent the spread of infection. They include, e.g. the use of gloves when directly handling a patient. Avoidance of needlestick injuries is important in the spread of blood-borne viruses;
- *Strict isolation*: this is required for highly infectious or dangerous pathogens. For high risk infections, e.g. Lassa fever, these patients need to be located in designated high-risk isolation hospitals.

Upper respiratory tract infections

Jonathan Sandoe
Leeds Teaching Hospitals NHS Trust and University of Leeds, Leeds, UK

Infections of the upper respiratory tract are very common, but vary greatly in aetiology, pathogenesis, anatomical site of infection and severity. The spectrum of severity ranges from self-limiting viral infections that resolve without medical consultation to life threatening systemic bacterial illness or acute airway compromise.

In this text, the 'upper respiratory tract' is separated from the 'lower respiratory tract' at the level of the vocal cords. Above the cords, the mucosal surfaces are colonised by bacteria, below the cords is normally maintained free of microorganisms by body defences. Infections of the upper respiratory tract therefore include those affecting the nose, pharynx, tonsils, sinuses, larynx and ears.

Viral infections

The common cold syndrome

Definition

An acute, self-limiting syndrome comprising coryza (clear nasal discharge), accompanied by other upper respiratory tract symptoms and signs.

Aetiology

Rhinoviruses are a frequent cause of common colds. Other associated viruses are adenoviruses, coronaviruses, enteroviruses, influenza viruses, metapneumoviruses, parainfluenza viruses and respiratory syncytial virus (RSV). A number of systemic viral infections may present with similar upper respiratory tract symptoms, e.g. measles, mumps and rubella. Re-infections are common as a result of antigenic diversity within each of the viral groups.

Epidemiology

- The common cold occurs worldwide.
- Peak incidence in temperate regions is in the winter, whereas in the tropics, incidence peaks during the rainy season.
- Transmission is by aerosol or large droplets or via virus-contaminated hands. Nasal discharge causes irritation and results in sneezing, facilitating spread.
- The usual incubation period is 1–3 days.

Clinical features

- The predominant symptom is coryza, which is often accompanied by cough, sneezing and

Medical Microbiology and Infection Lecture Notes, Fifth Edition. Edited by Tom Elliott, Anna Casey, Peter Lambert and Jonathan Sandoe.
© 2011 Blackwell Publishing Ltd. Published 2011 by Blackwell Publishing Ltd.

non-specific symptoms, such as headache and malaise; fever is not a prominent feature.

- Nasal blockage is common and sinusitis is part of the common cold syndrome. Nasal discharge may become purulent.
- The common cold should resolve spontaneously within 7–10 days.
- Secondary bacterial infection may result in bacterial sinusitis or otitis media (see below).
- Pharyngitis and conjunctivitis may occur, with enterovirus or adenovirus infection.

Investigations

Routine microbiological investigation of the common cold is not usually warranted, because it does not change management. In the hospital setting or in immunocompromised patients, nasopharyngeal aspirates can be examined for respiratory viruses by PCR. These results may be used to instigate therapy (immunocompromised patients) or to inform infection control procedures. When mumps, measles and rubella are suspected, serology can be useful (Chapter 15).

Treatment and prevention

In immunocompetent patients, antiviral agents are not indicated and symptomatic treatment only is used. In immunocompromised patients, antiviral agents are available for some viruses, e.g. influenza. Handwashing and using a tissue when sneezing can help prevent transmission.

Acute pharyngitis, tonsillitis (including glandular fever)

Definition

Acute inflammation of the pharynx and/or tonsils, usually caused by infection.

Aetiology

- *Viral*: Most cases of acute pharyngitis are caused by viruses. Many of the viruses associated with the common cold syndrome may also result in pharyngitis and include rhinoviruses, coronaviruses, enteroviruses, adenoviruses, influenza and parainfluenza viruses and RSV.

  Epstein–Barr virus (EBV) and cytomegalovirus (CMV) may also cause acute pharyngitis (glandular fever).

Bacterial infections

Streptococcus pyogenes and occasionally other β-haemolytic streptococci (groups C and G). Other bacteria (e.g. *Arcanobacterium haemolyticum*, *Neisseria gonorhoeae*) can uncommonly cause pharyngitis.

Epidemiology

- *Viral*: Transmission is by aerosol and direct contact;
- *Bacterial*: Approximately 5–10% of the population carry *Streptococcus pyogenes* in the pharynx; carriage rates are higher among children, particularly during the winter. Spread is by aerosol and direct contact, and is common within families. Epidemics of streptococcal pharyngitis may occur occasionally in institutions, e.g. boarding schools.

Clinical features

- There are no clinical features that reliably distinguish viral and bacterial causes.
- Acute pharyngitis is characterised by acute onset of sore throat.
- Sore throat may be mild or severe (stopping eating/and drinking).
- Fever and systemic symptoms may be present (e.g. influenza, group A streptococcal infection).
- Examination reveals pharyngeal inflammation, tonsillar enlargement, occasionally with an exudate (Figure 25.1).

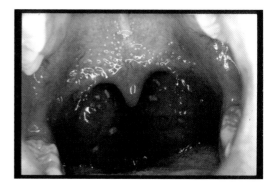

Figure 25.1 Pharyngitis.

- Vesicles on the soft palate suggest herpes simplex virus (HSV) or Coxsackie virus infection.
- Concurrent conjunctivitis suggests influenza or adenovirus infection.
- Glandular fever syndrome: persistent pharyngitis with tiredness, malaise and cervical lymphadenopathy. This syndrome may be associated with an enlarged liver and/or spleen and jaundice. A maculopapular rash may occur after ampicillin or amoxicillin.
- Peritonsillar abscesses (quinsy), scarlet fever; rheumatic fever; acute glomerulonephritis and Henoch–Schönlein purpura may complicate group A streptococcal pharyngitis.

Investigations

- Routine throat swabbing is not recommended.
- Direct antigen detection tests are available for rapid diagnosis of group A streptococcal pharyngitis, but are not recommended for routine use because of poor specificity.
- In suspected glandular fever, EBV and CMV infections may be diagnosed by specific serological assays.
- Throat swabs should be sent for culture when unusual pathogens are suspected, e.g. *Neisseria gonorrhoea*, and the laboratory informed.
- Serology (detection of anti-streptolysin O antibodies – 'ASO titres') may be useful in patients presenting with post-streptococcal complications (rheumatic fever, glomerulonephritis).

Treatment

For viral pharyngitis; symptomatic treatment only.

Specific bacterial pathogens may require antimicrobial therapy. Penicillin, or erythromycin for penicillin-allergic patients, is appropriate for group A streptococcal pharyngitis when treatment is required. Symptomatic treatment, including analgesia, is usually required.

Laryngotracheobronchitis (croup)

Definition

Acute inflammation of the larynx, trachea and bronchi caused by infection. Note: this infection involves the upper and lower respiratory tract.

Aetiology

The majority of cases are caused by viruses. Parainfluenza viruses are the most frequent cause of croup; other viruses associated with upper respiratory tract infections can occasionally cause croup.

Epidemiology

Transmission is by aerosol spread. Most cases occur in the autumn and winter and the infection is largely restricted to children aged less than 5 years.

Clinical features

Distinctive deep cough ('bovine cough'), frequently with inspiratory stridor, dyspnoea and, in severe cases, cyanosis.

Investigations

Virus isolation, antigen detection or PCR on nasopharyngeal aspirates.

Treatment

Symptomatic relief by mist therapy is often recommended, but there is no scientific proof of its effectiveness; antibiotics are of no benefit, except when croup is complicated by bacterial infection. In severe cases, hospitalisation is required and ventilatory support may be necessary.

Epiglottitis

Definition

Acute inflammation of the epiglottis caused by infection, usually bacterial.

Aetiology

Since the introduction of the Hib vaccine, this infection has become rare in the UK. Causes of epiglottitis include non-capsulated *H. influenzae*, *S. pneumoniae* and β-haemolytic streptococci.

Epidemiology/Pathogenesis

A rare infection, more common in children, usually less than 5 years. Adults are occasionally affected.

Direct infection of the epiglottis by pathogenic bacteria results in swelling of the epiglottis, which

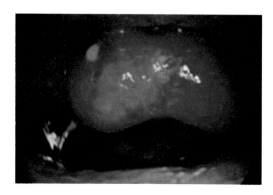

Figure 25.2 Epiglottitis.

can cause fatal airway obstruction and usually causes severe systemic illness.

Clinical features

There is acute onset of fever, sore throat and stridor or difficulty in breathing. Patients may be drooling, unable to swallow oral secretions. Examination of the pharynx is often normal. When epiglottitis is suspected, direct visualisation of the epiglottis should not be attempted, except where facilities for immediate intubation are available, because acute airway obstruction can be precipitated. When visualised, the epiglottis is inflamed and markedly swollen (Figure 25.2).

Investigations

Throat swabs should not be taken, because swabbing can precipitate acute airway obstruction. Epiglottic swabs for culture should be taken under direct vision by specialists. Blood cultures should also be sent. Lateral radiographs of the neck may show the enlarged epiglottis.

Treatment and prevention

Intubation and ventilation may be necessary. Intravenous antibiotic therapy should be instituted immediately; third-generation cephalosporins (e.g. cefotaxime) are the current treatment of choice. Ampicillin should not be used as sole therapy, because 10% of strains of *H. influenzae* produce β-lactamase. Family contacts of cases of *H. influenzae* b infection should be given rifampicin prophylaxis when there is a child in the family aged less than 5 years old.

Vincent's angina

This is an uncommon throat infection caused by a mixture of anaerobic bacteria (e.g. fusobacteria, spirochaetes) normally found in the mouth. As with acute ulcerative gingivitis, with which it may coexist, it is associated with poor oral hygiene and underlying conditions such as immunodeficiency.

Clinical features include pharyngitis with a necrotic pharyngeal exudate. Microscopy of the exudate shows typical fusobacteria and spirochaetes. Treatment is with penicillin or metronidazole.

Diphtheria

Definition

An acute upper respiratory tract or skin infection, caused by toxin-producing strains of *Corynebacterium diphtheriae* with central nervous system and cardiac complications.

Aetiology

Diphtheria is caused by toxigenic strains of *Corynebacterium diphtheriae*.

Epidemiology/Pathogenesis

- After the introduction of immunisation, diphtheria became rare in the developed world, but still common in developing countries.
- Diphtheria has occurred in intravenous drug users.
- The microorganism is transmitted by aerosol spread, but infected skin lesions can also act as reservoirs for infection.
- The microorganism colonises the pharynx, multiplies and produces toxin.
- The toxin produced by pathogenic strains of *C. diphtheriae* inhibits protein synthesis.
- It acts locally to destroy epithelial cells and phagocytes, resulting in the formation of a prominent exudate, sometimes termed a 'false membrane'.
- Cervical lymph nodes become grossly enlarged ('bull-neck' appearance).
- The membrane and swelling can cause airway obstruction and death.
- The toxin also spreads via the lymphatics and blood, resulting in myocarditis and polyneuritis.

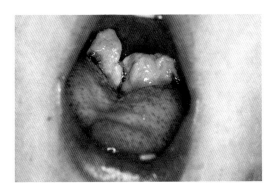

Figure 25.3 Case of diphtheria showing false membrane on tonsils.

Clinical features

Fever and pharyngitis with false membrane (Figure 25.3) that may cause airway obstruction; enlarged cervical lymph nodes; myocarditis with cardiac failure; and polyneuritis. In skin infections chronic ulcers with a membrane form and toxicity is mild.

Laboratory diagnosis

By isolation of the microorganism from throat swabs, followed by demonstration of toxin production by the Elek test, or more recently detection of toxin genes by PCR. PCR may also be used to detect toxin genes directly from throat swabs. Demonstrating toxin or the presence of the toxin gene is essential, because non-toxin-producing strains of *C. diphtheriae* do not cause diphtheria.

Treatment and prevention

Patients with suspected diphtheria should be isolated in hospital. In suspected cases, treatment should be commenced before laboratory confirmation and includes antitoxin and antibiotics (penicillin or erythromycin). Diphtheria is a notifiable infection in the UK. Close contacts should be investigated for the carriage of the microorganism, given prophylactic antibiotics (erythromycin) and immunised. Childhood immunisation with diphtheria toxoid has resulted in the virtual disappearance of diphtheria from developed countries.

Acute otitis media

Definition

Acute inflammation of the middle ear caused by infection.

Aetiology and pathogenesis

Upper respiratory tract infection may result in oedema and blockage of the eustachian tube, with subsequent impaired drainage of middle-ear fluid, predisposing to viral or bacterial infection (acute otitis media). About 50% are caused by respiratory viruses; common bacterial causes include *Streptococcus pneumoniae*, *H. influenzae*, group A beta-haemolytic streptococci and *S. aureus*.

Epidemiology

It occurs worldwide and is most common in children aged less than 5 years, with an increased incidence in winter months.

Clinical features

Fever and earache, aural discharge. The eardrum appears reddened and bulging and, if untreated, drum perforations with subsequent purulent discharge may occur.

Laboratory diagnosis

Acute otitis media is a clinical diagnosis, but if there is a purulent ear discharge, this can be cultured. Needle aspiration of middle ear fluid (tympanocentesis) is performed occasionally.

Treatment and prevention

Most infections are self limiting but antibiotics such as amoxicillin or erythromycin may be required. Follow-up is important, because residual fluid in the middle ear ('glue ear') can result in hearing impairment.

Otitis externa

Infections of the external auditory canal are frequently caused by *S. aureus* and *P. aeruginosa*. Topical treatment with antibiotic-containing eardrops may be required in severe cases. 'Malignant otitis externa' is a severe form, involving skull base and cranial nerves, systemic antimicrobial therapy is required in these cases.

Acute sinusitis

Acute sinusitis is often part of the common cold syndrome and resolves spontaneously. Secondary bacterial infection of the sinuses by pathogens such as *S. pneumonia* or *H. influenza* may complicate viral upper respiratory tract infections. It is also predisposed to by cystic fibrosis, nasal polyps, septal deviation and dental abscess. It presents with fever, facial pain and tenderness over affected sinuses; radiographs may show fluid-filled sinuses. Management is with antibiotics and occasionally sinus drainage is required.

Lower respiratory tract infections

Shruti Khurana
Central Manchester University Hospitals NHS Foundation Trust, Manchester, UK

As described in Chapter 25, the 'upper respiratory tract' is separated from the 'lower respiratory tract' at the level of the vocal cords. Lower respiratory tract infections (LRTI) therefore include those affecting the trachea, bronchi, bronchioles and lung parenchyma.

Pneumonia

Pneumonia is common, with a significant morbidity and mortality.

Definition

It is an infection of the lung substance with focal chest signs and radiological shadowing. The most clinically useful classification is:

- community-acquired pneumonia;
- hospital-acquired pneumonia;
- pneumonia in immunocompromised individuals;
- aspiration pneumonia.

Community-acquired pneumonia

Epidemiology

This is an important infection worldwide. It is most common in the winter months; the overall incidence may vary in relation to epidemics (e.g. *Mycoplasma* pneumonia and influenza).

Clinical features

Symptoms and signs: malaise, fever and shortness of breath, productive cough, pleuritic chest pain, tachypnoea and tachycardia, focal chest signs e.g. crackles, cyanosis, hypoxia and confusion. There can be a preceding history of viral infection. Severe cases lead to bloodstream infection and severe sepsis with circulatory collapse and multi-organ failure.

Complications

Lung abscess and empyema (infected pleural effusion).

Medical Microbiology and Infection Lecture Notes, Fifth Edition. Edited by Tom Elliott, Anna Casey, Peter Lambert and Jonathan Sandoe.
© 2011 Blackwell Publishing Ltd. Published 2011 by Blackwell Publishing Ltd.

Investigations

- Sputum specimens for culture and microscopy (Gram stain) – only occasionally useful, not routinely recommended;
- Blood cultures (positive in 15% of cases);
- Urine antigen detection for pneumococcal and *Legionella* infection;
- Polymerase chain reaction (PCR) now commonly replacing serology for viruses, *Mycoplasma*, *Chlamydophila* and *Coxiella* infections;
- Serology (viruses and *Mycoplasma*, *Chlamydia*, *Coxiella* and *Legionella* species);
- Bronchoalveolar lavage (BAL) specimens obtained by bronchoscopy for microscopy, culture and direct immunofluorescence tests;
- *Chest radiograph:* lobar, patchy or diffuse shadowing. Radiological changes often lag behind clinical course and are not predictive of the microbiological cause.

Treatment

Management of gas exchange, fluid balance and antibiotic therapy are important. Clinical judgement supported by objective severity scoring (e.g. CURB65 score) should guide management. Empirical antibiotics of choice are amoxicillin for non-severe, and clarithromycin plus co-amoxiclav for severe illness. Usual duration of antimicrobial therapy 7–14 days, depending upon severity.

Specific causes of community-acquired pneumonia

Streptococcus pneumoniae

The most common cause of community-acquired pneumonia (30–50%) and occurs in all age groups. Patients with chronic lung disease, splenectomised patients and immunocompromised individuals (including HIV infection) are most at risk. Chest radiograph may show lobar consolidation (Figure 26.1). Laboratory diagnosis is by sputum and blood culture and urine antigen detection. Clinically relevant antibiotic resistance is rare in the UK. Penicillin is the treatment of choice. Alternatives: a macrolide (e.g. clarithromycin) or tetracycline or a respiratory fluoroquinolone (levofloxacin or moxifloxacin).

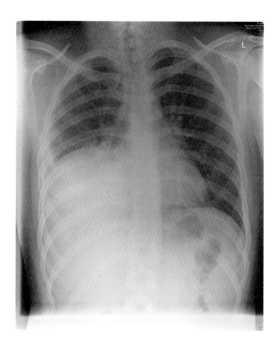

Figure 26.1 Right lower lobe consolidation on chest X-ray associated with *S. pneumoniae* pneumonia.

Conjugate vaccine is available for children and polysaccharide vaccine for other risk groups.

Mycoplasma pneumoniae

Incidence varies (<1–20%) as a result of epidemics; occurs primarily in young adults. Generalised symptoms may precede a dry cough, thus resembling influenza. Extrapulmonary complications can dominate the clinical findings (rash, arthralgia, myocarditis, meningoencephalitis). Laboratory diagnosis is by serology or PCR. Treatment includes macrolides or tetracycline or fluoroquinolones.

Haemophilus influenzae

H. influenzae type b (Hib) vaccine has considerably reduced this cause of pneumonia in all age groups. Most cases are now caused by non-typable strains. Laboratory diagnosis is by sputum culture. ß-lactamase production in 15–20% compromises the effectiveness of amoxicillin. Treatment: aminopenicillin, co-amoxiclav, tetracycline or fluoroquinolones.

Staphylococcus aureus

Most common after influenza and in intravenous drug users. An important cause of severe pneumonia. Strains producing *Panton-Valentine Leucocidin* (PVL) toxin cause severe illness. Laboratory diagnosis is by sputum and blood culture. Treatment is with flucloxacillin.

Legionella species

L. pneumophila serogroup 1 results in 95% of UK cases caused by this species. It is transmitted via aerosols from contaminated sources, e.g. air-conditioning systems or showers. Less than 5% of pneumonias are caused by *L. pneumophila* but incidence varies according to outbreaks. Hospital and community outbreaks may occur. Sporadic cases can be associated with recent travel. Smokers and the immunocompromised are particularly at risk. There are no reliable clinical indicators, but it should always be considered in severe pneumonia. Laboratory diagnosis is by urine antigen detection (*L. pneumophila* serogroup 1 only). Direct immunofluorescence on BAL specimens, sputum culture and serology may also be used. Treatment is with a fluoroquinolone or macrolide.

Chlamydophila pneumoniae

Its importance is uncertain due to lack of 'gold standard' for diagnosis. *C. pneumoniae* is transferred from person to person mainly in age groups of 5–35 years. Symptoms are similar to those of *Mycoplasma* pneumonia. Laboratory diagnosis is by serology. Treatment is with a macrolide, tetracycline or a fluoroquinolone.

Chlamydophila psittaci

This is associated with contact with infected birds, including pigeons and parrots. Laboratory diagnosis is by serology. Treatment is with a tetracycline or macrolide.

Coxiella burnetii

C. burnetii is a rare cause of pneumonia and is usually confined to farm workers and vets. Laboratory diagnosis is by serology. Treatment is with a tetracycline.

Mycobacterium tuberculosis

May mimic bacterial pneumonia, but patients usually have a longer duration of symptoms (Chapter 27).

Viral causes of community-acquired pneumonia

Primary viral pneumonia occurs mainly in children, elderly people and immunocompromised patients, with an increased incidence in winter. Underlying cardiopulmonary diseases are recognised as risk factors for viral pneumonia in children and adults.

Clinical manifestations in children vary considerably, but typically include fever, difficulty in breathing or apnoeic episodes in young infants, non-productive cough, wheezing or increased breath sounds. Common viral causes include Respiratory syncytial virus (RSV), Parainfluenza viruses, Influenza A and B, Adenoviruses, Measles and Human metapneumovirus. Influenza A subtype H1N1 presents with symptoms similar to those of seasonal influenza.

Primary viral pneumonia in adults is characterised by non-productive cough, cyanosis and hypoxia, fever, rhinitis, increased respiratory rate, wheezes and diffuse bilateral interstitial infiltrates on chest radiograph. Consider Varicella-zoster virus (VZV), if vesicular rash.

Diagnosis of viral pneumonia is by PCR or culture of viral agents in, e.g. nasopharyngeal aspirates, throat and nasal swabs and BALs. Viral antigens can be detected by immunofluorescence techniques.

Specific antiviral therapy is available for some of the viruses associated with viral pneumonia (see Chapter 22). Ribavirin is used for the treatment of some cases of RSV and Parainfluenza infections, and for Adenovirus infections in immunocompromised patients. The neuraminidase inhibitors (oseltamivir and zanamivir) are available for the treatment of Influenza A (including H1N1 subtype) and B infections.

Hospital-acquired pneumonia (HAP)

Aetiology

Commonly *Streptococcus pneumoniae* and *Haemophilus influenzae* in early-onset infections (first

4 days of admission), thereafter Gram-negative bacteria (e.g. *Escherichia coli*, *Klebsiella* and *Serratia* spp.) and in ventilator-associated pneumonia especially meticillin-resistant *Staphylococcus aureus* (MRSA) and multiresistant Gram-negative bacteria, including *Acinetobacter* and *Pseudomonas aeruginosa*.

Epidemiology

HAP is a pneumonia presenting two or more days after admission to hospital. Pneumonia is one of the most common nosocomial infections, affecting about 0.5% of hospitalised patients. Risk factors include endotracheal intubation and ventilation, immune compromise and pre-existing pulmonary disease.

Ventilator-associated pneumonia (VAP) is a subtype of hospital acquired pneumonia, which occurs in people who are on mechanical ventilation through an endotracheal or tracheostomy tube for at least 48 hours.

Investigations

Sputum and blood cultures. For VAP, bronchoscopically-collected respiratory secretions or blind bronchoalveolar lavage.

Treatment

Broad spectrum antimicrobial therapy usually required, because of large number of potential pathogens. Treatment usually guided by local antibiotic policies.

Pneumonia in immunocompromised patients

Immunocompromised means having an immune system that has been impaired by disease or treatment, resulting in an increased risk of infection. Patient immunity may be impaired temporarily or permanently as a result of either an immunodeficiency state (congenital or acquired) or induced immunosuppression, due to a disease state or its management using cytotoxic, immunosuppressive or radiation therapy.

Aetiology

These patients may become infected with classic chest pathogens, e.g. *S. pneumoniae*, *M. pneumoniae*, or the important opportunistic lung pathogens e.g. *Pneumocystis jirovecii* (formerly *carinii*), *Aspergillus fumigatus*, *Actinomyces israelii*, *Nocardia asteroides*, Cytomegalovirus, *Mycobacterium avium-intercellulare* and *Cryptococcus neoformans*.

Immunocompromised patients are at increased risk of severe viral pneumonia by viruses that are typical causes of upper respiratory tract disease in normal hosts (e.g. Rhinoviruses) and other more opportunistic viral pathogens. Cytomegalovirus (CMV) is the most frequent cause of pneumonitis in immunosuppressed patients, particularly transplant recipients. Other common causes include Herpes simplex virus (HSV), VZV, Adenoviruses, RSV, and Influenza A and B.

Investigations

Consider early bronchoscopy for BAL fluid to be examined by:

- microscopy (Gram and Ziehl–Neelsen stains);
- culture (bacteria, fungi, mycobacteria, viruses);
- direct immunofluorescence (*Pneumocystis jiroveci* and *Legionella* spp.);
- PCR for *Pneumocystis*, viruses and non-commensal bacteria;
- also urinary antigen (*Legionella* spp.), *serology* (e.g. *M. pneumoniae* and *L. pneumophila*), galactomanan enzyme immunoassay (Invasive aspergillosis) and CT chest.

Treatment

Effective treatment relies on deciphering the causative microorganism rapidly. In the absence of clear aetiology, empirical therapy is often required. The choice depends on clinical presentation, laboratory data, underlying disease and previous antibiotic therapy. Ganciclovir is frequently used for the treatment of CMV pneumonia, whereas acyclovir and foscarnet are used for HSV and VZV infections.

Aspiration pneumonia

Patients may aspirate oropharyngeal or gastric contents into their upper and lower airways. The initial insult is a chemical pneumonitis, but infection may develop later. It should be considered in pneumonia complicating vomiting, swallowing disorders or impairment of consciousness. Microbial cause seldom found, but oropharyngeal anaerobes probably important. Treat established pneumonia with antimicrobials appropriate for hospital acquired pneumonia. Antimicrobials are not usually indicated for acute aspiration.

Bronchiolitis

Bronchiolitis is caused by RSV, and to lesser extent by parainfluenza and influenza viruses, and results in obstruction of bronchioles by mucosal oedema. Infection occurs mainly in children aged less than 2 years; it is particularly severe in infants aged less than 6 months and with underlying cardiopulmonary disease. Spread is by droplets. Clinical manifestations include fever, cough, dyspnoea, respiratory distress and cyanosis. Laboratory diagnosis is by immunofluorescence or enzyme immunoassay for RSV antigen in nasopharyngeal aspirates, culture and PCR. Management is mainly supportive, but treatment with nebulised ribavarin is occasionally used.

Acute bronchitis

This is principally viral (rhinoviruses, coronaviruses, influenza and parainfluenza viruses); rarely caused by *M. pneumoniae*. Clinical manifestations include fever, malaise, dry cough, wheeze and dyspnoea. Allergens and irritants can produce a similar picture. Laboratory diagnosis is by PCR, culture or serology, but this is rarely performed. Treatment symptomatic; antimicrobials usually not helpful.

Infective exacerbation of chronic obstructive pulmonary disease

Aetiology

About 50% viral (rhinovirus, coronavirus) and 50% bacterial (*H. influenzae, S. pneumoniae, Moraxella catarrhalis*).

Clinical features

Usually mucoid sputum becomes purulent, often with increased dyspnoea and wheeze.

Investigations

Sputum culture for bacterial pathogens. Results need careful interpretation, because causative agents are also commensals.

Treatment

Antimicrobial treatment should be prescribed only if sputum purulent or severe illness. Amoxicillin (resistant *H. influenzae* is an increasing problem), tetracycline or co-amoxiclav.

Bronchiectasis

Underlying lung pathology leads to irreversible damage to the terminal bronchial and bronchiolar walls. The abnormal permanently dilated airways act as a site of chronic infection. Pathogens include *H. influenzae*, *S. pneumoniae*, *S. aureus*, *Moraxella catarrhalis*, *P. aeruginosa* and anaerobes. Clinical features are similar to chronic bronchitis but may also have halitosis, clubbing and haemoptysis; antibiotic therapy is guided by sputum results and the patient's clinical condition.

Whooping cough (pertussis)

Aetiology

This is caused by *Bordetella pertussis*.

Epidemiology

Transmission is by aerosol. It is principally an infection of childhood, but adults may occasionally be infected. Immunisation has dramatically reduced the incidence in many countries.

Clinical features

The initial catarrhal phase is indistinguishable from common upper respiratory tract infections. In the second phase, a severe cough develops; bouts of coughing are frequently followed by an inspiratory whoop.

Investigations

Culture of nasopharyngeal swabs, also PCR assay and antigen detection.

Treatment and prevention

Treatment is with macrolides, which reduce infectivity if given early, but has limited effect on the clinical course. The acellular component vaccine is given in childhood.

LRTI in cystic fibrosis patients

This is the most common autosomal recessive disease among Caucasians, with an occurrence of 1 case per 3,300 live births. In cystic fibrosis, there is an alteration in the viscosity and tenacity of mucous production at epithelial surfaces. This usually presents with bronchopulmonary infection and pancreatic insufficiency in childhood and early adult life.

Colonisation with pathogenic bacteria, including *H. influenzae, S. aureus, P. aeruginosa and Burkholderia spp.*, causes sinopulmonary disease. This presents as a chronic cough with sputum production, airway obstruction manifested by wheezing and air trapping, nasal polyps and digital clubbing. Regular physiotherapy, bronchodilators and intermittent antibiotic treatment (oral or intravenous) may be sufficient initially. For persistant infection with *Pseudomonas* spp., aerosolised antibiotics, e.g. colomycin or tobramycin are used.

Tuberculosis and mycobacteria

Sumeet Singhania
Central Manchester University Hospitals NHS Foundation Trust, Manchester, UK

Definition

Gram-positive bacilli; acid-fast; obligate aerobes; non-capsulated; non-motile; grow slowly on specialised media; cell walls have high lipid content.

Classification

- The genus includes: *Mycobacterium tuberculosis* and *M. bovis* (tuberculosis); *M. leprae* (leprosy); the environmental (atypical) mycobacteria, over 100 species including *M. avium-intracellulare*, *M. kansasii* and *M. marinum*.
- Mycobacteria stain poorly by Gram stain as a result of cell-wall mycolic acid. They are recognised by the Ziehl–Neelsen (ZN) stain (Figure 27.1).
- Mycobacteria grow slowly; visible colonies appear on solid media after 1–12 weeks depending on the species.
- Classification is based on culture characteristics, including nutritional requirements, rate of growth, pigmentation and biochemical properties.

M. tuberculosis

Commonly called the tubercle bacillus (primary host humans), is the usual causative agent for tuberculosis (TB).

Epidemiology

- One-third of the world's population is infected with *M. tuberculosis*.
- Increase in incidence is related to poverty, population displacement, HIV and drug resistance, mostly in Asia and Africa. In Western Europe and North America, the incidence had declined over the last 30 years as a result of improvements in nutrition, housing and preventive measures, including Bacille Calmette–Guérin (BCG) immunisation. More recently, this decline has reached a plateau, and in some developed countries there has been an increase. In the UK, about 8,400 new cases, with about 270 associated deaths, are recognised each year; infection is more common in Asian and African immigrants, drug addicts, alcoholics, HIV-infected and other immunocompromised patients.
- *M. tuberculosis* infections are spread usually by inhalation of 'droplet nuclei' (droplets containing mycobacteria, aerosolised by coughing or sneezing, dry in the air and remain suspended for long periods) and rarely by ingestion. Incubation period is 4–16 weeks. TB is highly infectious and outbreaks may occur.
- Mycobacteria are able to survive for long periods in the environment, because they withstand drying.

Medical Microbiology and Infection Lecture Notes, Fifth Edition. Edited by Tom Elliott, Anna Casey, Peter Lambert and Jonathan Sandoe.

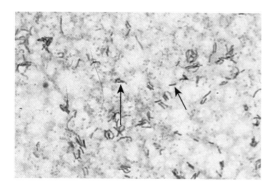

Figure 27.1 Ziehl-Neelsen stain of *Mycobacterium tuberculosis* (stained red, arrowed). Acid-fast slender rods, 3 μm × 0.3 μm.

Pathogenesis

- *Primary TB*: inhalation of *M. tuberculosis* results in a mild acute inflammatory reaction in the lung parenchyma, with phagocytosis of bacilli by alveolar macrophages. *M. tuberculosis*, in common with other mycobacteria, is an intracellular pathogen; its survival within macrophages is related to its ability to prevent phagosome-lysosome fusion. Bacilli survive and multiply within the macrophages and are carried to the hilar lymph nodes, which enlarge. The local lesion and enlarged lymph nodes are called the primary complex (referred to as the 'Ghon focus').
- The host response to mycobacterial infection is via the cell-mediated immune system and results in the formation of granulomata. Histologically, granulomas consist of epithelial cells and giant cells, which eventually undergo caseous necrosis. In many individuals, the immune system kills the bacteria and the complex becomes fibrotic and calcified. In a small number of cases, a defensive barrier is built round the infection but the TB bacteria are not killed and lie dormant. This is called latent tuberculosis; the person is not ill and is not infectious. In some patients, particularly immunocompromised individuals, microorganisms spread locally and via the bloodstream to other organs, causing widespread disease (miliary TB). Some sites become dormant and may reactivate years later.
- *Secondary TB*: may arise in two ways:
  1 Dormant mycobacteria may reactivate, often as a result of lowered immunity in the patient; reactivation occurs most commonly in the lung apex, but may occur in other organs (e.g. kidney, bone).
  2 A patient may become re-infected after further exposure to an exogenous source.

As with primary TB, local and distant dissemination may occur.

Clinical features

- *Pulmonary TB*: chronic cough, haemoptysis, weight loss, malaise and night sweats. Chest radiograph: apical shadowing, often with cavities
- *Extrapulmonary TB*:
  ○ *pleural tuberculosis*: pleural effusion, tuberculous empyema;
  ○ *lymph glands*: the most common site of non-pulmonary TB, typically cervical lymph nodes, particularly in children;
  ○ *genitourinary*: sterile pyuria, with haematuria, pyrexia and malaise;
  ○ *meningitis*: insidious onset, with high mortality;
  ○ *bone and joints*: most commonly affects the lumbar spine;
  ○ *abdominal*: pain and ascites;
  ○ *miliary*: multisystem involvement.

Laboratory diagnosis

Diagnosis of active infection:

- Microscopy of relevant specimens, including sputum, bronchoscopy material, pleural fluid, urine, joint fluid, biopsy tissue and cerebrospinal fluid. ZN stain – appearance as thin bacilli with beads (positive in <60% pulmonary; <25% extrapulmonary). A fluorescent rhodamine-auramine dye can also be used.
- Culture on special media for up to 12 weeks, e.g. Lowenstein–Jensen medium, which contains egg yolk, glycerol and mineral acids plus inhibitors, such as malachite green, to reduce growth of other bacteria. Specimens, e.g. sputum, contaminated with normal flora, are pre-treated with alkali to reduce microbial contamination. Liquid cultures are now preferred due to shorter turnaround time. Antibiotic sensitivity can be obtained in about 2 weeks using radiometric and non-radiometric automated systems. Biochemical tests, pigment production or DNA probes are used to confirm species identification and for rifampicin and isoniazid resistance detection.

Diagnosis of latent infection

1 *Tuberculin skin test* (e.g. *Mantoux test*): based on the inoculation of purified protein derivative (PPD), derived from tubercle culture filtrate, into the patient's skin to demonstrate cell-mediated immunity to *M. tuberculosis*. Relatively inexpensive and easy to perform, but false positives occur with prior BCG and environmental mycobacterial exposure.
2 *Interferon Gamma test*: measures the release of interferon-gamma from lymphocytes in whole blood in response to stimulation by specific tuberculous bacterial antigens. More specific than skin test, but predictive value for future active disease not yet known.

Treatment and prevention

- Combinations of up to four (used to prevent emergence of resistance) anti-mycobacterial drugs (e.g. rifampicin, isoniazid, pyrazinamide and ethambutol) for 2 months (initial phase), followed by 4 months (continuous phase) of rifampicin and isoniazid). However, multiple drug resistant strains of *M. tuberculosis* (MDRTB) are now emerging (<5% in the UK). Second-line anti-mycobacterial agents include fluoroquinolones, macrolides, cycloserine, amikacin, kanamycin and capreomycin. Treatment beyond 6 months is indicated for meningitis (usually 1 year), resistant strains and where any break in treatment has occurred. Directly observed therapy for non-compliant patients may be instigated 3 times weekly. Addition of steroids indicated in central nervous system, ureteric and pericardial disease.
- Strategies for prevention include improving living standards (housing, nutrition); immunisation with a live attenuated vaccine (BCG), and isolation plus prompt treatment of cases as appropriate, and chemoprophylaxis when latent infection is found.

M. bovis

Primary host is cattle. Human infection with *M. bovis* is acquired via contaminated milk.

- Infection is typically localised to bone marrow and cervical or mesenteric lymph nodes. Clinical picture, pathogenesis and treatment are similar to *M. tuberculosis*, although it is always pyrazinamide resistant.

- Infection is prevented by destruction of tuberculin-positive cattle and milk pasteurisation.

M. leprae

M. leprae (Hansen's bacillus) causes leprosy.

Epidemiology

- There are over 210,000 cases of leprosy worldwide, mainly in Asia, Africa and South America. Armadillos may be an animal reservoir in the USA.
- Transmission follows prolonged exposure to shedders of the bacilli via respiratory secretions or ulcer discharges. The incubation period is 2–10 years; without prophylaxis up to 10% develop the disease.

Morphology and identification

M. leprae is an acid-fast bacillus. It can be grown in the footpads of mice or armadillos, from tissue culture and on artificial media.

Associated infections

There are two major types of leprosy: lepromatous and tuberculoid, with various intermediate stages:

1 *Lepromatous*: progressive infection, resulting in nodular skin lesions (granulomata) and nerve involvement; associated with a poor prognosis.
2 *Tuberculoid*: a more benign, non-progressive form that involves macular skin lesions and severe asymptomatic nerve involvement. Spontaneous healing usually results after tissue and nerve destruction.

Laboratory diagnosis

Microscopy of scrapings from skin or nasal mucosa, or skin biopsies, examined by ZN staining.

Treatment and control

- Treatment: combination of dapsone plus rifampicin and/or clofazimine;
- Chemoprophylaxis is needed for close contacts of infected individuals, and is particularly important for young children in contact with adults with leprosy.

Table 27.1 Infections associated with environmental mycobacteria

Mycobacterium species	Associated infections
M. avium-intracellulare	Cervical lymphadenopathy in children; colonises damaged lungs and causes invasive infections in HIV infected patients
M. chelonei	Cutaneous abscesses; occasionally disseminated infection in immuno-compromised individuals
M. kansasii	Lung disease
M. marinum	Granulomatous skin lesions associated with cleaning fish tanks and swimming pools
M. ulcerans	Skin ulcers (tropics)

Environmental (atypical) mycobacteria

These grow at a variety of temperatures; some are rapid growing (3–4 days), whereas others are slower (>8 weeks). Some produce pigmented colonies in light (photochromogens) or in light and dark (scotochromogens).

They are transmitted to humans primarily from environmental or animal sources. Associated infections are listed in Table 27.1. Some species, e.g. *M. avium-intracellulare*, are resistant to first-line anti-mycobacterial agents.

Laboratory diagnosis

ZN positive and resemble *M. tuberculosis*. Distinction by gene probe or culture characteristics.

Treatment

Clinical response unrelated to *in vitro* antibiotic resistance pattern. Usually combination of rifampicin, ethambutol and clarithromycin continued until culture negative for one year.

Gastrointestinal infections

Tariq Iqbal
Consultant Gastroenterologist, University Hospitals Brimingham NHS Foundation Trust,
Birmingham, UK

This chapter outlines the common causes and pathogenesis of infective gastroenteritis and food poisoning. There is also a brief description of enteric fever which, although transmitted via the faecal-oral route, does not cause typical gastroenteritis. Finally, *Clostridium difficile* infection (CDI) is described. Which has become a major threat to the health of hospitalised patients in the Western world over the last decade.

Definitions

Infective gastroenteritis

This is an inflammation of the gastrointestinal (GI) tract caused by microorganisms. It is spread principally by the faecal-oral route, either directly or via vectors such as food or water. Infective gastroenteritis may result from the direct effect of microorganisms on the intestinal mucosa or from the indirect effect of toxins produced by these pathogens. Symptoms include diarrhoea, vomiting, abdominal pain and fever.

Food poisoning

This is an acute illness resulting from consumption of food contaminated with pathogenic microorganisms and/or their toxins. It mainly affects the GI tract, but can affect other sites (e.g. *Listeria monocytogenes* – meningitis; *Clostridium botulinum* – paralysis). In the UK, statutory notification of food poisoning is made to the Consultant in Communicable Disease Control (CCDC) for the area of residence of the affected patient.

It is difficult to distinguish with confidence, on clinical grounds alone, between microbiological aetiologies of either infective gastroenteritis or food poisoning. However, knowledge of risk factors and incubation periods may hint at the aetiology and are essential in public health management to prevent further cases.

Bacterial causes of infective gastroenteritis

Shigella spp.

Epidemiology

Shigella spp. are highly host adapted and infect only humans. The microorganism is spread by the faecal-oral route and the infective dose is very low; food is an occasional vector. The microorganism can be harboured by inanimate objects (e.g. toilet seats). In the developing world, both adults and children are affected (e.g. with *S. dysenteriae* and

Medical Microbiology and Infection Lecture Notes, Fifth Edition. Edited by Tom Elliott, Anna Casey,
Peter Lambert and Jonathan Sandoe.
© 2011 Blackwell Publishing Ltd. Published 2011 by Blackwell Publishing Ltd.

S. boydii). In developed countries, the disease predominantly affects children (typically outbreaks in nurseries) and the commonest strains are S. sonnei and S. flexneri.

Pathogenesis

Shigella spp. invade the colonic mucosa, causing inflammation and ulcers. S. dysenteriae produces a potent exotoxin, which disrupts absorption. Bacteraemia is rare.

Clinical features

The incubation period is 1–4 days. There is bloody diarrhoea with mucus with abdominal cramps and the frequent passage of small volume stools.

Complications

S. sonnei and S. flexneri cause a mild self-limiting disease; S. dysenteriae can lead to renal failure (the haemolytic uraemic syndrome), seizures, toxic megacolon and rarely (associated with HLA B27) reactive arthritis.

Salmonella spp. (other than s. typhi and s. paratyphi – see below-typhoid fever)

Epidemiology

Salmonella spp. are commonly carried by domestic and wild animals. Spread is by the faecal-oral route, with food and animals being the most important source and inadequate cooking of meat the main hazard. Salmonella spp. survive deep-freezing, so that inadequate thawing of meat prior to preparation is hazardous. Salmonella infections account for a small proportion of hospital admissions with diarrhoea. Institutional outbreaks can occur. Long-term carriage (biliary tract) may follow infection.

Pathogenesis

Salmonella spp. multiply in the gut and cause direct mucosal damage. The overall increased fluid loss causes diarrhoea.

Clinical features

The incubation period is 18–48 hours. Clinical features are diarrhoea (occasionally bloody) with abdominal pain. Headache, malaise and fever are common. The disease is usually self limiting, abating after a few days.

Complications

Dependant on severity. Elderly and immunocompromised patients in particular, may develop bacteraemia and (rarely) metastatic spread (e.g. to bone). Reactive large joint arthritis is HLA B27-associated.

Campylobacter spp.

Epidemiology and pathogenesis

See Chapter 11.

Clinical features

The incubation period is 2–3 days. Illness is characterised by diarrhoea with blood, mucous and pus. Fever and abdominal pain are prominent. May mimic appendicitis. Symptoms last for 5–7 days.

Complications

Guillain-Barre syndrome (rare).

Vibrio spp.

Epidemiology

Cholera (V. cholera) is one of the most devastating human diarrhoeal diseases. Although humans are the only host, the pathogen can survive in brackish water and is spread by the faecal-oral route due to contaminated water, shellfish and other seafood. Person-to-person spread is possible and individuals with blood group O are most susceptible. Outbreaks exhibit seasonality in endemic areas. V. parahaemolyticus is associated with the consumption of shellfish. This is a rare cause of a self-limiting febrile, diarrhoeal disease usually affecting travellers to endemic areas.

Pathogenesis

See Chapter 11.

Clinical features

The incubation period is 1–3 days. The majority of affected individuals have a mild diarrhoeal illness. However, severe cholera can develop abruptly (usually overnight), leading to the production of a copious volume (20 litres/day) of isotonic, mucous (rice-water) stool, initially associated with vomiting. Untreated the mortality rate is 20–50%, due to dehydration and acidosis.

Escherichia coli (E. coli)

Epidemiology and pathogenesis

Although *E. coli* is part of the normal flora of the colon, some strains can cause enteritis by a variety of mechanisms. It is an important pathogen causing diarrhoea in travellers. There are four main types of enteropathogenic *E. coli*, which cause enteritis by different mechanisms:

- *Enteropathogenic E. coli (EPEC)*: This causes direct damage to the intestinal wall and causes a diarrhoeal disease among infants, with bloody, mucous stools.
- *Enterotoxigenic E. coli (ETEC)*: An important cause of travellers' diarrhoea and in children in developing countries. It produces enterotoxins (heat stable-ST and heat labile-LT) which, similar to cholera toxin, produce profuse watery diarrhoea.
- *Enteroinvasive E. coli (EIEC)*: This produces a *Shigella*-like infection, with invasion of the intestinal mucosa, resulting in diarrhoea containing blood, pus and mucous.
- *Verocytotoxin-producing E. coli (VTEC)*: VTEC is harboured in the gastrointestinal tract of cattle and transmission is by undercooked beef, unpasteurised milk and contact with farm animals. The infective dose is very low, so person-person spread is common. Prolonged excretion is uncommon but can occur in children. The commonest serotype is 0157. The toxin is similar to that of *Shigella dysenteriae* type 1.

Clinical features of E. coli gastroenteritis

The incubation period is 3–4 days.

ETEC causes watery diarrhoea, up to 20 times per day. This is the most common presentation and the differential diagnosis in travellers includes diarrhoea due to *rotavirus*, norovirus or *Campylobacter* spp. EPEC (rarely-in children) EIEC or VTEC cause dysentery (blood and mucous) and the differential diagnosis in travellers includes *Shigella* spp., *Salmonella* spp. and *Campylobacter* spp. VTEC causes two distinct conditions: haemorrhagic colitis due to the action of the toxin locally on the gut or haemolytic uraemic syndrome in which the toxin causes haemolysis secondary to systemic microvascular angiopathy leading to renal failure. VTEC can also cause thrombocytopaenic purpura in adults.

Yersinia enterocolitica

Epidemiology

This is a comparatively rare cause of bacterial gastroenteritis. Pigs are the important reservoir of human disease. The microorganism can grow at $\leq 4\,^{\circ}C$, so prolonged refrigeration of pork is a risk factor.

Pathogenesis

The microorganism invades the epithelial lining of the terminal ileum and colon. The microorganism unusually does not produce iron-binding compounds and thus individuals with iron-overload are prone to infection.

Clinical features and complications

The incubation period is 4–10 days and may result in a self-limiting acute febrile bloody gastroenteritis or mesenteric adenitis, which mimics acute appendicitis. Bloodstream spread leading to extra-intestinal pyogenic syndromes may occur in immunocompromised individuals or those with iron overload. The infection can cause an (HLA B27 associated) reactive arthritis and erythema nodosum is not uncommon.

Diagnosis of bacterial causes of infective gastroenteritis

The diagnosis is established by stool culture on selective media. The microorganism can be further differentiated by typing, which may be useful in outbreak investigations. Cholera may be diagnosed 'in the field' using microscopy of stool samples to recognise vibrios.

Diagnosis of *Yersinia* species may be by culture of blood and stools and occasionally mesenteric nodes or peritoneal fluid. Correlation with elevated and falling serum antibody titres will prevent false positive diagnosis related to the incidental finding of non-pathogenic bacteria in stool.

Food poisoning

This is the illness resulting from consumption of food contaminated with pathogenic microorganisms and/or their toxins. The common causes are outlined below:

Staphylococcus aureus

Epidemiology

S. aureus contaminates foods (typically cooked meats and cream cakes) and produces an entero-toxin, which is responsible for the associated enteritis. The source of the contamination is often a food handler who is colonised with a toxigenic strain of S. aureus.

Clinical features

The incubation period is 1–6 hours. Severe abdominal pain and vomiting ensue (diarrhoea is rare). The severity of the illness is dependent on the amount of contaminated food and toxin ingested, individual susceptibility and the general condition of the patient. The illness lasts 12–24 hours with no long-term sequelae.

Diagnosis

Culture and also serological techniques to detect the presence of enterotoxin in the suspect food.

Clostridium perfringens

Epidemiology

C. perfringens is widely present in the environment, in the intestine of humans and domestic animals and can contaminate meat during preparation for consumption. Small numbers of microorganisms may survive subsequent cooking particularly in large pieces of meat, and multiply during the cooling down and storage resulting in food poisoning. A more serious but rare illness (necrotising enteritis or pig-bel disease) is caused by ingesting food contaminated with Type C strains.

Clinical features

The incubation period is 8–24 hours. The common form of the disease associated with diarrhoea and abdominal cramps is self-limiting and usually over in 24 hours. Necrotising enteritis (caused by ingestion of large numbers of the causative microorganism of Type C) is often fatal.

Diagnosis

Detection of toxin in faeces. Bacterial confirmation by isolating the causative microorganism in foods and/or faeces of patients.

Bacillus cereus

Epidemiology

The heat-resistant spores of B. cereus are widespread and contaminate rice and other cereals. After surviving boiling of rice, the spores germinate if left at room temperature. A heat-labile toxin can also be produced which can survive "flash frying".

Clinical features

There are two clinical syndromes produced by the heat stable or heat labile toxin:

1 *Heat stable toxin-vomiting disease*: Incubation period 0.5–6 hours followed by an illness similar to that due to S. aureus, although occasionally diarrhoea and cramps can occur. The illness is usually self-limiting and over in 24 hours
2 *Heat labile toxin*: Incubation period 6–15 hours followed by an illness similar to that seen with C. perfringens. The diarrhoea and abdominal cramps may be associated with nausea (vomiting is rare) but are over in 24 hours.

Diagnosis

This is by the isolation of B. cereus from the suspect food, as well as from the stool or vomitus of the patient.

Clostridium botulinum

Epidemiology

Spores of C. botulinum are widespread and heat resistant and can survive in foods that have been incorrectly or minimally processed. Canned foods are often implicated. The spores produce a potent neurotoxin which is heat-labile and can be destroyed if food is heated to 80 °C for $\geq$10 minutes.

Clinical features

Food-borne botulism is a rare but severe type of food poisoning caused by the ingestion of food containing the neurotoxin. After an incubation period of 18–36 hours there is marked lassitude weakness and vertigo followed by lower motor neuron dysfunction affecting first the cranial nerves (diplopia, dysphagia, dysarthria) and progressing caudally.

Diagnosis

The detection of botulinum toxin in serum, faeces and suspected food.

Treatment

Early administration of botulinum antitoxin and supportive treatment, which may require a period of assisted ventilation in an intensive care setting.

Listeria monocytogenes

Epidemiology

L. monoctyogenes is found widely in soil and carried by mammals, fish and birds. It is a hardy bacterium, which survives freezing, drying, heating and can grow at temperatures as low as 3 °C, hence being able to proliferate in refrigerated food. Sources of infection include raw milk, unpasteurised soft cheese, ice cream, raw vegetables, raw meat, raw and cooked poultry or smoked fish. Pregnant women are at risk, as are infants in the perinatal period and immunocompromised individuals.

Clinical features

Although healthy individuals will remain asymptomatic, the bacterium can cause bloodstream infection, meningitis, meningo-encephalitis in susceptible people and intra-uterine infections in pregnant women, which can lead to spontaneous abortion. Serious infections are variably preceded by nausea, vomiting and diarrhoea.

Complications

Listeria meningitis and perinatal infection has a high mortality rate. Penicillin is an effective treatment, often combined with gentamicin.

Management of bacterial causes of infective gastroenteritis and food poisoning

Maintenance of hydration is essential for all patients with diarrhoea. Most diarrhoea in small children is viral, hence antibiotics are rarely ever necessary. In most cases of bacterial gastroenteritis, antibiotic therapy only slightly shortens the duration of symptoms and might select for resistance. Ciprofloxacin therapy may be considered for patients with continuing severe diarrhoea, caused by *Shigella*, *Salmonella* or *Campylobacter* spp., particularly if there are systemic symptoms such as fever, or in immunocompromised patients. However, many strains of these microorganisms have developed resistance to quinolones and other antibiotics. Antibiotics are indicated for invasive salmonellosis (ciprofloxacin) and cholera (ciprofloxacin or tetracycline reduces duration of symptoms and excretion). Antibiotics do not influence the outcome of uncomplicated yersinia enteritis.

Antibiotics should not be used in the treatment of disease due to VTEC, as patients with this infection are more likely to develop associated serious complications if so treated. This is because antibiotic exposure causes a 'stress' response in VTEC, which results in increased toxin production.

Bacterial pathogens causing food poisoning usually result in a self-limiting disease and only supportive measures are required. An exception is botulism, for which early administration of antitoxin has a beneficial effect on outcome. Parenteral penicillin is used for serious listeria infections.

Anti-motility drugs should be avoided, except perhaps for pragmatic reasons as a short course in travellers' diarrhoea when abroad. Anti-motility drugs should particularly be avoided in young children, as they can allow pathogens to proliferate.

Prevention of bacterial causes of infective gastroenteritis and food poisoning

Providing safe drinking water, proper disposal of sewage and food hygiene, are very important in preventing gastrointestinal infections. Raw and cooked food should be handled separately, frozen food thawed thoroughly and previously prepared food reheated thoroughly. Careful attention should be given to the preparation and storage of canned foods and meat should not be kept refrigerated for long periods.

When patients are symptomatic, high standards of personal hygiene and providing hand-washing facilities are essential to prevent secondary cases. Travellers should be advised to take precautions, such as avoiding tap water, ice, uncooked fruit and vegetables and to consider the use of water purification tablets. In hospitals, patients should be put in 'source isolation' until asymptomatic for 48 hours. Similarly, in the community, cases should be excluded from work or school until asymptomatic for 48 hours. Food handlers should have three negative consecutive stool samples at weekly intervals, before being allowed to resume work.

In the UK, statutory notification of food poisoning, other causes of gastroenteritis and typhoid is made to the local Consultant in Communicable Disease Control (CCDC). The CCDC will coordinate the investigation of cases, and advise on the management of outbreaks and exclusion criteria for affected people.

Immunisation does not have a major role to play in the prevention of gastrointestinal infection. Parenteral, killed, whole-cell cholera vaccines provide short-lived protection in only a proportion of recipients and are of little practical use. Oral cholera vaccines, suitable for use by travellers, have recently been developed.

Viral causes of infective gastroenteritis

Viruses frequently result in gastroenteritis, particularly in children; in the developing countries, they are a major cause of death. Up to a million infants worldwide die of viral gastroenteritis every year. There is no specific treatment, except fluid replacement. In small children in developing countries, oral fluid replacement with electrolyte solutions is an extremely important part of management.

Laboratory diagnosis is by electron microscopy, by the direct detection of virus particles by immunoassays, e.g. ELISA or PCR, depending on the virus being detected.

Rotaviruses

Epidemiology

Many different serotypes exist. Different serotypes cause diarrhoeal disease in other mammals, including cats, dogs, cattle, sheep and pigs. The infecting dose is small and spread is generally person to person. It is most common in children between 6 and 24 months old, but elderly people can be affected. Rotavirus infections are most common in the winter, with epidemics occurring occasionally in nurseries, elderly care homes and hospitals.

Pathogenesis

Rotaviruses damage jejunal enterocytes and disrupt enterocyte transport mechanisms, resulting in loss of water and electrolytes and diarrhoea.

Clinical features

The incubation period is 1–2 days. Vomiting and watery diarrhoea occur, often preceeded by upper respiratory tract symptoms. Infections are self-limiting and there is no specific treatment, apart from fluid replacement.

Noroviruses and sapoviruses

Epidemiology

Cause 'winter vomiting disease'. Humans are the only reservoir of infection. Both sporadic infections and outbreaks are common, but clinical cases are usually diagnosed in outbreaks. Outbreaks occur year round but more frequently during the winter months in temperate climates. Outbreaks can be associated with contaminated water supplies and food. They develop rapidly in institutions, including hospitals and affect patients and staff. The vomiting caused by these viruses results in direct spread by aerosol and indirectly by environmental contamination. The viruses are very stable in the environment. Control of outbreaks requires good hygiene and environmental cleaning.

Pathogenesis and clinical features

Infects mainly the small intestinal villi, but the exact mechanism of diarrhoea production is unknown. The hallmark of infection is the acute onset of vomiting and diarrhoea. Duration of the illness is from 12–60 hours. Treatment is symptomatic.

Other viral causes

Adenoviruses (types 40 and 41)

This is the second most common cause of acute diarrhoea in young children. Incubation period is 8–10 days. Diarrhoea is milder but of longer duration compared with rotavirus gastroenteritis. Fever and vomiting are common. Transmission to family contacts is rare. Diagnosis is by electron microscopy (EM), enzyme immunoassay (EIA) and PCR. Treatment is symptomatic.

Astroviruses

These viruses have a distinctive star-like surface appearance by electron microscopy. They have worldwide distribution. The peak incidence of infection is during the winter months in temperate climates. Transmission is by contaminated water or food. The incubation period is 24–36 hours. It is a common cause of diarrhoea in infants and young children, and in elderly and institutionalised patients. Diarrhoea may be accompanied by fever, vomiting or abdominal pain. The illness lasts for 2–3 days. Diagnosis is by EM, EIA and PCR. Treatment is symptomatic.

Protozoal causes of infective gastroenteritis

Giardia lamblia

Epidemiology

G. lamblia has a worldwide distribution. It is spread by the faecal-oral route and is frequently associated with drinking water contaminated with cysts. These cysts may persist for months in water or soil surviving many environmental hazards outside the host. Person to person spread in institutions is can occur.

Host-parasite interactions

The life cycle of *Giardia lamblia* is described in Chapter 18. Trophozoites attach to the mucosa of the small intestine: epithelial cells are damaged, affecting transport mechanisms, impairing absorption and resulting in diarrhoea.

Clinical features

Infants and children are most susceptible to infection. The incubation period is 1–3 weeks. Infection can lead to an asymptomatic chronic carrier state, an acute self-limiting diarrhoea, mild abdominal pain lasting 7–10 days or, in compromised individuals, a chronic infection with malabsorption, progressive weight loss and anorexia.

Laboratory diagnosis

Microscopy of stool samples, duodenal aspirates or duodenal mucosal biopsies.

Treatment and prevention

Treatment is with metronidazole. Public health measures are important in prevention by ensuring clean drinking water.

Cryptosporidium hominis

Aetiology

Cryptosporidium hominis is a well-recognised cause of diarrhoea in farm (especially calves) and wild animals. It also infects humans. The parasite's complex life cycle has asexual and sexual phases of development in the same host (see Chapter 18).

Epidemiology

Transmission is by the ingestion of cysts acquired either from direct contact with farm animals or infected cases, or via contaminated water or milk.

Clinical features

Diarrhoea is normally mild and lasts several weeks. It can be severe in immunocompromised patients, particularly patients with acquired immune deficiency syndrome (AIDS), and can continue for months or be fatal. An asymptomatic carrier state may occur.

Laboratory diagnosis

By microscopy of faecal samples stained by a modified acid-fast stain.

Treatment and prevention

There is no recognised effective treatment for cryptosporidial diarrhoea. Prevention includes care with personal hygiene when handling farm animals. As the cysts are not killed by chlorination, filtration is important in preventing contamination of drinking water supplies. Cysts will be killed if drinking water is boiled.

Entamoeba histolytica

Infections with *E. histolytica* are endemic in sub-tropical and tropical countries. The life cycle and associated infections are described in Chapter 18.

Typhoid and paratyphoid fever (enteric fever)

These infections, although not primarily gastrointestinal infections, are acquired by the faecal-oral route. Although the causative microorganisms, *Salmonella serotype Typhi* and *Salmonella serotype Paratyphi* belong to the genus *Salmonella*, they are distinguished from other *salmonellae* by the nature of the infection that they cause.

Epidemiology

Enteric fever is prevalent in the developing world, reflecting the poor standards of water supply and sanitation; paratyphoid is endemic in southeast Europe. In developed countries, enteric fever is mostly imported. Humans are the source of the infection and transmission is through food or water contaminated by faeces or urine. Raw fruit and vegetables are important sources in countries in which human faeces is used as a fertiliser. Shellfish from sewage-polluted water are also an important source of infection. Person to person spread is rare. Long-term carriage may occur.

Pathogenesis

The microorganisms invade the intestine and spread to local lymph nodes and then to the liver and spleen where they multiply. The infection enters a bacteraemic phase that coincides with the start of a fever. During this phase, in addition to the monocyte-macrophage system (Peyer's patches, liver, spleen, bone marrow) the gall bladder becomes involved. After recovery, the biliary tract may become the site of chronic carriage, although the urinary tract can also harbour the microorganism. Inflammation and ulceration of Peyer's patches result in diarrhoea and may lead to haemorrhage and perforation. Abscesses in bone or the spleen may occur.

Clinical features

The first week of typhoid produces non-specific symptoms associated with the bacteraemia (headache, fever, constipation, relative bradycardia). The spleen is palpable towards the end of the first week. Although diarrhoea can be a feature from the onset, generally gastrointestinal features appear during the second week. They include diarrhoea, abdominal distension and the characteristic "rose spots" on the skin of the lower chest and upper abdomen. The patient also usually has a cough. During the third week, the "typhoid state" characterised by apathy, toxaemia, delirium and perhaps coma is seen and gastrointestinal complications of bleeding and perforation may occur. During the fourth week, the temperature settles and the patient improves. Paratyphoid results in a much milder infection.

Laboratory diagnosis

Definitive diagnosis is from blood culture during the bacteraemic phase; cultures being positive in 90% of cases in the first week. Stool and urine cultures may be positive in the second week when the gastrointestinal tract is affected but, because of the possibility of chronic carriage, must be interpreted in light of the clinical picture.

Treatment and prevention

Multi-drug resistant salmonella are endemic in Southeast Asia. The use of ciprofloxacin (empirical and first choice) or ceftriaxone should be guided by sensitivity tests. Amoxicillin, co-trimoxazole or chloramphenicol are cheaper alternatives when microorganisms are sensitive. Surgery may be needed for perforation. Chronic carriage may be cured by ciprofloxacin for 1 month. Typhoid and paratyphoid are notifiable infections in the UK. Three vaccines are available: killed whole cell (systemic side effects common), Vi capsular polysaccharide and the oral attenuated Ty21a vaccine.

Clostridium difficile

Although *C. difficile* is a normal component of the human colon, overgrowth of enterotoxin-producing *C. difficile* causes CDI, which has become a serious cause of morbidity and mortality in hospitalised people in the Western world. Recently the emergence of virulent strains (NAP1/BI/027) has led to a dramatic increase in the prevalence, severity and refractoriness of CDI.

Epidemiology

C. difficile is spread indirectly via the faecal-oral route through spores left on surfaces. Intestinal colonisation of *C. difficile* is facilitated by disruption of normal microflora due to antimicrobial treatment. The most common antibiotics implicated are clindamycin, penicillins, cephalosporins and fluoroquinolones. Following germination *C. difficile* produces at least two distinct cytotoxins (A and B), which are both enteropathic. They bind to receptors on intestinal epithelial cells and cause inflammation which leads to diarrhoea. Although CDI can affect healthy individuals who have not used antibiotics, the condition is seen typically in institutions where antibiotics are used and where the environment is contaminated by spores. Predisposing factors apart from prior antibiotic use include malignancy, immune-suppression, chronic obstructive pulmonary disease and renal failure. Peri-partum women and individuals on long-term proton pump inhibitors are at increased risk.

Clinical features

The incubation period is 48–72 hours with the diarrhoea typically occurring 4–9 days after discontinuation of the antibiotic, although the typical watery diarrhoea can occur much longer after an antibiotic has been used (2–3 months). The diarrhoea is profuse and watery but can become bloody with the development of pseudomembranous colitis.

Complications

Fulminant colitis develops in about 5% and is associated with high mortality. A toxic megacolon and bowel perforation can occur.

Laboratory diagnosis

The diagnosis is made by detecting an enterotoxin in a stool sample from a patient with diarrhoea. Usually both toxins A and B are detectable in a patient with CDI. Flexible sigmoidoscopy with biopsy may be useful if there is high clinical suspicion in the presence of a negative stool toxin result. Often typical pseudomembranes are seen, usually in the sigmoid colon.

Treatment

Stop antibiotics for other clinical indications where possible. Metronidazole is first line; vancomycin being used for metronidazole failures and severe CDI. Approximately 20% of cases of CDI will relapse after treatment. Metronidazole may be used for first recurrence.

In the case of the development of a toxic megacolon or acute abdomen, early surgical treatment can be life-saving, although this is associated with a high mortality especially in the elderly.

Recent trials with faecal bacteriotherapy using faeces from healthy individuals to replace the abnormal flora in those with recurrent CDI have shown promise in reducing the likelihood of recurrence.

29

Liver and biliary tract infections

David Mutimer
University Hospitals Birmingham NHS Foundation Trust, Birmingham, UK

The liver has an important role in removing micro-organisms and their products from the circulation. Patients with chronic liver disease often have impaired immune defences and are more susceptible to infection.

Cholecystitis is infection of the gallbladder; cholangitis is infection of the bile duct; there is often an overlap between these two infections. Hepatitis is infection of the liver parenchyma, while a liver abscess is a focal suppurative (pus-forming) process within the liver.

The liver may become infected via the bloodstream (the dual blood supply of the liver via the hepatic artery and the portal vein results in the liver being particularly vulnerable to blood-borne infection) or via the common bile duct, particularly when bile drainage is obstructed. It may be involved in infection as a primary site (e.g. viral hepatitis) or as part of a multi-system infection (e.g. miliary tuberculosis, metastatic abscesses). Liver dysfunction (indicated by jaundice and deranged liver enzymes) may be a feature of severe sepsis arising at other sites.

Aetiology and host–parasite interactions

Cholecystitis and cholangitis

The incidence of cholecystitis and cholangitis increases with age and is more frequent in women, as a result of an association with gallstones. Other factors predisposing to cholangitis are biliary surgery or instrumentation (e.g. endoscopic retrograde cholangio-pancreatography (ERCP)), biliary stricture or tumour, and pancreatitis. Obstruction of the bile duct results in stagnant bile, which becomes infected with commensal bacteria from the intestinal tract. Coliforms and enterococci are the most common microorganisms isolated; infections are frequently mixed and may include anaerobes.

Some parasites (see Chapters 18 and 19) are associated with biliary tract infection. *Fasciola hepatica* may cause biliary obstruction and cirrhosis. Schistosome eggs may lodge in the liver,

Medical Microbiology and Infection Lecture Notes, Fifth Edition. Edited by Tom Elliott, Anna Casey, Peter Lambert and Jonathan Sandoe.

resulting in liver fibrosis and subsequent portal hypertension.

Liver abscess – bacterial and amoebic

Bacterial liver abscesses may result from spread via the systemic circulation, via the bile duct (i.e. secondary to cholangitis), or via the portal vein (e.g. complicating appendicitis or diverticulitis). There are multiple abscesses present in about a third of cases.

Amoebic abscess is a complication of intestinal amoebiasis caused by *Entamoeba histolytica* (see Chapter 18). Severe intestinal disease allows microorganisms to spread to the liver via the portal vein. The abscess increases in size and liver tissue is destroyed; amoebae are present at the margin of the abscess, the centre being filled with blood-stained pus. Abscesses are often single and more commonly in the right lobe of the liver.

The dog tapeworm, *Echinococcus granulosus*, may infect humans and result in hydatid cysts, frequently developing in the liver (see Chapter 19).

Viral hepatitis

Viruses that primarily affect the liver are described as hepatotropic viruses. Currently five are recognised: hepatitis A, B, C, D and E. Viral hepatitis is a notifiable infection in the UK (see Chapter 16).

Hepatitis A virus (HAV)

HAV is an RNA virus and a member of the picornaviridae family.

Epidemiology

HAV is transmitted by the faecal-oral route. It is excreted in the faeces about 1 week before symptoms appear and up to 1 week after the appearance of jaundice. Outbreaks have been associated with infected food handlers and ingestion of contaminated shellfish.

Incidence is highest in the areas of the world with poor sanitation. In these locations the virus is ubiquitous and infection is likely to occur in childhood.

Clinical features

An incubation period of 2–6 weeks is followed by malaise, anorexia, nausea and right upper quadrant pain.

Jaundice appears during the second week and normally lasts several weeks, but may be prolonged. Many infections do not cause jaundice (called anicteric infection). Infections during childhood are generally asymptomatic and symptoms are more severe in older patients. Fulminant liver failure occurs in about 0.1% of cases. Chronic infection does not occur, so chronic liver disease (and progression to cirrhosis) is not seen with HAV infection.

Laboratory diagnosis

Liver function tests show markedly elevated serum levels of liver enzymes (aminotransferases) and bilirubin.

Diagnosis is confirmed by the detection of serum IgM antibodies to HAV. Measurement of anti-HAV IgG is used to confirm immunity to HAV (representing past infection or immunisation).

Treatment and prevention

There is no specific antiviral treatment and hospitalisation is rarely necessary. A killed hepatitis A vaccine is very effective. For those who are unresponsive or allergic to vaccination, passive immunisation with normal immunoglobulin provides protection for about 6 months.

Hepatitis E virus (HEV)

HEV is an RNA virus, formally unclassified but considered a calicivirus.

Epidemiology

Endemic in the Indian subcontinent, Southeast Asia, Middle East, North Africa and central America. Spread by the faecal-oral route, often via water; large waterborne epidemics have occurred in India. It is rare in the developed world, except in travellers from endemic areas. Infection is increasingly observed in the developed world in the absence of travel and without an obvious source of exposure. Phylogenetic analysis of isolates suggests that pigs may be the responsible source.

Clinical features

The incubation period is up to 6 weeks, followed by mild hepatitis. Severe fulminant HEV hepatitis may occur in pregnant women (10–20% of cases). Infections do not become chronic.

Diagnosis

Detection of IgG and IgM antibodies and by nucleic acid detection.

Treatment and prevention

Treatment is symptomatic. The results of vaccination appear promising, though a vaccine is not yet commercially available.

Hepatitis B virus (HBV)

HBV is a DNA virus and a member of the hepadnaviridae family.

Epidemiology

Transmission of HBV is by percutaneous and permucosal routes. There are three important mechanisms of transmission:

1 *Maternal–infant transmission*: across the placenta or during delivery (on a global scale, this is the most important means of transmission and accounts for the majority of infection).
2 *Contact transmission*: via bodily secretions (e.g. blood, semen and vaginal fluid). This is the most common means of acute infection in Western society.
3 *Percutaneous transmission*: at-risk groups include parenteral drug abusers and healthcare workers involved in needlestick injuries. Infection via transfusion of contaminated blood products is rare in most countries, because of screening of blood donors.

Prevalence patterns of HBV infection vary. In developed countries, prevalence is less than 1%, but in some endemic areas (e.g. North Africa, Asia) prevalence of the carrier state may be as high as 20%. Migration from areas of high prevalence is increasing the prevalence of hepatitis B infection in countries that previously had a low incidence and prevalence.

In high prevalence areas, maternal-infant transmission is important, whereas, in areas of low prevalence, percutaneous and sexual routes are more important modes of transmission.

Clinical features and complications

An incubation period of 6 weeks to 6 months is followed by malaise, anorexia and jaundice. Symptoms associated with immune complex disease occur rarely, e.g. arthralgia, vasculitis, glomerulonephritis. Acute infection may cause fulminant liver failure (<1% of cases). Infection may be asymptomatic. Likelihood of symptoms increases with age, so asymptomatic infection may be observed in more than 90% of children but fewer than 50% of adults. Infection may become chronic. Risk for chronicity depends on the age at time of infection. Infection of the infant (vertical infection) is very likely to become chronic. Infection in adulthood is likely to resolve without chronicity.

Laboratory diagnosis in acute and chronic infection (Table 29.1)

Three HBV antigens and the corresponding antibodies are used in the diagnosis of acute and chronic HBV infection:

1 *Hepatitis B surface antigen (HBsAg)*: the first serological marker of acute HBV infection, appearing several weeks before symptoms. HBsAg is always present in the serum of patients with chronic infection. Presence of antibody to HBsAg (anti-HBs) indicates past infection with HBV or previous immunisation.
2 *Hepatitis B 'e' antigen (HBeAg)*: appears soon after HBsAg and disappears early in the recovery from acute hepatitis B. In chronic hepatitis B, the detection of HBeAg in serum is associated with very high viral titres.
3 *Hepatitis B core antigen*: never detectable in the serum. Serum antibodies to core antigen (anti-HBc) simply indicate that a patient has been exposed to hepatitis B at some time. Anti-HBc will be detectable in the serum of individuals with past resolved acute infection, and in the serum of patients with acute or chronic hepatitis infection. Anti-HBc of IgM class indicates recently acquired infection.

Treatment and prevention of acute hepatitis B

Antiviral treatment is not indicated for acute hepatitis B. The majority of infections diagnosed at this stage will resolve without clinical sequelae. A minority becomes chronic. Prevention is by screening

Table 29.1 Serological profiles according to the stage and activity of hepatitis B virus infection

| | Acute HBV | Chronic HBV (carrier) | | | Immune to HBV (past exposure) |
		'Healthy carrier'	HBeAg-positive hepatitis	HBeAg-negative hepatitis	
HBsAg	Positive	Positive	Positive	Positive	Negative
Anti-HBs	Negative	Negative	Negative	Negative	Positive
Anti-HBc	Positive	Positive	Positive	Positive	Positive
IgM anti-HBc	Positive	Negative	Negative	Negative	Negative
HBeAg	Pos or neg	Negative	Positive	Negative	Negative
Anti-HBe	Pos or neg	Positive	Negative	Positive	Positive
HBV DNA (virions/ml)	10^6 (falls quickly)	Undetectable	$>10^7$	$>10^5$ (fluctuates)	Undetectable

of blood donors and products, use of disposable needles and other instruments and efficient sterilisation of re-usable medical instruments. A recombinant HBsAg vaccine is available and should be given to at-risk groups, including healthcare workers. Specific immunoglobulin (passive immunisation) may be given to non-immunised people exposed to HBV (e.g. in a needlestick injury) and to babies born to HBeAg-positive carrier mothers.

Chronic hepatitis B

Some patients develop chronic infection following exposure to hepatitis B. The risk for chronic infection depends upon the age at time of infection. For instance, neonatal exposure to hepatitis B will result in chronic infection in more than 90% of cases. Adult-acquired infection seldom becomes chronic. By definition, infection that persists for longer than 6 months is called 'chronic'.

Clinical features and outcome

The outcome of chronic infection varies enormously. The risk for chronic liver damage depends mainly on the level of viral replication. Prolonged periods of high-level replication will cause significant liver damage. Chronic hepatitis causes liver fibrosis, which can progress to cirrhosis. Cirrhosis can lead to liver failure and can be complicated by the development of primary liver cancer (hepatocellular carcinoma). The long-term prognosis of chronic hepatitis B is gender-dependent. Fifty percent of males with chronic hepatitis B will die

(after ~50 years of infection) as a consequence of cirrhosis and/or liver cancer. A much smaller proportion of chronically infected women will suffer the same fate.

Laboratory diagnosis of chronic infection

HBsAg is present in serum. HBeAg may also persist and indicates high levels of viral replication and increased infectivity. Patients with HBeAg-negativity may have very low levels of virus (sometimes called a 'healthy carrier'), though some have sufficient levels to cause liver damage (so-called 'HBeAg-negative hepatitis'). Serum hepatitis B DNA measurement gives an exact indication of the level of viral replication and of the future risk of clinical complications.

Management

Specific treatment is with antiviral agents, which suppress viral replication and prevent the development of liver damage in patients with chronic infection. Treatment options include α-interferon (given by subcutaneous injection) or nucleoside analogues (see Chapter 22). Liver transplantation may be indicated for patients with end-stage liver failure and/or liver cancer.

Hepatitis C virus (HCV)

HCV is an RNA virus of the flaviviridae family. There is high genome variability with at least six different genotypes (1–6) and several subtypes (1a, 1b, 2a, 2b, etc.).

Epidemiology

Infection is typically acquired via the parenteral route. In Western countries, the commonest mode of transmission is intravenous drug use. In developing countries with limited healthcare resources, the commonest mode of transmission is via needle re-use by healthcare practitioners. Though vertical transmission and sexual transmission may explain a minority of cases, these modes of infection are numerically much less important.

Clinical features

The incubation period is 2–6 months. Most infections are asymptomatic (80%) and in symptomatic cases the hepatitis is often mild. In contrast with the natural history of adult-acquired hepatitis B infection (which seldom becomes chronic), approximately 70% of cases of acute hepatitis C infection will become chronic. Chronic infection causes chronic liver damage and can progress to cirrhosis after many years (at least 20 years). Cirrhosis can be complicated by the development of primary liver cancer.

Laboratory diagnosis

This is by serology, for the presence of antibody to HCV and molecular techniques for the detection of HCV RNA.

Treatment and prevention

Avoidance of needle re-use by drug users and in the healthcare setting is the mainstay of prevention. A vaccine has not been developed. Treatment is with α-interferon and ribavirin for up to 12 months, and will cure infection (permanent eradication of infection) in 50% of cases. HCV genotypes, in addition to other factors, can determine the response to treatment: genotype 1 is the least responsive. New and potent HCV-specific drugs are in development.

Hepatitis D virus (HDV)

The hepatitis D virus or delta agent is a defective RNA virus that can replicate only in HBV-infected cells. Transmission is via infected blood and sexual intercourse. HDV accentuates HBV infection, resulting in more severe liver disease. Laboratory diagnosis is by HDV antibody detection and infection can be confirmed by HDV RNA detection. Treatment is with α-interferon, but response to treatment is disappointing. Prevention of hepatitis B (by vaccination) will also prevent HDV infection (since HDV can only infect HBV-positive cells).

Other causes of viral hepatitis

- Ebstein-Barr virus (EBV) can cause hepatitis during acute infectious mononucleosis. Usually a mild self-limiting infection, but can be severe.
- Cytomegalovirus (CMV) can cause hepatitis during acute infections or reactivation of latent virus in immunocompromised patients.
- Human herpesvirus 6 (HHV6) can cause hepatitis in acute infections or following reactivation of latent virus in immunocompromised patients.
- Herpes simplex virus (HSV) can cause hepatitis in generalised infection in neonates or immunocompromised patients.
- Varicella-Zoster virus (VZV) causes hepatitis as a complication of chickenpox or disseminated zoster in immunocompromised patients.
- Rubella can cause hepatitis in congenital or acquired infections.
- Viral haemorrhagic fever viruses can cause hepatitis (Yellow fever, rift valley fever virus, Ebola and Marburg viruses, Lassa fever virus, Junin and Machupo viruses).

Urinary tract infections

Chris Catchpole
Worcestershire Acute Hospitals NHS Trust, Worcester, UK

Clinical definitions

There are three clinical syndromes associated with urinary tract infection (UTI).

Lower UTI (frequency dysuria syndrome)

The clinical features of lower UTI commonly include dysuria (pain on passing urine), urinary frequency, urgency and fever. Non-specific symptoms, including confusion, unsteadiness, irritability and poor weight gain, may predominate in children and the elderly. These symptoms are caused by one of the following:

- Bacterial cystitis with bacteriuria (the presence of bacteria in urine), often associated with pyuria and haematuria due to acute inflammation.
- Abacterial cystitis ('urethral syndrome') where no microbial cause is identified. Some cases may be associated with microorganisms that are not cultured by routine laboratory methods (Chapter 14). Unlike urethritis caused by sexually transmitted infections, this syndrome is not associated with urethral discharge.

Lower UTI, if untreated, may resolve spontaneously; however, infection may progress to, or be complicated by, pyelonephritis (see below), bloodstream infection, epididymitis or prostatitis.

Upper UTI (acute bacterial pyelonephritis)

This condition is caused by infection of the kidney, and clinical presentation includes loin pain and tenderness, pyrexia and symptoms of lower UTI accompanied by bacteriuria and pyuria. This potentially serious infection may progress to peri-nephric abscess formation or bloodstream infection and, in chronic cases, to scarring and renal failure.

Asymptomatic (covert) bacteriuria

This is defined as significant numbers of bacteria present in the urine of apparently healthy people, with no associated symptoms. Urinary catheterisation is commonly associated with this finding, and does not usually require antibiotic therapy. Asymptomatic bacteriuria may, however, be of clinical importance in childhood and pregnancy, where treatment may be warranted to prevent complications should infection develop.

Microbial aetiology and host–parasite interactions

The bacteria that commonly cause UTI are commensals (normal flora) of the perineum or lower

Medical Microbiology and Infection Lecture Notes, Fifth Edition. Edited by Tom Elliott, Anna Casey, Peter Lambert and Jonathan Sandoe.

Table 30.1 Common bacterial causes of UTI (approximate percentage)

Microorganism	Community acquired (%)	Hospital acquired (%)
Escherichia coli	75	40
Proteus mirabilis	3	10
Other enterobacteriaceae	5	25
Pseudomonas aeruginosa	1	5
Enterococcus faecalis	5	8
Staphylococcus saprophyticus	5	1
Staphylococcus epidermidis	2	3

intestine, and include *Escherichia coli* (the most common cause), *Proteus mirabilis* (associated with urinary tract stones) and other enterobacteriaceae (e.g. *Klebsiella* spp. *Enterobacter* spp. and *Serratia* spp.) Other microorganisms are associated with particular patient groups, e.g. *Staphylococcus saprophyticus* with sexually active young women, and *Pseudomonas aeruginosa* with urethral catheterisation (Table 30.1). Non-bacterial causes of UTI are shown in Table 30.2.

Bacterial virulence factors include:

- *Fimbriae*: certain serotypes of *E. coli* have specific fimbriae (pili) that facilitate colonisation

Table 30.2 Non-bacterial causes of UTI

Group	Microorganism	Infection
Viruses		
	Adenoviruses	Haemorrhagic cystitis
	Human polyoma virus	Infections in kidney and ureter
Parasites		
	Trichomonas vaginalis	Urethritis
	Schistosoma haematobium	Bladder inflammation
Fungi		
	Candida albicans	UTI in immunocompromised patient

and adherence to the periurethral areas, urethra and bladder wall;
- *Capsules*: some strains of *E. coli* produce a polysaccharide capsule that inhibits phagocytosis and these are associated with the development of pyelonephritis.

Host factors

Defence mechanisms, which protect against UTI, include:

- *hydrodynamic forces*: the flow of urine removes microorganisms from the bladder and urethra;
- phagocytosis of microorganisms by polymorphs on the bladder surface;
- the presence of IgA antibody on the bladder wall;
- a mucin layer on the bladder wall prevents bacterial adherence;
- urinary pH.

The following are important host risk factors for UTI:

- *Short urethra in females*: sexual intercourse facilitates the passage of microorganisms up the urethra ('honeymoon cystitis');
- *Structural and functional abnormalities*: causing outflow obstruction (e.g. prostatic enlargement, pregnancy, tumours, neurogenic bladder). These result in residual urine in the bladder, which can act as a focus for infection. Reflux of urine from the bladder up the ureter (vesicoureteric reflux) into the kidney can also result from anatomical abnormalities and cause pyelonephritis and renal scarring. Renal stones can also be associated with pyelonephritis;
- *Increasing age*: post-menopausal increase in vaginal pH and shift of normal vaginal flora to coliforms, bladder prolapse and prostatic disease.

Other host risk factors for UTI include:

- diabetes mellitus;
- immunosuppression (e.g. steroids, cytotoxic drugs);
- instrumentation (e.g. surgery or the use of urinary catheters); bacteria may be introduced into the bladder on catheter insertion, or may migrate up the catheter into the bladder at a later stage. UTI associated with urinary catheterisation is an important cause of healthcare associated infection.

Sample collection

For non-catheterised patients, a well taken mid-stream specimen of urine (MSSU) should be collected, avoiding perineal contamination, into a sterile universal container. Samples taken from catheterised patients should be collected directly from the catheter tubing, not from the drainage bag. In infants, an adhesive bag or supra-pubic aspiration (SPA) may be used. Ideally samples should be processed as soon after collection as possible, to prevent bacterial overgrowth. If a delay in processing is unavoidable, samples should be refrigerated at 4°C, or transported in boric acid or (agar-coated) dipslide collection bottles.

Laboratory diagnosis

The use of commercial dipstick tests is popular as a point of care test (POCT) for screening for UTI. Infection can be confidently excluded in samples that test negative for both leucocyte-esterase and nitrites on dipstick testing, but positive results should be confirmed by microscopy and culture if clinically indicated.

The mainstay of laboratory diagnosis of UTI is assessment for the presence of:

- white and red blood cells, epithelial cells and casts by microscopy or flow cytometry; and
- bacteriuria by semi-quantitative culture of a freshly collected urine sample.

However, results should always be interpreted in the context of the clinical picture.

Significant bacteriuria is commonly defined as the presence of $\geq 10^5$ bacteria/mL (equivalent to $\geq 10^8$ bacteria per litre) of an MSSU sample; occasionally, urine from patients with UTI symptoms may have fewer microorganisms, possibly as a result of dilution. Bacteriuria between 10^4 and 10^5 microorganisms/mL should be correlated with clinical symptoms, antibiotic use, and fluid intake to determine whether infection is likely. When bacteriuria of $<10^4$ microorganisms/mL is detected, in patients who are not receiving antibiotics, infection is unlikely.

White blood cells at a concentration of 10/mL or greater indicates significant pyuria; however, neutropaenic patients may not produce high numbers of cells in urine.

The presence of epithelial cells indicates perineal/peri-urethral contamination, which may give a false positive culture result. Sample contamination should also be suspected when culture yields more than two bacterial species.

Blood cultures should also be taken, if pyelonephritis or bloodstream infection is suspected.

Antibiotic sensitivity tests are undertaken on bacterial isolates, which are considered to be of potential clinical significance. The results of these tests should be used as a guide to appropriate therapy.

Management

Non-antibiotic management includes increasing fluid intake to 'flush out' microorganisms. In uncomplicated lower UTI, a short course (e.g. 3 days) of first-line empirical oral antibiotic therapy should be considered, and choices should take account of local susceptibility patterns; options may include trimethoprim or nitrofurantoin. Therapy should then be amended as required, based on the results of antibiotic sensitivity tests. Patients with upper UTI or UTI associated bloodstream infection may require parenteral therapy initially, and a more prolonged course of antibiotics is indicated (7–10 days). Failure to respond to apparently appropriate therapy is an indication to repeat urine culture.

As with all antibiotic therapy, choice of agent should be guided by causative microorganism, history of known drug allergy, presence of other underlying medical conditions, and risk of antibiotic adverse effects or drug interactions, particularly in the elderly, e.g. *Clostridium difficile* infection.

It is also important to recognise that the presence of bacteriuria and/or pyuria is common, particularly in the elderly, and that it does not always indicate an infection that requires antibiotic therapy. However, in pregnancy, asymptomatic bacteriuria should be treated to prevent complications, which include pyelonephritis and preterm delivery.

Sterile pyuria (routine urine culture is negative in the presence of significant numbers of white blood cells) may require further investigation: causes include concomitant antibiotic therapy, inflammatory renal disease, the presence of foreign bodies, tumours or infection with uncommon bacterial (e.g. *Mycoplasma* spp.) or non-bacterial pathogens (Table 30.2).

31

Genital infections

Kaveh Manavi
University Hospitals Birmingham NHS Foundation Trust, Birmingham, UK

This chapter outlines some of the more common genital infections.

Vaginitis

Definition

The term applies to inflammation of vaginal mucosa that may extend to the vulva and is commonly associated with a white or yellow discharge. Occasionally vaginitis may be associated with dysuria and dyspareunia.

Clinically the term mainly applies to unusual vaginal symptoms (i.e. unusual discharge or any form of abnormal vaginal sensation) with or without mucosal inflammation. Many women seek medical treatment for these symptoms; however, a large number are treated incorrectly in the absence of appropriate laboratory diagnosis.

The most common causes of vaginal symptoms are bacterial vaginosis, *Trichomonas* vaginitis and candidiasis. Less common causes of vaginitis, including foreign bodies, lichen planus, chemical irritation and atrophic vaginitis are not discussed in this chapter.

Bacterial vaginosis (BV)

Aetiology

- BV is believed to be the result of reduction of vaginal lactobacilli and colonisation of vaginal mucosa by groups of abnormal microorganisms rather than one single pathogen. Some of the bacteria associated with BV include *Gardnerella vaginalis*, anaerobes such *Bacteroides* spp., and *Peptostreptococcus* spp., *Mycoplasma hominus*, and *Ureaplasma urealyticum*.
- BV is not associated with inflammation of vaginal mucosa.
- BV has been reported to facilitate HIV acquisition.

Epidemiology

- BV is the most common cause of vaginal discharge.
- It has been estimated that a third of women may develop BV sometime in their life.
- In 2008, more than 110,000 BV episodes were diagnosed in GUM clinics in England.
- Young age, smoking, vaginal douching, and having multiple sexual partners have been separately associated with BV.

Medical Microbiology and Infection Lecture Notes, Fifth Edition. Edited by Tom Elliott, Anna Casey, Peter Lambert and Jonathan Sandoe.
© 2011 Blackwell Publishing Ltd. Published 2011 by Blackwell Publishing Ltd.

- BV is not a sexually transmitted infection (STI) and there is no equivalent entity in men.

Clinical features

- Malodorous 'fishy' vaginal discharge has been proposed as characteristic of BV in the past. However, this is not the case, as many women with BV may not complain of such discharge.
- Most women with BV are asymptomatic; up to 75% of women with BV deny any foul smelling discharge.
- BV has been associated with post-partum endometritis, chorioamnionitis, pre-term labour and pelvic inflammatory disease (PID).

Diagnosis

- Diagnosis of BV relies on clinical and microscopic findings; no single clinical manifestation can reliably assist.
- Amsel's criteria have been used by many clinicians; BV requires the presence of three of the four criteria:
  1 Viscid abnormal vaginal discharge;
  2 Positive 'whiff test'; fishy odour of vaginal fluid after addition of 10% potassium hydroxide;
  3 Presence of clue cells (epithelial cells embedded with bacteria with unidentified border) on microscopy of vaginal fluid;
  4 Vaginal fluid pH of more than 4.5.
- Hay–Ison Criteria; a new diagnostic system for BV and includes the following:
  ○ Grade 1: normal lactobacilli, Grade 2: mixed flora with some lactobacilli, and *Gardenerella*; Grade 3: mostly *Gardnerella*
  ○ In symptomatic women, grades 2, or 3 are consistent with BV.
  Presence of more than one polymorphonuclear cell (PMN) in microscopy of vaginal fluid raises the possibility of TV or cervicitis (gonococcal or chlamydial).

Treatment and prevention in adults

- Oral metronidazole (multiple or single dose);
- Clindamycin or metronidazole cream are alternatives;
- Prolonged oral metronidazole for recurrent BV;
- Prolonged metronidazole gel use for recurrent BV.

Trichomonas vaginitis (TV)

Aetiology

- The protozoan parasite *Trichomonas vaginalis* is the cause of TV
- TV facilitates HIV acquisition and has been reported to be strongly associated with other STIs.
- Men infected with *Trichomonas vaginalis* are mostly asymptomatic; mild dysuria may be reported by some infected men.
- During pregnancy, TV can cause pre-term delivery and low birth weight. Because treatment of TV during pregnancy with metronidazole has been reported to be associated with similar unfavourable outcomes, routine screening of asymptomatic women for TV is not currently recommended.

Epidemiology

- In GUM clinics in England, 5,600 episodes of TV were diagnosed in 2008.
- Worldwide, 170 million cases of TV are reported each year.
- *Trichomonas vaginalis* is transmitted by sexual intercourse, hence it is an STI.

Clinical features

- Most women with TV are believed to be asymptomatic.
- Abnormal vaginal discharge, vulval and peri-anal itching are the most common symptoms.
- Erythema of vagina with diffuse petechiae on the cervix (strawberry cervix) have been considered pathognomonic for TV. Strawberry cervix is not commonly observed in women with symptomatic TV.

Diagnosis

- Wet mount microscopy of vaginal fluid shows motile *Trichomonas vaginalis.*
- Vaginal fluid of women with TV may also have PMN with a pH of higher than 4.5
- Inoculation of vaginal fluid for *Trichomonas vaginalis* culture has higher sensitivity and should be performed for women considered at risk of infection.
- Use of nucleic acid amplification assays for diagnosis of TV has been approved. These assays have higher sensitivity and specificity than TV culture and may be used as a standard test in future.

Treatment and prevention in adults

- Multiple or single dose of oral metronidazole;
- Sexual partners of women with TV need to be treated as well;

Vulvo-vaginal candidiasis (VC); ('Thrush')

Aetiology

- VC is caused by *Candida albicans* in the majority of cases. Infections with *C. glabrata* or *C. tropicalis* often result in recalcitrant VC.
- VC is a common cause of vaginitis.
- Immunosuppression (secondary to HIV, or immunosuppressive agents), diabetes mellitus, pregnancy, use of broad spectrum antibiotics can each predispose women to VC.
- Many women incorrectly relate their vulvo-vaginal symptoms to VC.

Epidemiology

- More than 70,000 cases of VC were diagnosed in GUM clinics in England in 2008.
- The number of episodes treated for assumed VC by over the counter medicines remains unclear.
- VC is not a STI and affects most women at least once in their life time.

Clinical features

- Itching and irritation, vaginal discharge, dyspareunia and dysuria are the most common complaints patients present with.

Diagnosis

- Microscopical examination of vaginal fluid (wet mount, or Gram stained) reveals yeasts.
- Yeast culture is the gold standard method for diagnosis of candidiasis and species identification. Yeast culture should only be performed in symptomatic women.

Treatment and prevention in adults

- Topical azole antifungal agents (as pessary or creams) can be used; clotrimazole, miconazole;
- A single oral dose of fluconazole is an alternative treatment option. This is contraindicated for pregnant women.

Urethritis and cervicitis

Gonococcal urethritis and *cervicitis*

Epidemiology

- The gonococcus, *Neisseria gonorrhoea* is an obligate human parasite;
- Many women are asymptomatic and may act as a reservoir of infection;
- Highly transmissible by sexual contact;
- Occurs worldwide;
- Infections are most common among sexually active young adults.

Pathogenesis

See Chapter 7.

Clinical features

- Urethral discharge in men and cervicitis in women;
- Complications include epididymitis, prostatitis, urethral stricture, Bartholin's abscess, pelvic inflammatory disease and infertility.

Laboratory diagnosis

- A diagnosis can be confirmed by microscopy, culture and/or molecular analysis (nucleic acid amplification tests, NAAT) of pus and secretions from various sites (depending upon the infection): cervix, urethra, rectum, conjunctiva, throat and synovial fluid.
- Clinical samples are cultured on enriched selective media.
- Specimens requiring culture should be rapidly transported to the laboratory, because gonococci die readily on drying.
- Blood cultures should be sent before antimicrobial therapy is commenced when disseminated infection is suspected, e.g. in sexually active patients with septic arthritis, concurrent with NAAT.
- Serology is not helpful in the diagnosis of gonococcal infection.

Treatment and prevention

Resistance to penicillins, tetracyclines and quinolones is common in the UK and worldwide. Most strains remain susceptible to third-generation cephalosporins (e.g. ceftriaxone or cefixime). Single-dose therapies are recommended to increase patient compliance. Prevention of gonorrhoea includes sex education, promotion of public awareness and the use of condoms. Contact tracing is essential in preventing further spread and the disease. No vaccine is available.

Non-gonococcal urethritis and cervicitis

Chlamydia trachomatis (see Chapter 14)

Epidemiology

- *C. trachomatis* is the most common bacterial STI in the UK and the world.
- It has been estimated that 10% of women and 13% of men younger than 25 years in the UK may be infected with chlamydia.
- The majority of infected (70% of female and 50% of male) patients are asymptomatic.
- Untreated chlamydial infection can cause pelvic inflammatory disease (PID) in 10–40% of women.
- Each year a substantial amount of health budgets around the world are spent on management of the long-term consequences of untreated chlamydial infections.

Pathogenesis

See Chapter 14.

Clinical features

Female genital tract

In women, chlamydial infection can cause symptomatic cervicitis (Figure 31.1), but most cases are asymptomatic. It is likely that a significant proportion of infected women may develop PID. PID can cause infertility, ectopic pregnancy and chronic pelvic pain syndrome in affected women.

Male genital tract

C. trachomatis is the most common cause of urethritis in men. Persistent chlamydial infection in men can lead to epididymo-orchitis, painful swelling of the epididymis that is mostly unilateral.

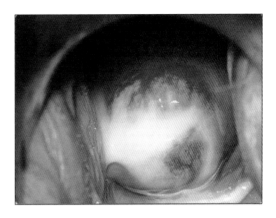

Figure 31.1 Chlamydial cervicitis.

Sexually acquired reactive arthritis (SARA)

One of the auto-immune manifestations of persistent chlamydial infection presents as pain of lower limb joints mostly in asymmetrical fashion. The symptoms commonly start within 30 days of sexual contact. Box 31.1 summarises the clinical manifestations of SARA.

BOX 31.1 Clinical presentations of sexually acquired reactive arthritis (SARA)

- Circinate balanitis or vulvitis (typical psoriatic lesions of the glans penis or labia)
- Guttate cutaneous psoriasis
- Pustular psoriasis on the soles of the feet
- Psoriasiform rash
- Subcutaneous nodules
- Geographical tongue
- Nail dystrophy
- Conjunctivitis
- Enthesopathy (pain at the sites of tendon or fascia attachments, especially the Achilles tendon and plantar fascia attachments to the calcaneum).
- Tenosynovitis (tenderness over tendon sheaths of the lower limbs).
- Sacroiliitis (low back pain and stiffness)
- Pericarditis and aortic valve disease
- Thrombophlebitis of the lower limbs
- Renal pathology (proteinuria, haematuria and aseptic pyuria)
- Nervous system involvement including meningo-encephalitis and nerve palsies

Laboratory diagnosis

- NAAT are the most sensitive and specific tests for detection of *C. trachomatis* infections. These assays can be used on self-collected specimens (urine or vaginal swabs) enabling patients to be tested for *C. trachomatis* infection without the need for genital examination.
- Polymerase chain reaction, transcription mediated amplification and strand displacement amplification are some of the NAAT available for detection of *C. trachomatis*.

Treatment and prevention

Uncomplicated *C. trachomatis* can be treated with tetracyclines, macrolides or quinolones (except ciprofloxacin). At least one week of treatment with any of those agents is required. Treatment of complicated chlamydial infection (PID, epididymo-orchitis or LGV) require longer duration of antibiotic therapy. Treatment of chlamydial infection has been significantly simplified with the advent of azithromycin. A single dose of azithromycin will be adequate for treatment of uncomplicated chlamydial infection. The most effective method for prevention of genital transmission of chlamydial infection is consistent use of male latex condoms. Partners of patients with chlamydial infection need chlamydial screening and treatment.

Other causes of urethritis

Ureaplasma spp., *Mycoplasma hominis*, TV and Herpes simplex virus may also cause urethritis.

Genital ulcers

There are generally three main causes for genital ulcer disease (GUD); infections, inflammatory diseases and malignancies. In the developed countries, herpes simplex virus (types 1 or 2) and syphilis are the most common infectious causes of GUD. Chancroid caused by *Haemophilus ducreyi* is another infectious cause of GUD, mostly diagnosed in developing countries.

Herpes simplex virus (HSV) infection

Aetiology

- Although classically HSV-2 has been associated with genital herpes, HSV-1 has become the main cause of genital herpes in developed countries.
- HSV results in a chronic infection that may cause recurrent episodes.

Epidemiology

- HSV is the most common cause of GUD in the world.
- HSV is transmitted through direct skin to skin contact.
- It is believed that a significant number of patients infected with HSV remain undiagnosed, as their symptoms are short-lived and atypical.
- Viral shedding can occur without active ulceration.
- With use of nucleic acid amplification tests, more cases of HSV have been diagnosed.

Clinical features

- *Primary HSV episode*: patients without prior HSV infection may develop systemic illness with genital blisters. The systemic illness manifests as flu like symptoms, fever, lymphadenopathy, aseptic meningitis and atonic bladder.
- *Herpetic blisters*: can appear in clusters, dry out over 2 weeks and develop a crust. Finally the ulcers heal without scarring.
- *Initial HSV episode*: the first clinical presentation of genital herpes. Patients mostly complain of painful genital blisters and herpetic blisters.
- *Recurrent HSV episode*: the subsequent episodes of herpes attacks are manifested with herpetic ulcerations that heal within 3–5 days. Patients report milder symptoms during recurrent herpes episodes.
- The number of recurrent herpes episodes is highest in the first year.
- Patients with frequent herpes attacks may benefit from suppressive therapy.

Laboratory diagnosis

- Use of polymerase chain reaction (PCR) assays has become the standard method of diagnosis in recent years. This testing method has high sensitivity and specificity. Herpes PCR can also confirm the type of HSV as well.

- HSV culture is still considered the gold standard method of HSV diagnosis, but is no longer used in most diagnostic laboratories. It is not as sensitive as PCR and therefore may miss a number of positive cases.
- HSV-serology is generally not helpful in the diagnosis of genital HSV. Type specific HSV serology can diagnose previous infections with HSV-2 and may be useful in asymptomatic patients.

Treatment and prevention

- HSV-DNA polymerase inhibitors (aciclovir, valaciclovir, famciclovir) used systemically are highly effective in controlling HSV episodes. These agents do not eradicate infection.
- Aciclovir is used for recurrent episodes.
- For patients with frequent HSV recurrence episodes (more than 5 episodes a year), suppressive therapy can be initiated. This includes acyclovir or valaciclovir once a day. The duration of suppressive therapy is 12 months.
- Use of condoms reduce rate of HSV transmission but does not completely prevent it. Counselling of sexual partners of patients is an important component of prevention of HSV transmission strategy.

Syphilis

Aetiology

Syphilis is an infection caused by the spirochete, *Treponema pallidum*.

Epidemiology

- Syphilis is mainly an STI.
- The number of patients with primary and secondary syphilis (see Pathogenesis) in the UK has increased significantly since 2000; more than 12,500 cases have been diagnosed between 2004 and 2008.
- Globally, syphilis has been increasingly diagnosed in countries with a high rate of HIV infection. Syphilis significantly increases the rate of HIV transmission; its diagnosis and treatment may therefore be an important strategy for prevention of HIV infection.

- Pregnant women with untreated syphilis can also pass infection to their foetus at any point during pregnancy or delivery.
- If a pregnant woman is in the early stages of infection, her foetus is at greatest risk of congenital syphilis unless treated for syphilis.
- The rate of congenital infection significantly reduces if the mother is treated before the 16th week of pregnancy.

Pathogenesis

T. pallidum is a spirochaete capable of movement within extra cellular human tissues. It is able to penetrate skin or mucosa through micro-abrasions. Once inside the dermal or sub-mucosal tissues, it replicates rapidly and enters the circulation.

The majority of syphilitic presentations are related to plasma cell infiltration of infected sites that leads to permanent occlusion of small arterioles responsible for feeding the wall of main arteries and nervous system.

Clinical features

Untreated syphilis is an illness with clinically recognisable stages. The first two years are called 'early syphilis' and includes primary, secondary and early latent stages of infection. Infection after the second year is known as the late stage of syphilis:

- *Primary syphilis*: 3–6 weeks after exposure; punched out ulcers with an indurated edge develop (chancre) at the site of inoculation. This period is called primary syphilis. Syphilitic chancres are typically painless, however super-infection or concomitant herpes ulcers may make them tender. Chancres are highly infectious. Although chancres resolve completely after 4–6 weeks, *T. pallidum* remains in the body.
- *Secondary syphilis*: 4–6 weeks after resolution of the chancre, secondary syphilis develops as the result of widespread treponemal replication throughout the body. This stage can present as any of multitude of signs (Table 31.1), including a widespread macular rash and palmar rash (Figures 31.2 and 31.3). These signs also resolve spontaneously after 4–6 weeks.
- *Early latent syphilis*: After the secondary stage, infection becomes mostly asymptomatic.
- *Late syphilis*: presents as late latent (asymptomatic), neurosyphilis, cardiovascular disease and parenchymal diseases of syphilis.

Table 31.1 Summary of clinical stages of syphilis if untreated in chronological order

Stage of syphilis	Clinical manifestation	Duration
Incubation	None	3–6 weeks
A. Primary syphilis	*Typical lesions*: single painless indurated genital ulcer, with local lymphadenopathy *Variants*: multiple painful purulent destructive extragenital (mainly oral) ulcers Severe syphilitic balanitis of Follman Asymptomatic neurosyphilis: abnormal CSF with no signs/symptoms; unknown significance	4–6 weeks
Asymptomatic stage		4–6 weeks
B. Secondary syphilis		4–6 weeks
B.1. Skin manifestations	*Typical presentation*: maculopapular lesions symmetrically distributed over the body, may involve palms, soles and oral mucosae *Atypical presentation*: papulo-squamous or pustular lesions (resembling psoriasis) that can be itchy *Condylomata latum* (Figure 31.3): painless, highly infectious wart-like, grey-white lesions that develop in warm, moist sites (e.g. peri-anal skin). They are mistaken as peri-anal wart by the untrained eye *Patchy alopecia*: including scalp, facial hair and eye brows '*Split pea*' *lesions*: non-tender lesions in the inter-triginous areas: mouth, nasolabial folds, post. Auricular *Mucosa*: patches, husky voice, snail track ulcers	
B.2. Systemic presentations of secondary syphilis	*Lymphadenopathy*: non-tender, rubbery Fever, malaise *Eye*: uveitis, iritis: clinical in 5–10%; sub-clinical in >50% *CNS*: meningitis, cranial nerve palsies, meningovascular disease, A*symptomatic neurosyphilis*: abnormal CSF with no signs/symptoms; unknown significance *Musculoskeletal*: painful osteitis, arthralgia, myalgia *Gastrointestinal*: hepatitis, syphilitic jaundice, splenomegaly *Renal*: nephritis (proteinuria, haematuria)	
C. Asymptomatic (Early latent)		Up to 2 years
D. Asymptomatic (Late latent)	*D.1 Asymptomatic neurosyphilis*: abnormal CSF with no signs/symptoms; unknown significance	After 2 years
	D.2 Meningovascular syphilis: focal arteritis inducing infarction/meningeal inflammation	After 2 years
	D.3 General paresis of insane: Gradual decline in memory and cognitive functions, emotional lability, personality change, psychosis and dementia. Seizures and hemiparesis can be late complications	2–7 years
	D.4 Tabes dorsalis: Plasma arteritis of arteries feeding spinal dorsal column/nerve roots; lightening pains, areflexia, paraesthesia, sensory ataxia, Charcot's joints, mal perforans, optic atrophy, pupillary changes (e.g. Argyll Robertson pupil)	10–20 years
	D.5 Cardiovascular: aortitis (ascending usually); asymptomatic, substernal pain, aortic regurgitation, heart failure, coronary ostial stenosis, angina, aneurysm	15–25 years
	D.6 Gummatous: Granulomatous destructive lesions that can occur in any organ, but most commonly affect bone and skin	10–30 years

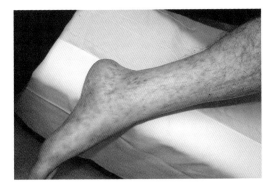

Figure 31.2 The rash of secondary syphilis.

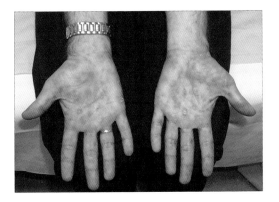

Figure 31.3 The palmar rash of secondary syphilis.

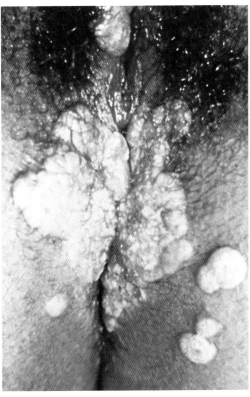

Figure 31.4 Condylomata lata. Courtesy of CDC.

in any of the two stages of congenital syphilis, early or late (Table 31.2). If untreated, the infection may cause deafness, blindness, crippling or death.

Nearly 50% of infants infected with syphilis *in utero*, die before or shortly after birth. Pulmonary haemorrhage is the most common cause of death. Surviving infants infected with syphilis may present

Laboratory diagnosis

Dark ground microscopy, polymerase chain reaction and serology (see Chapter 12).

Table 31.2 Summary presentations of congenital syphilis

Stage	Clinical manifestations	Age of child
Early	Vesiculobullous lesions, snuffles, haemorrhagic rhinitis, osteochondritis, periostitis, pseudoparalysis, mucous patches, perioral fissures, rash, condylomata lata, hepatosplenomegaly, haemolysis, thrombocytopenia, generalised lymphadenopathy, non-immune hydrops, glomerulonephritis, neurological or ocular involvement (Figure 13.4)	0–2 years
Late	Interstitial keratitis, Clutton's joints, Hutchinson's incisors, mulberry molars, high palatal arch, short maxilla, protuberance of mandible, saddlenose deformity, rhagades, deafness, frontal bossing, sterno-clavicular thickening, paroxysmal cold haemoglobinuria, neurological or gummatous involvement	>2 years

Treatment and prevention

Any ano-genital ulcer should be considered as syphilitic, unless proven otherwise. Penicillin remains the treatment of choice of syphilis. Benzathine penicillin G intramuscular, single injection, or procaine penicillin G intramuscular, daily for 10 days, are treatments of choice for early syphilis. Doxycycline or ceftriaxone are alternative antibiotics for treatment of syphilis. Treatment of neurosyphilis or late latent syphilis requires a longer duration of penicillin therapy.

Infants with congenital syphilis must be treated for syphilis, although most of the developmental signs will be permanent.

Sexual transmission of syphilis occurs with direct skin-to-skin contact. In this respect, male latex condoms may prevent transmission of syphilis as long as they cover the infected skin/site. It is likely that consistent use of male latex condoms may prevent some but not all cases of syphilis. Congenital syphilis can be effectively prevented with diagnosis and treatment of infected mothers at early stages of pregnancy.

Genital warts

Epidemiology

- In the UK, more than 90,000 new cases of genital warts were diagnosed between 2008 and 2009.
- Genital warts are a common diagnosis amongst patients attending genitourinary medicine clinics. They are considered as the most common viral STI in the UK. They affect both sexes equally and are mostly diagnosed in patients aged 16–30 years.
- Genital warts are caused by infection with human papilloma virus (HPV), which is transmitted through close skin contact.

Pathogenesis

- HPV is a double stranded DNA virus.
- There are more than 200 types of HPV; more than 40 are mostly transmitted sexually. The role of HPV in causing cervical cancer is well established. Because of their strong association with malignancy, HPV types 16, 18, and 31 are considered high risk.
- The virus infects basal layer cells of the epidermis through skin micro-abrasions. After a latency of 3 weeks to 9 months, the infected cell starts

production of viral particles. Infected cells undergo changes that result in koilocyte formation; a dysplastic squamous formation.
- E6 and E7 genes of high risk HPV types code for proteins that block host cells' tumour suppressing genes p53, p21 and RB. Over time, because of eratic mitosis, some infected cells will develop cancerous mutants that may lead to development of cancer, if untreated.

Clinical features

- Warts can affect any part of ano-genital skin, in addition to the anal canal and cervical mucosa. HPV types 6 and 11 are responsible for more than 80% of genital warts. It is important to note that the site of infection may not relate to sexual practice; peri-anal warts should not be considered as an evidence of history of receptive anal intercourse.
- Genital warts may present in different numbers and sizes. They are mostly asymptomatic but may cause itching. Genital warts are caused by low risk HPV types (6 or 11) in more than 85% of cases. They therefore do not cause long-term complications.
- Warts caused by high risk HPV types (16 or 18) may evolve in pre-cancerous and cancerous skin lesions. Cervical warts should be referred for colposcopical examination and treatment.
- HPV infections of genital skin may also present as bowenoid papules or seborrheic keratoses.
- Because the majority of humans infected with HPV do not present with genital warts, partner notification for genital warts is not recommended.

Diagnosis

Diagnosis of warts is clinical. They are occasionally diagnosed after microscopy examination of biopsy of skin lesions.

Although HPV typing can be performed for wart lesions, this is not commonly used.

Treatment

Patients should be advised that treatment of warts does not eradicate HPV and they may therefore experience recurrences in future. There are different treatment options for genital warts, none of which is considered superior.

Medical therapy of genital warts can be achieved by topical application of podophyllotoxin (twice daily, 3 days a week for a maximum of 5 weeks), or imiquimod (alternative nights for maximum of 4 months). Because topical therapy of warts can be applied by patients, they are the treatment of choice for many.

Podophyllotoxin is an anti-mitotic agent through inhibition of tubulin polymerisation.

Imiquimod is a topical activator of toll-like receptor 7 (TLR-7), leading to local production of interleukin 6, tumour necrosis factor and interferon alpha. However, the anti-tumour activation of imiquimod may not be related to its immune activation feature. Upgrade in opioid growth factor receptor is considered to be imiquimod's anti-neoplastic activity.

Ablation therapy with cryotherapy (liquid nitrogen), laser or surgical excision are other treatment options for warts.

32

Infections of the central nervous system

Erwin Brown
North Bristol NHS Trust, Bristol, UK

- *Meningitis* is an infection of the meninges, the membranous covering of the brain and spinal cord.
- *Encephalitis* is infection of the brain tissue, frequently accompanied by inflammation of the meninges (meningoencephalitis).
- Brain abscess is a focal (or, less frequently, multifocal) pus-forming process that develops within the brain parenchyma.
- Infection may occur:
  - following direct inoculation of the brain during trauma, neurosurgery or invasive diagnostic or therapeutic interventions, e.g. needle biopsy;
  - by spread from infection outside the central nervous system (CNS), either from a contiguous focus, e.g. mastoiditis, or by haematogenous dissemination to the choroid plexus (as in meningitis);
  - directly to the brain parenchyma from a distant focus (as in abscesses secondary to septic embolism); or by invasion via nerves, e.g. herpes simplex virus.
- Infections of the CNS may result in long-term sequelae (e.g. cranial nerve damage, epilepsy, deafness), as inflammatory changes and/or raised intracranial pressure can cause irreversible damage to neuronal tissue.

Bacterial meningitis

The principal causes of bacterial meningitis are shown in Table 32.1.

Major causes of bacterial meningitis

Neisseria meningitidis

Epidemiology (see Chapter 7)

- Upper respiratory tract colonisation occurs in approximately 10% of healthy individuals; this may increase during epidemics.
- Spread is by the respiratory route (droplets).
- Invasion of the meninges follows bacteraemia/or bloodstream infection.
- There is a small increase in risk of infection among close contacts of patients with meningococcal meningitis.
- Infections occur principally in children and young adults, occasionally elderly people are affected.

Medical Microbiology and Infection Lecture Notes, Fifth Edition. Edited by Tom Elliott, Anna Casey, Peter Lambert and Jonathan Sandoe.

Table 32.1 Causative microorganisms of acute bacterial meningitis according to age group

Age	Causative microorganism
<1 month	Group B β-haemolytic streptococcus, *E. coli*, *Citrobacter* spp., *Klebsiella* spp., *Enterobacter* spp., *P. aeruginosa*, *L. monocytogenes*, *S. aureus*, *S. epidermidis*
1–23 months	Group B β-haemolytic streptococcus, *E. coli*, *H. influenzae*, *S. pneumoniae*, *N. meningitidis*
2–50 years	*S. pneumoniae*, *N. meningitidis*
≥50 years	*S. pneumoniae*, *N. meningitidis*, *L. monocytogenes*, aerobic Gram-negative bacilli (coliforms)

- In the USA and Europe, cases of meningococcal meningitis are sporadic and caused mainly by serotype B; epidemics of *N. meningitidis* serotypes A and C occur in Africa and South America.

Clinical features

- Usually rapid onset, headache, fever and meningism (neck stiffness, irritability, photophobia). Typical petechial rash, which may become haemorrhagic – this clinical feature is not pathognomonic of meningococcal disease, a similar rash occurs in asplenic patients with overwhelming *Streptococcus pneumoniae* or *Haemophilus influenzae* type b infections. Other clinical features include signs of cerebral dysfunction (confusion, delirium or a falling level of consciousness –ranging from lethargy to coma), focal neurological deficits, including cranial nerve palsies (particularly III, VI, VII and VIII), hemiparesis and papilloedema.
- In fulminant cases, endotoxin release results in shock, with disseminated intravascular coagulopathy and multi-organ failure. In a minority of cases, haemorrhagic necrosis of the adrenal glands and intracranial bleeding, which is invariably fatal (Waterhouse–Friderichsen syndrome) may occur.
- Presentation in the elderly may be insidious with lethargy or obtundation, confusion, no fever and variable signs of meningeal inflammation.

Treatment and prevention

- Intravenous penicillin; cefotaxime or ceftriaxone (chloramphenicol may be used in penicillin-allergic patients).

- In the developed world epidemics are rare; however, related cases in families or institutions can occur and prophylaxis with rifampicin or ciprofloxacin is recommended for close contacts.
- Healthcare workers in contact with cases are not at increased risk, but prophylaxis is recommended for those who have administered mouth-to-mouth resuscitation.
- A vaccine is available for protection against serotypes A and C, and is recommended for prophylaxis of close contacts of meningococcal cases caused by these serotypes.

Haemophilus influenzae type b

Epidemiology (see Chapter 9)

- Occurs principally in children aged <5 years.
- Spread is by the respiratory route and symptomless upper respiratory colonisation is common.
- Cases are often sporadic, but small outbreaks, particularly in nurseries, may occur.
- Number of cases has decreased dramatically since introduction of *H. influenzae* type b vaccine.

Clinical features

Similar to meningococcal meningitis, except that onset is often less acute (1–2 days) and, although a petechial rash can occur rarely, it is much less common.

Treatment and prevention

Antibiotic therapy with cefotaxime, ceftriaxone or amoxicillin (if the strain is susceptible) or chloramphenicol. Rifampicin is used for prophylaxis of close contacts. A vaccine is available and should be considered for at-risk household contacts.

Streptococcus pneumoniae

Epidemiology

- Pneumococci are common commensals of the upper respiratory tract.
- Infection is most common in young (<2 years of age) and elderly individuals.
- Asplenic patients (including those with sickle cell disease) are at particular risk.
- Meningitis may be secondary to pneumococcal pneumonia and bloodstream infection or skull fracture (direct spread).
- Patients with pneumococcal meningitis.

Clinical features

Similar to other causes, but *S. pneumoniae* infection may be acute or insidious in presentation. Complications (e.g. deafness) are more common than with other pathogens.

Treatment and prevention

- Strains with a reduced susceptibility to penicillin have emerged. Patients should therefore receive either cefotaxime or ceftriaxone empirically, but they can be converted to benzylpenicillin, if the strain is subsequently found to be susceptible.
- Contacts of cases of pneumococcal meningitis are not at increased risk and prophylaxis with antibiotics is not recommended.
- A vaccine against many of the pneumococcal serotypes is available and is recommended for splenectomised and other immunocompromised

patients and those with base of skull fractures/cerebrospinal fluid (CSF) leaks.

Laboratory diagnosis of bacterial meningitis

Meningitis is a medical emergency and laboratory investigations are urgent:

- Blood cultures should ideally be obtained before administration of empirical antibiotic therapy.
- Lumbar puncture (LP) is usually performed after raised intracranial pressure has been excluded by neuroimaging. Typical features of CSF microscopy are a raised polymorph count, although a predominance of lymphocytes can occur, especially in Gram-negative bacillary meningitis in neonates and in patients with meningitis caused by *Listeria monocytogenes*. A low glucose (compared with blood glucose) and an increased protein concentration occurs (Table 32.2). Gram staining may reveal the causative microorganism; culture is important for confirmation.
- Note: a normal CSF white blood cell count may be seen in patients who present within 12 hours of the onset of the disease, in some cases of neonatal meningitis and in neutropenic patients.
- Antigen detection tests are available.
- PCR can detect DNA of *Neisseria meningitidis* and *Streptococcus pneumoniae*.

Table 32.2 Typical CSF changes in meningitis

		Meningitis		
	Normal	**Bacterial**	**Tuberculous**	**Viral**
Leukocytes (cells/μL)	<5	100–10,000	<500	50–500
Polymorphs (%)		>80	20[a]	5[a]
Lymphocytes (%)		10	80	95
Protein (g/L)	0.2–0.45	↑↑ (>50)	↑↑↑ (>50)	↑
Glucose (mmol/L)	4.5–8.5[b]	↓↓[c]	↓↓[c]	Normal

[a]Polymorphs may predominate in the early stages
[b]About 80% of blood glucose level
[c]<40% of blood glucose level

- Blood cultures are positive in about 40% of cases.
- Serology may give a retrospective diagnosis of meningococcal meningitis, but is rarely used in clinical practice.

Treatment of bacterial meningitis

The fundamental principle in the treatment of bacterial meningitis is early, parenteral antibiotics in high dosages. Intramuscular penicillin administered early by primary care physicians has been shown to reduce the incidences of morbidity and mortality associated with meningococcal meningitis. Antibiotic therapy for common causes of bacterial meningitis in children and adults is shown in Table 32.3. There is some evidence that steroids, when initiated immediately before or concurrent with antimicrobial therapy, are beneficial.

Neonatal meningitis

Aetiology

Predominantly caused by *Escherichia coli* and occasionally other coliforms, *Pseudomonas aeruginosa*, group B β-haemolytic streptococci, *Listeria monocytogenes*, *Staphylococcus epidermidis* and *Staphylococcus aureus*. Bacteria which colonise the upper respiratory tracts of neonates – *S. pneumoniae*, *H. influenzae* and *N. meningitidis* may also cause this infection.

Epidemiology

Acquisition is normally from the maternal genital or alimentary tract, at or around the time of delivery:

- *E. coli* is a common gut commensal and frequently contaminates the perineal area.
- Group B streptococci are part of the vaginal and perineal flora of about 30% of mothers.
- *L. monocytogenes* is a gut commensal in a small proportion of healthy mothers.
- Neonates with prolonged hospital stay may acquire these microorganisms from nosocomial sources. Prematurity, low birth weight and prolonged ruptured membranes are important risk factors for neonatal meningitis.

Clinical features

Neonates do not usually exhibit meningism or other signs referable to the CNS, the clinical features tend to be those of sepsis. Diagnostic clues include temperature instability (hypothermia or hyperthermia), listlessness, lethargy, irritability, failure to feed, weak suck, jaundice, vomiting, diarrhoea and respiratory distress. A bulging fontanelle is seen in 33% (late in the course of the illness) and seizures in 40% of cases.

Treatment

Early empirical therapy is imperative. Commonly-used regimens include a combination of penicillin and an aminoglycoside (e.g. gentamicin) or cefotaxime and amoxicillin.

Table 32.3 Antimicrobial therapy for common causes of bacterial meningitis

Microorganism	Treatment
Aetiology unknown[a]	Benzylpenicillin; or cefotaxime/ceftriaxone or chloramphenicol
N. meningitidis	Benzylpenicillin (chloramphenicol or cefotaxime/ceftriaxone if penicillin allergic)
H. influenzae type b	Cefotaxime/ceftriaxone or chloramphenicol
S. pneumoniae	Benzylpenicillin (cefotaxime/ceftriaxone or chloramphenicol if penicillin allergic or if isolate is resistant to penicillin)

Note: that rifampicin is given for 48 h or ciprofloxacin (single dose) to patients with meningitis caused by *N. meningitidis* or *H. influenzae* to eliminate nasopharyngeal carriage.
[a]Empirical treatment will be directed by the most likely causative microorganism and local antimicrobial sensitivity pattern.

Post-operative meningitis

The incidence of bacterial meningitis complicating neurosurgical procedures is low. *E. coli*, *Klebsiella pneumoniae*, *P. aeruginosa*, *Acinetobacter* spp. and *S. aureus* are the most common aetiological agents. In patients with defects of the dura and CSF leaks (rhinorrhoea or otorrhoea), who have not received prophylactic antibiotics, *S. pneumoniae* is the predominant pathogen. Post-operative meningitis usually presents within the first 7–10 days following surgery and the clinical features are often indistinguishable from those of community-acquired meningitis. In some cases the onset is insidious and it may be difficult to distinguish meningitis from any underlying neurological disease or post-operative condition. Examination of the CSF is the definitive diagnostic procedure. A CT scan is frequently performed to determine that a lumbar puncture is safe. When a lumbar puncture is considered unsafe, a ventricular puncture or empirical treatment may be considered. The CSF protein concentration and leukocyte count are usually elevated. The glucose concentration is normally depressed in the presence of infection, but a Gram's stain may be negative in up to 70% of patients with culture-positive infections. However, the CSF parameters (both cellular and biochemical) may be altered in the post-operative period due to the surgery, especially in the presence of subarachnoid haemorrhage.

Isolation of a pathogen from the CSF of post-operative neurosurgical patients remains the definitive diagnostic test. All patients who develop post-operative meningitis should therefore receive empirical therapy with a broad-spectrum antibiotic. If the CSF is subsequently shown to be sterile (usually after 2–3 days), antibiotic treatment can be discontinued. Third-generation cephalosporins (cefotaxime or ceftriaxone) are often used for empirical therapy; meropenem or ceftazidime may be required for more resistant pathogens.

Tuberculous meningitis

- *Mycobacterium tuberculosis* is a rare cause of bacterial meningitis in developed countries, but remains an important complication of tuberculosis (TB) in many areas of the world.
- It is a complication of either primary TB (normally pulmonary) or post-primary reactivation.
- The disease tends to run an indolent course:
  - *Stage I*: Patients typically present with non-specific prodromal signs and symptoms of 2–8-weeks' duration, e.g. malaise, fatigue, anorexia, headache, nausea and vomiting.
  - *Stage II*: Patients develop signs and symptoms of meningeal irritation, with fever and minor focal neurological deficits (e.g. cranial nerve palsies).
  - *Stage III*: In the final stage, patients are severely ill and present with gross neurological deficits (pareses), stupor or coma, behavioural changes or involuntary movements. Seizures, which may be focal, temporal or generalised, can occur at any stage, more frequently in children than in adults.
- Both the peripheral white blood cell count and the ESR may be normal or only minimally elevated. Hyponatraemia may occur.
- In a patient with lymphocytic meningitis, radiological evidence of active pulmonary tuberculosis is of diagnostic importance. However, if absent, the diagnosis depends almost entirely on examination of CSF. Lumbar puncture is safe in patients with tuberculous meningitis and can be carried out, even in the presence of papilloedema. The CSF is typically clear or slightly opalescent. A pleiocytosis is an almost invariable finding, with cell counts usually less than $500/mm^3$ and uncommonly more than $1,000/mm^3$. Counts can occasionally be normal in severely ill patients, those who are immunocompromised and those who are receiving steroids. Lymphocytes characteristically predominate, although the majority of cells in the early stage of infection may be polymorphonuclear leukocytes. The glucose concentration is typically low and the protein concentration is typically moderately elevated (Table 32.2). The identification of acid-fast bacilli in CSF is diagnostic. Immunodiagnostic techniques have proved promising in terms of facilitating more rapid diagnosis and higher diagnostic yields. Of these tests, conventional PCR and a technique based on the amplification of ribosomal RNA derived from *M. tuberculosis*, followed by recognition using a gene probe, are the latest diagnostic tools.
- Treatment follows the principles of anti-tuberculous triple therapy (rifampicin, isoniazid and pyrazinamide).
- If untreated, it is virtually always fatal. Patients presenting with more advanced disease (stage III) at the onset of treatment have a much worse

prognosis than do those in whom treatment is initiated in the early stage (stage I). Early diagnosis and initiation of therapy are therefore important prognostic factors. Long-term complications are frequent because of the dense fibrous exudate; steroids appear to reduce the risk of complications.

Viral meningitis

Viral meningitis, the most common form of meningitis, is often mild and full recovery is usual.

Aetiology

Important causes are enteroviruses (echoviruses, Coxsackieviruses, polioviruses, enterovirus 71, see Chapter 16), mumps in countries without routine childhood immunisation coverage (MMR), herpes simplex virus, particularly in association with primary genital herpes (4–8% of cases) and arboviruses in countries where they are endemic (see Chapter 42).

Clinical features

Influenza-like illness, followed by meningism (neck stiffness, headache and photophobia).

Investigations

Lumbar puncture: CSF microscopy, which shows a lymphocytosis (Table 32.2); viral nucleic acid detection by molecular techniques (e.g. PCR). Viral culture of CSF, stool and throat swabs is undertaken less frequently.

Treatment

There is no specific antiviral therapy, except aciclovir for herpes simplex virus.

Fungal meningitis

Fungal meningitis occurs principally in immunocompromised patients, but can occur rarely in immunocompetent patients. Pathogens include *Cryptococcus neoformans*, *Aspergillus* spp. and *Candida* spp.

Protozoal meningitis

Very rarely, the free-living amoeba, *Naegleria fowleri*, causes meningitis. Patients normally have a history of swimming in warm, brackish water 1–2 weeks before presentation. Direct invasion of the meninges via the cribriform plate results in severe meningitis with a high incidence of mortality. Amoebae may be seen in unstained CSF preparations. Treatment is with amphotericin B.

Encephalitis

Encephalitis is mainly caused by viruses, but other microorganisms are occasionally responsible (Table 32.4). Clinical signs include fever and vomiting, followed by decreased level of consciousness, focal neurological signs and eventually coma. Some important causes are outlined below; other causes are described in chapters dealing with individual pathogens.

Herpes simplex virus (HSV)

Epidemiology

- Encephalitis is an uncommon complication of HSV infection. The incidence is increased in immunocompromised patients, neonates and elderly individuals.
- HSV encephalitis may complicate primary (infancy) infection or follow viral reactivation (adults). Invasion of the temporal lobe is a prominent feature.

Investigations

CSF may contain a few lymphocytes, but culture for HSV is often negative. PCR is probably the most useful diagnostic test for HSV encephalitis. Brain biopsy is the definitive diagnostic test, but is difficult to justify.

Electroencephalographic (EEG) studies and computed tomography (CT) may be helpful.

Treatment and prevention

Treatment is with intravenous aciclovir. Neonatal HSV encephalitis is normally acquired from the maternal genital tract during labour and pregnant women with active genital lesions at term should undergo caesarean section. Immunocompromised patients, particularly transplant recipients, often receive aciclovir prophylaxis to prevent invasive HSV disease.

Table 32.4 Principal causes of encephalitis and meningoencephalitis

Cause	Comments
Viruses:	
Herpes simplex virus	Most common cause of viral encephalitis
Mumps virus	Rare complication of mumps parotitis
Varicella-zoster virus	Complication of chickenpox and zoster
Cytomegalovirus	Immunosuppressed patients (e.g. AIDS, transplant recipients)
Human herpesvirus 6	Rare complication of primary infection in young children and after primary infection or reactivation in immunocompromised patients
Polio- and other enteroviruses	Important cause in developing world
Measles virus	Rarely in acute measles; disease develops 6–8 years later, causing subacute sclerosing panencephalitis (SSPE)
Rabies virus	Zoonosis
Arboviruses	Important cause of meningitis and encephalitis in endemic areas
Retroviruses HTLV-I and HIV	Endemic in some areas of the world; must be distinguished from other causes in AIDS patients
Bacteria:	
Treponema pallidum	Tertiary syphilis
Mycoplasma pneumoniae	Rare complication of mycoplasma pneumonia
Borrelia burgdorferi	Part of multisystem infection (Lyme disease)
Protozoa and fungi:	
Toxoplasma gondii	Immunocompromised individuals
Cryptococcus neoformans	Meningoencephalitis, mainly immunocompromised individuals
Plasmodium falciparum	Cerebral malaria
Trypanosomes	
Toxocara	Larvae in brain; granulomata form

Brain abscesses

It is the second most common infection of the CNS after bacterial meningitis and is the most common space-occupying infection of the CNS. It is a relatively rare disease and occurs more frequently in immunocompromised patients, particularly those with Acquired Immunodeficiency Syndrome (AIDS, see Chapter 41).

Aetiology

Nearly half of all brain abscesses are caused by more than one microorganism. The range of pathogens reflects the broad spectrum of primary sources of infection. Streptococci are the most commonly recovered microorganisms, Aerobic bacteria have been isolated from most lesions and anaerobes from 25–50%. Abscesses that are secondary to penetrating trauma are caused by *S. aureus*, coliforms or *P. aeruginosa*. *Proteus* spp. and *P. aeruginosa* are also common pathogens in patients with otogenic brain abscesses. A broad range of other bacterial species are occasionally isolated, particularly in immunocompromised patients, and include mycobacteria, *L. monocytogenes*, *Actinomyces* spp. and *Nocardia* spp. Often they are culture-negative, either because the patient has already received antibiotics or use of suboptimal laboratory techniques.

Pathogenesis

Brain abscesses develop as consequences of implantation in the brain of bacteria or bacterial emboli from either local or distant septic foci. In the majority of cases, microorganisms gain access by direct spread from contiguous infected foci, e.g. sinusitis, acute or chronic otitis media (with or without mastoiditis), dental infections and, rarely, meningitis. Microorganisms may also gain access to the brain following a penetrating wound of the head, which may be traumatic or iatrogenic, e.g. following neurosurgery. Most abscesses (75–90%) are solitary, whereas multiple lesions, which account for 5–25% of abscesses, are almost always metastatic.

Clinical features

The clinical manifestations of brain abscesses range from fulminating to indolent and can vary in duration from hours to weeks. Headache is the most common symptom, but nausea and vomiting, fever, dizziness, impaired consciousness, papilloedema, focal neurological signs, coma, generalised seizures, behavioural disturbances or confusion may occur. Meningism may be secondary to concomitant meningitis or rupture of the abscess into a ventricle or the subarachnoid space. Other clinical features may reflect the extracranial underlying disease, e.g. ear or nasal discharge.

Investigations

The principal diagnostic procedures are radiological and culture of an aspirate of the abscess. The peripheral white blood cell (WBC) count is raised in 30–60% of patients and the serum CRP concentration will be markedly elevated in many cases; however, normal values of these parameters should not rule out the diagnosis. Blood cultures are positive in 10–20% of patients and are essential investigations if a systemic focus is suspected; they may be particularly helpful in patients with multiple (metastatic) abscesses.

Treatment

Excision or drainage of the lesion(s) and empirical antibiotic therapy, which should be reviewed following culture and antibiotic susceptibility test results.

Encephalopathy associated with scrapie-like agents

- Degenerative diseases caused by abnormal prion proteins. Prions are proteins found in normal cells but, in genetically predisposed individuals, they transform into a pathogenic abnormal form. Prions resist heat and chemicals, including formaldehyde.
- The infectious agent infects a range of mammals, including humans, scrapie in sheep and bovine spongiform encephalopathy (BSE) in cattle, and replicates slowly with a long incubation period.
- Diagnosis is based on histological changes in the brain. No treatment or vaccine is available.

Creutzfeldt–Jakob disease (CJD)

This is a rare encephalopathy of humans with an uncertain mode of transmission. Transmission has been associated with corneal grafts, neurosurgery and human growth hormone preparations. Variant CJD (vCJD), first reported in the UK, is thought to have resulted from transmission of infection from BSE in cattle to humans via contaminated beef. Prions are not destroyed by normal sterilisation cycles in autoclaves; killing requires 134 °C for 18 min or exposure to sodium hydroxide.

Kuru

Transmission is from human to human by cannibalism and recorded mainly in Papua New Guinea.

Tetanus

- Tetanus toxin is produced by *Clostridium tetani* in infected wounds. The toxin is carried to the peripheral nerve axons and CNS where it blocks inhibition of spinal synapses, resulting in overactivity of motor neurons with exaggerated reflexes, muscle spasms, lock-jaw (trismus), neck stiffness and opisthotonos (spasm of muscle of back, causing arching of trunk).
- Treatment is with anti-tetanus immunoglobulin and penicillin, and excision of the wound. Respiratory support is needed and the incidence of mortality is high.
- Prevention is by immunisation with toxoid vaccine.

Chronic meningitis

- Diagnosed when the neurological symptoms and signs persist or progress for more than 4 weeks.
- Causes include amoebae, *Brucella* spp., *Cryptococcus neoformans*, Lyme disease, syphilis and

TB; partially-treated bacterial meningitis may also present as chronic infection.

- Discrete (focal) lesions in the brain can occur with certain infections, including toxoplasmosis and aspergillosis.

- Non-infectious diseases can also give a similar clinical appearance, including: neoplastic meningitis, sarcoidosis, connective tissue diseases and chronic lymphocytic meningitis.

Bacteraemia and bloodstream infection

Tom Elliott
University Hospitals Birmingham NHS Foundation Trust, Birmingham, UK

Definitions

Bacteraemia

The presence of bacteria in the bloodstream; there is no implication of clinical significance. A patient with a bacteraemia may or may not have symptoms or signs of infection. Note: activities of daily life (such as tooth-brushing) can cause a bacteraemia, which is not usually associated with any symptoms.

Bloodstream infection

The presence of bacteria in the bloodstream associated with symptoms or signs of infection. These may be systemic (e.g. tachycardia, fever, sweats, confusion, hypotension) or localised (e.g. signs of pneumonia or osteomyelitis).

Note: consensus definitions of the more severe manifestations of infection have been developed to facilitate communication and research in this area.

Systemic inflammatory response syndrome (SIRS)

The presence of two or more of:

- temperature $>38\,°$ C or $<36\,°$C;
- pulse rate >90 beats per minute;
- respiratory rate >20 breaths per minute;
- white cell count $>12 \times 10^9$/L peripheral blood.

Many conditions can cause a systemic inflammatory response, e.g. infection, myocardial infarction, pancreatitis.

Sepsis

SIRS caused by infection.

Severe sepsis

Sepsis with evidence of end-organ hypoperfusion (e.g. acute kidney injury).

Septic shock

Sepsis with hypotension not responding to fluid resuscitation.

Medical Microbiology and Infection Lecture Notes, Fifth Edition. Edited by Tom Elliott, Anna Casey,
Peter Lambert and Jonathan Sandoe.

Aetiology

The common causes of bloodstream infection and the likely microorganisms are shown in Tables 33.1–33.4. Isolation and identification of bacteria from the blood is an important aid to the diagnosis of infection and enables directed antimicrobial therapy (see Chapter 20).

Table 33.1 Causes of bloodstream infection: Gram-positive cocci

Microorganism	Common focus of infection	Notes
Staphylococcus aureus	Deep abscesses, osteomyelitis, septic arthritis, intravascular catheter infection, endocarditis	
Coagulase-negative staphylococci (e.g. Staphylococcus epidermidis)	Intravascular catheter infection; other prosthetic device infections	Frequent contaminant of blood cultures, therefore assessment important in confirming diagnosis
	Endocarditis	Often post-cardiac valve replacement
β-haemolytic streptococci group A	Cellulitis, necrotising fasciitis (NF), puerperal sepsis, pharyngitis	NF can have a severe acute presentation; high mortality
β-haemolytic streptococci group B	Sepsis; meningitis	Important pathogen in neonatal period
β-haemolytic streptococci groups C/G	Cellulitis	
Streptococcus anginosus group	Deep abscesses	Particularly liver, intra-abdominal, lung and brain
Streptococcus pneumoniae	Pneumonia, otitis media, meningitis	More frequent in splenectomised patients
'Viridans streptococci'	Endocarditis	Often subacute presentation

Table 33.2 Causes of bloodstream infection: Gram-positive bacilli

Microorganism	Common focus of infection	Notes
Diphtheroids	Prosthetic device infection	Less common than Staphylococcus epidermidis
Listeria monocytogenes	Primary focus often unknown, meningitis	Important in neonates and immunocompromised patients
Clostridium perfringens	Gas-gangrene, anaerobic cellulitis	Uncommon, sometimes associated with diabetes mellitus

Table 33.3 Causes of bloodstream infection: Gram-negative cocci

Microorganism	Common focus of infection	Notes
Neisseria meningitidis	Sepsis (without focus), meningitis	Often acute and severe with purpuric rash; endotoxic shock a common feature
Neisseria gonorrhoeae	Genital infection	Sepsis is rare (<3% of cases of gonorrhoea) associated with arthritis and skin rash

Table 33.4 Causes of bloodstream infection: Gram-negative bacilli

Microorganism	Common focus of infection	Notes
Escherichia coli and other coliforms	Urinary tract infection; intra-abdominal sepsis (e.g. appendicitis, cholangitis); nosocomial pneumonia	
Pseudomonas aeruginosa	Nosocomial infections	Pneumonia in ventilated patients
Haemophilus influenzae type b	Meningitis, epiglottitis	Formerly in children < 5 years; now uncommon with Hib immunisation
Salmonella serotypes Typhi and Paratyphi	Primary focus often unknown	Rare in UK, cases normally imported
Other *Salmonella* spp.	Enteritis	Complication of salmonella enteritis; associated with HIV infection
Brucella spp.	Primary focus often unknown, vertebral osteomyelitis	Chronic illness often presenting as a pyrexia of unknown origin

Pathogenesis and epidemiology

A bacteraemia may be transient, intermittent or constant.

Transient bacteraemias are short-lived (<1 hour) and can occur as a result of normal activities of daily living (such as tooth brushing); may be caused by medical investigations (e.g. colonoscopy) or as a result of infection (e.g. flushing a colonised vascular catheter). Some infections, e.g. abscesses or pneumonia result in intermittent bacteraemia, while infections, such as endocarditis, result in a constant bacteramia.

Bloodstream infection is almost invariably a complication of localised infection (e.g. pneumonia). Invasion of bacteria from a localised focus of infection into the bloodstream is often a marker of more severe infection. The presence of microorganisms or their components in blood can stimulate a systemic inflammatory response.

Exposure to lipopolysaccharide (or endotoxin, see Chapter 1), a component of the cell walls of Gram-negative bacteria, can result in septic shock (also known as endotoxic shock). The presence of endotoxin leads to activation of various inflammatory cascades. Release of cytokines results in vasodilatation and increased vascular permeability, causing a fall in blood pressure (septic shock). Activation of the clotting cascade may result in disseminated intravascular coagulopathy (DIC), with bleeding and thrombosis occurring simultaneously.

Endotoxaemia can occur in the absence of culturable bacteria in the bloodstream, e.g. from Gram-negative bacteria causing infection elsewhere. The lipoteichoic acid in the cell walls of Gram-positive microorganisms, e.g. pneumococci, can also activate an inflammatory cascade to produce septic shock. Improved understanding of the immunological pathways leading to endotoxic shock have led to the design of monoclonal antibodies and drugs that may block the development of endotoxic shock.

The relative incidence of microorganisms causing bloodstream infection varies in different countries and with patients' age and circumstances, e.g.:

- *Coagulase-negative staphylococci (CoNS).* most frequent blood culture isolate in hospitalised patients in developed countries; related to frequent use of intravascular catheters;
- *Staphylococcus aureus.* usually in the top five causes of bloodstream infection in hospitalised patients;
- *E. coli.* frequent cause of bloodstream infection in elderly patients with urinary tract infection;
- *Salmonella* spp. uncommon in developed countries, but an important cause of bloodstream infection in developing countries.

Clinical diagnosis

The symptoms of bloodstream infection include fevers, chills, sweats (including night sweats), vomiting, confusion and the clinical manifestations of sepsis, severe sepsis and septic shock.

- Fungi, e.g. *Candida* spp., can also cause sepsis and be grown from blood cultures.

Laboratory diagnosis

- Blood for culture should be obtained aseptically. Bacteria that are part of the normal skin flora (e.g. CoNS) may contaminate blood cultures therefore careful sampling technique is mandatory to reduce contamination. Contaminating bacteria must be distinguished from true infection by clinical assessment.
- The length of time before growth is detectable depends on the type of microorganism, the volume of blood cultured, the number of bacteria present and whether antibiotics were in the original sample; most blood cultures become positive within 48 hours. Sampling the correct volume of blood is critical, to avoid both false negative and false positive results.
- A variety of automated blood culture instruments are now available that detect bacterial growth by various techniques, e.g. the detection of carbon dioxide by radiometric or optical methods.
- When bacterial growth is detected, Gram staining of the blood culture gives a presumptive indication of the likely microorganism. Further identification and antibiotic susceptibility testing are carried out after the microorganism has been grown.

Management

Management of bloodstream infection involves supportive therapy (e.g. intravenous fluids to prevent shock) and antimicrobial agents, which must be commenced without delay. The choice of antimicrobial treatment depends on a number of factors:

- the clinical symptoms and signs suggesting the likely focus and cause of infection;
- the patient's underlying condition;
- the blood culture results, including the Gram stain (after initial incubation);
- the severity of the patient's condition;
- patient allergies;
- severely ill patients require high-dose broad-spectrum antibiotics to cover a range of likely pathogens, including those that may be antibiotic resistant.

Antibiotic therapy can be adjusted according to the results of culture, bacterial identification and antibiotic susceptibility. The therapy may also need altering if a patient is in renal or liver failure and depends on how the antimicrobial is metabolised or excreted.

Device-related infections

Tom Elliott
University Hospitals Birmingham NHS Foundation Trust, Birmingham, UK

Clinical practice increasingly involves the use of temporary or permanent medical devices inserted into patients (Figure 34.1). Medical devices are foreign bodies and are associated with specific infectious complications. Microorganisms may gain access to the device during implantation, or after implantation e.g. via haematogenous spread from a distant focus. Medical devices widely used in clinical practice are shown in Table 34.1.

Pathogenesis of device-related infection

Device-related infections (DRI) result from a combination of bacterial, host and device factors:

- *Bacterial factors*: access to the device by a microorganism is the first stage in development of DRI. After access, the microorganism needs to adhere to the device. Some bacteria are able to produce molecules, e.g. glycoproteins and/or have specific bacterial structures, e.g. pili, fimbriae, which may assist adhesion. Other bacteria, e.g. *Staphylococcus epidermidis*, secrete a polysaccharide 'slime' (glycocalyx) that facilitates adhesion and cell aggregation. Bacteria growing on devices commonly form a biofilm, which consists of microorganisms, the polysaccharide they produce and host derived components, such as fibronectin. The microorganisms associated with DRI are shown in Table 34.2.
- *Host factors*: may increase risk of DRI; include immunosuppression, diabetes, site of prosthesis.
- *Device factors*: these include: type of device material, e.g. synthetic, biomaterial, those made from antimicrobial materials, e.g. silver containing intravascular catheters; surface of device, e.g. textured or smooth.

Examples of device-related infections

Intravascular catheter-related infection, including central venous catheters (CVC) and peripheral catheters

Pathogenesis

Microorganisms can gain access to intravascular catheters predominantly via the external or internal surfaces of the device.

Clinical features

Localised (at site of catheter insertion - see figures 34.2 and 34.3) and/or systemic infection.

Medical Microbiology and Infection Lecture Notes, Fifth Edition. Edited by Tom Elliott, Anna Casey, Peter Lambert and Jonathan Sandoe.

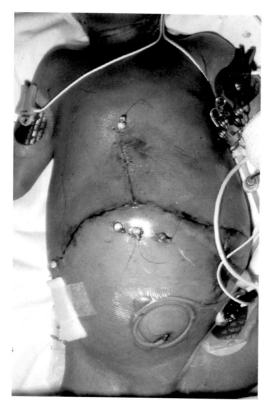

Figure 34.1 Liver transplant patient with numerous intravascular and drainage catheters.

Localised infection

Pain, oedema, erythema and purulent discharge at the catheter exit site (Figures 34.2–34.3).

Systemic infection

Fever, often low grade (≤38.5 °C), rigors on flushing catheter, no other obvious focus of infection.

The clinical diagnosis of intravascular catheter-related infection may be difficult to establish as a result of the non-specific clinical presentation.

Laboratory diagnosis

- *Localised infection*: culture of exit site swab (high negative predictive value);
- *Systemic infection*: semi-quantitative/quantitative culture of explanted CVC tip. If systemic CVC infection is suspected, paired blood cultures (via separate peripheral venepuncture and CVC) should be taken for analysis.

Treatment

Depends on causative microorganism; if *Staphylococcus aureus, Candida albicans or* coliforms, then appropriate antimicrobial therapy and catheter removal; if coagulase-negative staphylococci (CoNS), may attempt antibiotic treatment without catheter removal.

Prevention

Good aseptic technique pre- and post-insertion aids in reducing intravenous catheter infection.

Table 34.1 Examples of medical devices frequently used in medicine

Medical device	Example of clinical use
Central venous catheters	Administration of drugs, fluids, chemotherapy; venous blood sampling; total parenteral nutrition
Peripheral venous catheters	Drug and fluid administration
Continuous ambulatory peritoneal dialysis (CAPD) catheters	Renal dialysis
Urinary catheters	Maintenance of urine flow
Prosthetic joints	Replacement joints, e.g. hip, knee
Prosthetic heart valves	Replacement of failing heart valves
CSF shunts	Intracranial pressure control
Epidural catheters	Administration of fluids, e.g. anaesthetic, steroids
Endotracheal tubes	Provision of artificial ventilation

Table 34.2 Examples of microorganisms frequently associated with device-related infections

Device	Pathogens
Catheters (CVC, peripheral, CAPD)	Coagulase negative staphylococci (CoNS), *Staphylococcus aureus*
Urinary catheter	Coliforms eg *Escherichia coli*, *Candida albicans*
Prosthetic heart valves	CoNS, *Staphylococcus aureus*, α-haemolytic streptococci
Prosthetic joints	CoNS, *Staphylococcus aureus*
CSF shunts	CoNS
Epidural catheters	CoNS, *Staphylococcus aureus*
Endotracheal tubes	Coliforms including *Escherichia coli* and *Klebsiella pneumoniae*. Also *Pseudomonas aeruginosa* and *Staphylococcus aureus*

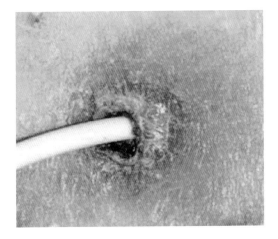

Figure 34.2 Localised exit site infection showing erythema and exudate.

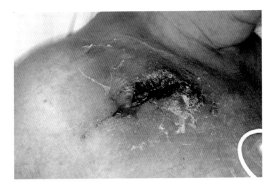

Figure 34.3 Infection of a tunnelled central venous catheter.

Continuous ambulatory peritoneal dialysis (CAPD) catheter infection

Pathogenesis

Microorganisms gain access to CAPD catheters, as with intravascular catheters (see above).

Clinical features

Localised infection at catheter insertion site may include pain, oedema, erythema, sometimes associated with purulent discharge. If associated with peritonitis, may present with abdominal pain, cloudy dialysate, pyrexia, nausea, vomiting and tachycardia. Usually have a raised dialysate white cell count (WCC $> 100/\text{mm}^3$)

Laboratory diagnosis

Localised infection; exit site swab culture. Systemic infection; culture peritoneal dialysis fluid (PDF); WCC in PDF usually elevated.

Treatment

Depends on causative microorganism and its antibiotic sensitivity. Examples include vancomycin (intraperitoneal) if CoNS; piperacillin–tazobactam for sensitive coliforms.

Prevention

Strict aseptic technique during CAPD catheter insertion and subsequent care.

Catheter-related urinary tract infection

Pathogenesis

Predominantly caused by coliforms present in the periurethral area gaining access to the urinary bladder, usually via the catheter's internal surface.

Clinical features

Urinary tract infection (see Chapter 30).

Laboratory diagnosis

See Chapter 30.

Treatment

Removal/replacement of catheter and appropriate antimicrobial treatment (see Chapter 30).

Prosthetic joint infection

Pathogenesis

See Chapter 36.

Clinical features

Joint or bone pain, tenderness, inflammation with or without oedema, fever. Complications may include loosening of the prosthetic joint, sinus formation, bloodstream infection, or chronic infection unless the prosthesis is removed.

Clinical diagnosis

To differentiate prosthetic joint infection from mechanical loosening is difficult.

Laboratory diagnosis

Non-specific laboratory tests: elevated peripheral blood WCC, raised C-reactive protein (CRP) and erythrocyte sedimentation rate (ESR). Microscopy and Gram stain of joint material (aspirates) or, if undergoing operative procedures, tissue, e.g. acetabular, capsular, femoral tissue for hip operations. Culture: joint fluid, multiple tissue samples are preferable (if available) and blood cultures. As many pathogens are derived from skin flora, at least two consecutive positive cultures from different tissues or aspirates assist in establishing the diagnosis.

Treatment

Requires antibiotic therapy for several weeks and usually removal of prosthesis. Antibiotic therapy may include, e.g. vancomycin for flucloxacillin-resistant CoNS.

Prevention

Appropriate antibiotic prophylaxis for implant surgery. Pre-existing infections (skin, urinary tract, oral cavity) may result in prosthetic joint infection via haematogenous seeding post-operatively and therefore require treatment before surgery. Intra-operative measures to prevent microbial contamination at the surgical site are paramount (e.g. ultra-clean filtered air; surgical gowns; aseptic techniques, including impervious drapes and double gloving).

Prosthetic heart valve infection

Pathogenesis

Microorganisms can gain access to valves at the time of surgery or subsequently from various sources, e.g. poor dental hygiene via haematogenous spread.

Clinical features

Endocarditis may occur. Symptoms include fever, chills, anorexia, weight loss and night sweats.

Clinical diagnosis

Made using Duke's criteria (includes presence of vegetation on heart valve and positive blood cultures). Infection may be associated with the presence of intravascular catheters.

Laboratory diagnosis

Non-specific laboratory tests, ESR, CRP, WCC, proteinuria and microscopic haematuria. Blood cultures: a minimum of at least three sets of blood cultures should be taken before antibiotic therapy. Commonly, several sets are culture positive. Detection of microbial DNA on explanted valves from patients with suspected endocarditis is being increasingly used to identify causative pathogens.

Cardiological investigation

Echocardiogram.

Treatment

Depends on causative pathogen, usually CoNS.

Prevention

Strict intra-operative measures (as for prosthetic joint infection); prophylaxis for specific procedures.

Epidural catheter-associated infection

Pathogenesis

Associated with epidural injections. Immunosuppression (diabetes, HIV, alcoholism) is a predisposing factor for infection. Epidural infection may cause extensive damage to the associated structures. Spinal epidural abscesses may occur.

Clinical features

Early presentation may be subtle and clinical diagnosis difficult to establish. Symptoms include fever, localised back pain, neurological deficit.

Laboratory diagnosis

Non-specific tests (CRP, ESR, WCC) and blood cultures.

Treatment

Commonly associated with CoNS that require intravenous vancomycin therapy if resistant to flucloxacillin.

Prevention

Good aseptic technique on insertion. Antibiotic treatment to eradicate existing infections, which may lead to haematogenous seeding of the device.

CSF shunt infection

Pathogenesis

See Chapter 32.

Clinical features

CSF shunts are commonly inserted via the ventriculoperitoneal (VP) route or rarely through the ventriculoatrial (VA) route. Average incidence of infection is approximately 10%.

VP infection may present within a few months of operation. Symptoms include vomiting, headache and visual disturbance, sometimes accompanied by abdominal distension.

VA shunt infections often do not appear for months or years after insertion. Early cases are characterised by fever, tachycardia and rigors. Delayed cases may present with intermittent/ rare fever, rash arthralgia, anaemia and muscle aches.

Laboratory diagnosis

Blood culture; cerebrospinal fluid (CSF) for microscopy and culture. Non-specific laboratory tests, including CRP and ESR, may provide supporting evidence of infection.

Treatment

Shunt removal and treatment with antimicrobials according to causative pathogen.

Prevention

Aseptic techniques on insertion and antimicrobial prophylaxis; antimicrobial shunts are also being used in some centres.

35

Cardiovascular infections

Richard Watkin
Heart of England NHS Foundation Trust, Sutton Coldfield, West Midlands, UK

Infective endocarditis

Definition

Infection of the endocardium, usually involving the heart valves.

Epidemiology

The incidence in the UK is estimated at between 1.0 and 7.0 per 100,000 population per year. In hospital, mortality is 20%. Up to 50% of patients require valvular surgery. Risk factors for developing infective endocarditis include congenital and acquired structural cardiac defects and intracardiac prostheses.

Pathogenesis

The characteristic manifestation of infective endocarditis is the vegetation. A vegetation forms when bacteria from the blood colonise microthrombi present on damaged endothelium on the valve surface. Endothelial damage occurs due to abnormal intracardiac jets and the presence of prosthetic material. The mitral and aortic valves are most commonly involved. Right-sided infective endocarditis occurs in up to 10% of cases and is more common in intravenous drug users.

Clinical features

Often symptoms of infective endocarditis are non-specific. They include fever, night sweats, malaise and dyspnoea. The clinical course may be indolent, or 'subacute', but often is rapidly progressive with considerable valvular destruction and regurgitation. Clinical signs may include a heart murmur, signs of left ventricular dysfunction, splenomegaly, splinter haemorrhages, digital clubbing, Osler's nodes (painful nodular lesions in the pulps of the fingers), Janeway lesions (painless petechiae on the palms and soles) and Roth's spots (retinal haemorrhages). Pyrexia often will not settle for at least 72 hours after treatment initiation. Complications of infective endocarditis include embolic phenomena, which can be fatal when involving the cerebrovascular system. Glomerulonephritis is common and causes microscopic haematuria.

Aetiology

Infective endocarditis is commonly caused by Gram-positive microorganisms. Staphylococci are the commonest causative microorganisms (both *Staphylococcus aureus* and coagulase negative

Medical Microbiology and Infection Lecture Notes, Fifth Edition. Edited by Tom Elliott, Anna Casey, Peter Lambert and Jonathan Sandoe.
© 2011 Blackwell Publishing Ltd. Published 2011 by Blackwell Publishing Ltd.

staphylococci), followed by 'viridans' streptococci and *Enterococcus* spp. Culture negative infective endocarditis occurs in up to 20% of cases when there is failure to identify a causative microorganism by blood culture. This is commonly caused by prior antibiotic administration or when infection is due to fastidious microorganisms.

Laboratory diagnosis

- *Non-specific tests.* Inflammatory markers are almost always elevated, including C reactive protein (CRP) and erythrocyte sedimentation rate (ESR), neutrophilia is common.
- *Cardiac tests.* Transthoracic and transoesophageal echocardiography visualise vegetations and evaluate valvular integrity.
- *Microbiological tests.* Blood cultures are extremely important. As the number of bacteria circulating in the blood is small, it is important to inoculate the maximum permitted amount of blood into each culture bottle to optimise the yield. Three sets of blood cultures should be obtained within the first 24 hours. Serological assays need to be used to diagnose infective endocarditis caused by *Coxiella burnettii*, *Brucella* spp. and *Bartonella* spp. Histology and molecular analysis (e.g. broad range polymerase chain reaction) of explanted heart valve tissue may also aid in the identification of microorganisms. The diagnosis of infective endocarditis is established using the Duke criteria, which is based mainly on culture results and presence of a vegetation.

Management

Synergistic bactericidal antibiotics are needed for prolonged periods of time (4–6 weeks). Clinical response to therapy should be monitored through measurement of CRP. Surgical debridement and valvular surgery may be required when response to treatment is poor or valvular destruction is extensive.

Prevention

Previously antibiotics have been recommended for all those considered to be at risk of infective endocarditis prior to bacteraemia producing procedures and operations. Currently, most guidelines recommend antibiotic prophylaxis for only those patients at the very highest risk (previous endocarditis, prosthetic heart valves, and complex congenital heart disease), although limited evidence exists supporting ongoing antibiotic prophylaxis for any at risk group.

Pacemaker and device related infection

Definition

Infection of pacing leads, device or within the device 'pocket'. Vegetations may be visible on echocardiography, adherent to the intracardiac portion of pacing leads.

Epidemiology

Intracardiac device infection occurs in 1–2% of implanted devices per year. It is associated with significant morbidity and mortality.

Pathogenesis

It is likely that device related infections are caused by bacteria being introduced during implantation. Adherence of blood-borne bacteria to devices *in situ* is less likely.

Clinical features

Clinical features vary from non-specific signs such as fever, malaise and night sweats to those associated with infective endocarditis.

Aetiology

Device related infections are most commonly caused by coagulase negative staphylococci and *S. aureus*.

Laboratory diagnosis

Frequently, blood cultures are negative as are wound swabs, usually due to prior antibiotic use. The CRP is usually elevated, as is the white cell count.

Management

Antibiotic treatment is as for infective endocarditis. The pacing leads and device usually need explantation.

Myocarditis

Definition

Infection or inflammation of the heart muscle.

Clinical features

Myocarditis is often preceded by a 'flu-like' illness. Symptoms are often non specific but include chest pain and fever. Left ventricular dysfunction will cause breathlessness and orthopnea. Cardiac arrhythmia can precipitate palpitations and collapse.

Aetiology

Myocarditis is commonly viral in origin, although toxic myocarditis occurs in diphtheria and chronic myocarditis is a feature of trypanosomiasis and chlamydial infection. Coxsackie B is the commonest causative agent, although Epstein-Barr (EBV), mumps virus, parvovirus B19 and human herpes virus 6 can also cause myocarditis.

Laboratory diagnosis

A viral aetiology can only be proved if virus is detected in altered myocardium through endocardial biopsy or at necropsy. This usually requires detection of viral nucleic acid by molecular methods. Echocardiography may demonstrate left ventricular dysfunction. Cardiac enzymes and troponins may be elevated.

Management

This is usually supportive with heart failure treatments. Cardiac transplantation is occasionally necessary. Prognosis is usually good in the long term.

Pericarditis

Definition

Infection or inflammation of the pericardium.

Clinical features

Sharp localised chest pain, which may be altered by posture. A pericardial friction rub may present. Signs of right-sided heart failure (raised JVP, peripheral oedema and ascites) may indicate significant pericardial effusion. The ECG shows global 'saddle'-shaped ST elevation. Secondary myocarditis may cause left ventricular dysfunction. Chest X-ray may demonstrate an enlarged globular heart.

Aetiology

Acute pericarditis has many causes, although frequently none is found. Infective causes are predominantly viral (EBV, enteroviruses, CMV), bacterial (localised spread from primary lung infection, haematogenous spread from a distant primary infection, tuberculosis) or fungal (histoplasma, aspergillus, *Candida* spp.). Fungal pericarditis occurs predominantly in immunocompromised individuals.

Laboratory diagnosis

- *Viral*: nucleic acid detection or isolation from pharyngeal washings, faeces or pericardial fluid (see Chapter 16);
- *Bacterial*: Culture of pericardial fluid and blood;
- Echocardiography may show a bright pericardium and the presence of pericardial fluid.

Management

Acute treatment is with analgesia with non-steroidal anti-inflammatory drugs. Clinical or echocardiographic features of cardiac tamponade require emergency pericardiocentesis. Antifungal and antibacterial drugs should be given, depending on the causative microorganism.

Bone and joint infections

Jonathan Sandoe
Leeds Teaching Hospitals NHS Trust and University of Leeds, Leeds, UK

Osteomyelitis

Definition

Infection of bone is termed osteomyelitis.

Aetiology

Staphylococcus aureus is the most common cause of osteomyelitis, but other microorganisms can be important in certain patients groups or situations. The microbial aetiology of osteomyelitis is shown in Table 36.1.

Pathogenesis and epidemiology

Osteomyelitis can occur in a wide variety of patient groups and any bone can be affected, but a relatively small number of pathogens are involved. Some patient groups are susceptible to infections in particular bones (Table 36.2).

Bone infection can result from:

- haematogenous spread (following transient bacteraemia or from a source of infection elsewhere, e.g. endocarditis);
- direct spread from infected tissue ('contiguous focus' osteomyelitis, e.g. tarsal osteomyelitis in a diabetic patient with foot ulcers (Figure 36.1));
- direct inoculation (e.g. trauma, such as open fracture or surgery involving bones).

There are no clear definitions of acute or chronic osteomyelitis. In acute ostemyelitis, symptoms are usually present for days or a few weeks, but chronic osteomyelitis usually refers to cases where infection has persisted for months or years in spite of antimicrobial therapy (and sometimes surgery); dead bone is often present. Frequently, this situation results from inadequately treated acute osteomyelitis.

Clinical features

- Clinical findings vary with the age of the patient and location of infection.
- Osteomyelitis can present acutely or develop slowly over a period of weeks to months, or even years.
- Pain and fever are the most common presenting features.
- If the affected bone is close to the skin there may be swelling, pain, erythema and tenderness over the affected area.
- In infants and young children, reduced use of an affected limb is an important sign.
- The duration of symptoms often varies with the virulence or growth characteristics of the causative microorganism (e.g. symptoms may be present for many months in patients with *Mycobacterium tuberculosis* osteomyelitis, but just a few days if *Staphylococcus aureus* is the cause).
- Discharging sinuses from the infected bone to the skin may occur in chronic *Staphylococcus aureus* osteomyelitis.

Medical Microbiology and Infection Lecture Notes, Fifth Edition. Edited by Tom Elliott, Anna Casey, Peter Lambert and Jonathan Sandoe.
© 2011 Blackwell Publishing Ltd. Published 2011 by Blackwell Publishing Ltd.

Table 36.1 Microbial causes of osteomyelitis and their treatment

Microorganism	Common treatment	Comment
Staphylococcus aureus (meticillin susceptible and resistant, MRSA)	Flucloxacillin (vancomycin for MRSA)	Most common cause of acute and chronic osteomyelitis
coagulase negative staphylococci	Vancomycin	Common cause of device-related infection, occasional cause of haematogenous infection
Beta-haemolytic streptococci (Group A,B,C)	Benzylpenicillin	Children and intravenous drug users (IVDU)
Enterococci and streptococci	Amoxicillin or benzylpenicillin	Cause haematogenous infection e.g. secondary to endocarditis
Anaerobes	benzylpenicillin, metronidazole	Following trauma
Kingella kingae	Amoxicillin	Children
Haemophilus influenzae type b	Cefotaxime	Rare since Hib vaccine
Pseudomonas spp.	Ceftazidime	Neonates and intravenous drug users
Enterobacteriaceae	According to susceptibilities, e.g. ciprofloxacin	Neonates, adults with recurrent urinary tract infections, IVDU
Salmonella spp.	According to susceptibilities	Uncommon but seen more often in patient with sickle cell disease
Mycobacterium tuberculosis	Isoniazid, rifampicn, ethambutol and pyrazinamide	Causes an indolent infection
Brucella spp.	Doxycycline and rifampicin	In areas where Brucella spp. are endemic
Actinomyces spp.	Benzylpenicillin	Cause of mandibular osteomyelitis secondary to periodontal infection
Fungi	Varies with species.	Immunocompromised patients

Table 36.2 Examples of bones affected by osteomyelitis in different patient groups

Patient group/scenario	Bone(s) affected
Diabetic patient with foot ulcers (Figure 36.1)	Tarsals, metatarsals and digits
Neonates and children	Long bones
Post sternotomy for cardiac surgery (Figure 36.2)	Sternum
Patients with endocarditis	Vertebral bodies (and intervertebral discs)

Investigations

- Peripheral blood white cell count (WCC), erythrocyte sedimentation rate (ESR) and C-reactive protein (CRP) may be raised, but all these tests lack sensitivity and specificity.
- Blood cultures are positive in approximately 40–60% of cases.
- Radiological investigations are important in confirming a diagnosis; plain X-rays, computed tomography (CT) and magnetic resonance imaging (MRI) can all be useful.
- Radiological changes are often delayed, even with MRI, the most sensitive investigation.
- Radiologically-guided or operative bone samples for culture are the diagnostic procedures of choice.
- A Gram's stain and Ziehl–Neelsen staining (for mycobacteria) of biopsy samples may be helpful.
- Routine culture, mycobacterial culture and fungal culture of operative or biopsy samples is necessary.

Treatment

Antibiotic treatment is normally for at least 6 weeks. Some commonly used regimens are shown in Table 36.1. Surgery, to allow drainage of pus and débridement of dead bone, may be necessary, particularly in chronic osteomyelitis. Antibiotic treatment depends on the causative microorganism, highlighting the need for appropriate microbiological investigation.

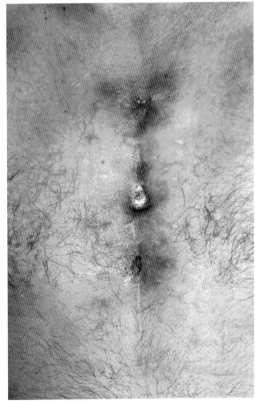

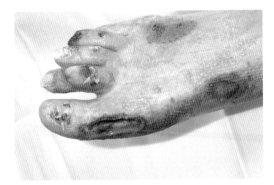

Figure 36.1 'Contiguous focus' osteomyelitis: tarsal osteomyelitis in a diabetic patient with foot ulcers.

Figure 36.2 Sternal osteomyelitis secondary to cardiac surgery.

Septic arthritis

Infection of joints is known as septic arthritis. Infection may affect native (natural) joints or prosthetic joints and these are discussed separately because of differences in pathogenesis, aetiology and management.

Septic arthritis of native joints

Aetiology

The microbial causes of septic arthritis are shown in Table 36.3.

Pathogenesis and epidemiology

Native joint infection can result from:

- haematogenous spread (following transient bacteraemia or from a source of infection elsewhere, e.g. endocarditis);
- direct inoculation (e.g. trauma, surgery or joint injection).

Some factors predisposing to native joint infection are:

- rheumatoid arthritis;
- trauma;
- intravenous drug use;
- immunosuppressive disease.

Synovial tissue is highly vascular and lacks a basement membrane – this may facilitate passage of bacteria from the blood into a native joint. Infection causes cartilage erosion, which results in joint space narrowing and impaired function.

Clinical features

Any joint can be affected. Usually patients present with a rapid onset of hot, swollen, painful joint (Figure 36.3), with reduction in movement and variable systemic signs of infection such as fever. Tuberculous arthritis presents insidiously with a cold swollen joint.

Investigations

Joint aspiration for microscopy and culture. Blood cultures (positive in ~30% of cases).

Treatment

Antibiotic therapy is required according to the causative microorganism, together with joint washout.

Table 36.3 Microbial causes of native and prosthetic joint infection, differences are highlighted in yellow

Native joint infection	Prosthetic joint infection
Staphylococcus aureus (meticillin susceptible and resistant, MRSA)	Staphylococcus aureus (meticillin susceptible and resistant, MRSA)
Beta-haemolytic streptococci (Group A,B,C,G)	Coagulase negative staphylococci
Streptococcus pneumoniae	Beta-haemolytic streptococci (Group A,B,C)
Enterobacteriaceae	Enterococci and other streptococci
Haemophilus influenzae type b (rare)	Diphtheroids
Neisseria meningitidis	Propionibacteria
Neisseria gonorrhoeae	Pseudomonas spp
Kingella kingae (children)	Enterobacteriaceae
Pseudomonas spp	Anaerobes
Anaerobes	Fungi
Mycobacterium tuberculosis	
Fungi	

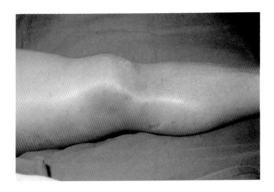

Figure 36.3 Septic arthritis of the knee.

Prosthetic joint infection

Aetiology

The causes of prosthetic joint infection are shown in Table 36.3.

Pathogenesis

Prosthetic joint infection can result from:

- haematogenous spread (following transient bacteraemia or from a source of infection elsewhere, e.g. endocarditis);
- microbial contamination of the prosthesis at implantation;
- surgical wound infection following implantation.

Any type of prosthesis can become infected. Microorganisms capable of attaching to man-made materials and forming an adherent film of bacteria (called biofilm) are most important.

Clinical features

Can present acutely with a hot, swollen, painful joint with reduction in movement and variable systemic signs of infection such as fever, but more commonly presents insidiously with pain and loss of function.

Investigations

- Joint aspiration for microscopy and culture and multiple tissue samples at the time of definitive surgery for culture. These help to distinguish between skin contaminants and causative microorganisms.
- Blood cultures are positive in less than 50% of cases.
- Plain X-rays may show loosening of the prosthesis.

Treatment

Prosthetic joint infection usually requires prosthesis removal. A new prosthesis may be implanted at the time of removal (single-stage procedure), but higher success rates can be achieved by removing the prosthesis followed by a period of antimicrobial therapy (usually 6 weeks) and then implantation of a new prosthesis at a later date (two-stage procedure). Antibiotic therapy can be administered systemically or locally in cement spacers or beads.

Reactive arthritis

This is immunologically mediated, resulting from infection at a distant site, e.g. *Yersinia enterocolitica* gastroenteritis or non-specific urethritis caused by *Chlamydia trachomatis*. Usually, more than one joint is affected.

Viral arthritis

A number of viruses may cause arthritis as part of a generalised infection, e.g. hepatitis B virus, HIV, rubella virus, mumps virus and parvovirus.

37

Skin and soft-tissue infections

Supriya Narasimhan[1] and Rabih Darouiche[2]
[1]Drexel University, Pittsburgh, USA
[2]Baylor College of Medicine, Houston, Texas, USA

Normal flora of skin

The normal skin is colonised mainly by Gram-positive microorganisms (especially coagulase-negative staphylococci and diphtheroids), some Gram-negatives and yeasts, which can survive the relatively harsh conditions – dryness, acidity and the presence of fatty acids, sebum and salt. The normal skin flora protects against infection by other microorganisms that must compete to survive in this ecological niche.

Pathogenesis of skin and soft-tissue infections

- Superficial skin infections affect the epidermis and dermis, e.g. impetigo and erysipelas.
- Deeper infections affect the subcutaneous tissue, e.g. cellulitis (Figures 37.1 and 37.2) and fasciitis.
- Infections of skin structures cause carbuncles and folliculitis (Figure 37.3).

- Infections may arise from pathogens that gain entry through damaged skin (streptococcal cellulitis) or via haematogenous spread (meningococcal skin rash).
- Bacterial toxins produced by infections at other sites may also result in skin changes (group A streptococci causing scarlet fever).

Skin and soft-tissue infections (SSTI)

Classification

There are many classifications. One such scheme is as follows:

- *Uncomplicated SSTI:* have a *low risk* for life- or limb-threatening infection and many can be treated with empiric oral antibiotics, with occasional surgical drainage (folliculitis, furuncles, carbuncles, acne, impetigo, erysipelas and cellulitis). Severe infections require IV antibiotics.
- *Complicated SSTI:* have a *high risk* for life- or limb-threatening infection, and often necessitate

Medical Microbiology and Infection Lecture Notes, Fifth Edition. Edited by Tom Elliott, Anna Casey, Peter Lambert and Jonathan Sandoe.

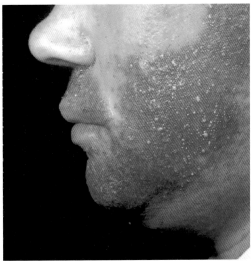

Figure 37.3 Staphylococcal folliculitis.

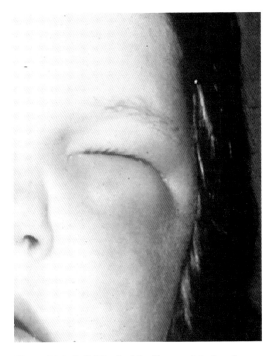

Figure 37.1 Cellulitis of orbit with associated erythema.

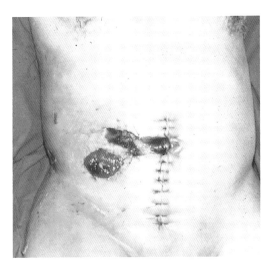

Figure 37.2 Post-operative cellulitis.

hospital admission, surgical debridement, along with broad-spectrum antibiotic therapy (synergistic bacterial gangrene, clostridial cellulitis, and fasciitis).

It is also crucial to differentiate necrotising soft tissue infections (NSTI) from non-necrotising infections, because all NSTI are complicated and warrant prompt aggressive surgical debridement. Clinical clues indicative of NSTI may include erythema, tense oedema, grey or discoloured tissue, bullae, skin necrosis or crepitus, with severe pain disproportionate to physical findings, fever, reduced skin sensation, tachycardia, hypotension and/or altered mental status.

Folliculitis, furuncles and carbuncles

Aetiology

These are commonly caused by *Staphylococcus aureus*, but perianal lesions are often caused by a mixture of faecal microorganisms (including *Escherichia coli*, *Pseudomonas aeruginosa*, anaerobes and the *Streptococcus anginosus* group).

Pathogenesis

Folliculitis is a minor infection of a hair follicle. It may expand into a furuncle (boil). Boils may rupture and drain pus or develop into a carbuncle (large loculated abscess), particularly in diabetics. Perianal abscesses are especially problematic in neutropenic patients.

Complications

- Local spread to bones, joints and other deep structures;
- Haematogenous spread, causing abscesses in various organs.

Laboratory diagnosis

Culture of aspirated pus.

Treatment

Drainage and sometimes antimicrobials (e.g. flucloxacillin for *S. aureus*; metronidazole for anaerobes). Whenever methicillin-resistant *S. aureus* (MRSA) is suspected, antibiotics such as vancomycin, linezolid, cotrimoxazole, clindamycin or daptomycin might be required.

Impetigo

Impetigo is a superficial infection of the skin, involving the epidermis.

Aetiology

Group A β-haemolytic streptococci, or *S. aureus*, sometimes both.

Epidemiology

Principally associated with childhood, poor socio-economic conditions and overcrowding.

Clinical features

Honey-coloured crusted lesions develop mainly on the face around the nose and spread by auto-inoculation. Fomite-borne transmission can also occur.

Laboratory diagnosis

Culture of swabs of lesions.

Treatment

Topical treatment often sufficient, when systemic antimicrobials are necessary: flucloxacillin, or macrolide (e.g. clarithromycin or erythromycin).

Acne

Acne lesions occur within sebaceous follicles with keratin plugs blocking the sebaceous canal, resulting in 'blackheads'. *Propionibacterium acnes* present in the inspissated sebum induces inflammation. Treatment of severe cases is tetracycline combined with topical antiseptics.

Erysipelas

Erysipelas is a rapidly spreading infection of the epidermis and dermis with prominent lymphangitic spread.

Aetiology

Group A β-haemolytic streptococci, occasionally other β-haemolytic streptococci (e.g. group B, C and G) or *S. aureus*

Epidemiology

Mainly in infants, young children and elderly patients.

Pathogenesis

Pathogen gains entry through skin breaks.

Clinical features

Affects mostly the lower limbs and face (particularly the cheeks and periorbital areas), and causes marked erythema and oedema, with a clear line of demarcation that helps distinguish erysipelas from cellulitis. Fever is common.

Laboratory diagnosis

Being mostly an intradermal infection, isolation of streptococci from superficial swabs is often unsuccessful; blood cultures and skin aspirates may be positive in approximately 25% of patients. Serological evidence (e.g. anti-streptolysin O (ASO) titre) of streptococcal infection is sometimes helpful.

Treatment

Benzylpenicillin or a macrolide (e.g. erythromycin or clarithromycin) or clindamycin.

Cellulitis

Cellulitis is an infection of the dermis and subcutaneous tissues, which can be localised or severe with bloodstream infection.

Aetiology

- Group A β-haemolytic streptococci and *S. aureus* are the most common cause.
- Other β-haemolytic streptococci may also cause cellulitis.

- *S. aureus* may produce cellulitis associated with wounds (Figure 37.2) or abscess formation.
- *Haemophilus influenzae* type b commonly caused cellulitis in children aged less than 5 years prior to the introduction of Hib vaccination.
- Facial and orbital cellulitis may follow sinusitis and involve respiratory pathogens (e.g. *Streptococcus pneumoniae*)
- *Erysipelothrix rhusiopathiae*, an unusual cause of cellulitis, seen in meat and fish handlers.
- Non-cholera vibrios (e.g. *Vibrio vulnificus*) are a rare cause of cellulitis complicating wounds contaminated with seawater, particularly in patients with underlying medical problems (e.g. cirrhosis, diabetes).
- Anaerobic cellulitis can complicate bites (oral anaerobes) or devitalised tissue (clostridia) in presence of trauma, diabetes mellitus or vascular insufficiency and in intravenous drug users (Figure 37.4).

Pathogenesis

Bacteria gain entry through inapparent skin breaks to incite infection. Lymphatic obstruction (e.g. after lymph node resection for breast cancer) is a predisposing factor in some cases.

Clinical features

Erythematous, hot, swollen skin with a poorly defined edge (contrast with erysipelas), along with fever and regional lymphadenopathy. Anaerobic cellulitis may be foul smelling, with skin crepitus and necrosis.

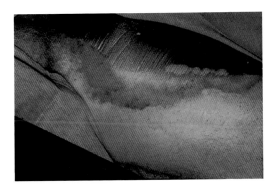

Figure 37.4 Gas gangrene of the leg.

Laboratory diagnosis

Cultures of skin swab/aspirate (positive in ~25% of cases) and blood (occasionally positive). Skin swabs are of limited value, particularly when the skin is unbroken.

Treatment

- High-dose flucloxacillin (active against streptococci and staphylococci) is appropriate empirical therapy, unless risk factors for unusual pathogens (e.g. bite or MRSA colonisation);
- Penicillin for streptococci/*Erysipelothrix* species;
- Flucloxacillin/vancomycin for staphylococci. Clindamycin, an alternative in penicillin-allergic patients, is especially useful in decreasing toxin production;
- Anaerobes can be treated with metronidazole and débridement of devitalised tissue;
- *H. influenzae* type b is treated with cefotaxime.

Synergistic bacterial gangrene

This is an infection of superficial fasciae and subcutaneous fat, but not muscles. It may involve the abdominal wall or male genitalia (Fournier's gangrene).

Aetiology/pathogenesis

Frequently, mixed infection involving *S. aureus*, microaerophilic or anaerobic streptococci and, occasionally, Gram-negative anaerobes (e.g. *Bacteroides* spp.). Predisposing conditions include local trauma, abdominal and genital surgery, and diabetes mellitus.

Clinical features

Rapidly spreading cellulitis with black necrotic areas, pain, fever and systemic toxicity.

Laboratory diagnosis

Culture of affected tissue or pus.

Treatment

Radical excision of necrotic tissue plus antibiotic therapy with flucloxacillin (*S. aureus*), penicillin (streptococci) and/or metronidazole (anaerobes). Broad-spectrum Gram-negative coverage (gentamicin or ciprofloxacin) is needed, especially in diabetics.

Necrotising fasciitis

Life-threatening infection of skin, subcutaneous tissue, deeper fascia and potentially muscles.

Aetiology

- *Type I*: caused by mixtures of non-group A aerobic streptococci, aerobic Gram-negative bacilli and anaerobes. Often complicates deep surgical and traumatic wounds with compromised vascular supply;
- *Type II*: monomicrobial, classically caused by Group A β-haemolytic streptococci. Rarer causes include *Vibrio vulnificus*, *Aeromonas hydrophila* and *S. aureus*.

Pathogenesis

Bacteria produce enzymes and toxins that cause local tissue destruction and systemic toxicity. Diabetes mellitus confers high risk.

Clinical features

Rapidly spreading cellulitis with necrosis, fever, systemic toxicity, hypotension and shock; high mortality.

Laboratory diagnosis

Cultures of tissue, pus or blood.

Treatment

Urgent extensive debridement of affected tissues plus broad-spectrum antibiotics, including combinations of high-dose benzylpenicillin, gentamicin (or ciprofloxacin) and metronidazole or carbapenems; clindamycin is an alternative to penicillin in allergic patients.

Clostridial cellulitis and clostridial myonecrosis (gas gangrene)

Epidemiology

Now rare in developed countries. Peripheral vascular disease and diabetes mellitus are important risk factors.

Pathogenesis

Contamination of traumatic or surgical wounds by clostridia, especially *C. perfringens*, results in gas gangrene or myonecrosis. Clostridia produce enzymes and exotoxins that facilitate rapid spread through tissue plains and result in haemolysis and septic shock.

Clinical features

Cellulitis with necrotic areas, bullae with foul-smelling drainage and gangrene (Figure 37.4). Tissue crepitus due to gas production, fever and toxaemia evolve as myositis develops.

Laboratory diagnosis

Isolation of clostridia from cultures of tissue/swabs or blood. However, isolation of clostridia from wounds does not necessarily indicate gas gangrene, because clostridia can contaminate wounds without infection. Gas gangrene is primarily a clinical diagnosis.

Treatment

Early intervention when suspected is vital. Extensive surgical débridement of devitalised tissue and penicillin and/or metronidazole.

Prevention

Wounds with devitalised tissue should be débrided thoroughly and carefully monitored during healing. Prophylactic antibiotics (e.g. penicillin) should be prescribed for patients undergoing amputations for peripheral vascular disease.

Venous ulcers/pressure sores

Various conditions (diabetes mellitus, peripheral vascular disease, venous insufficiency, and continuous pressure) can reduce cutaneous blood supply and predispose to formation of cutaneous ulcers. Ulcers commonly develop around the foot and ankle (e.g. diabetic foot ulcers and venous ulcers, respectively) or at pressure areas in bedridden patients ('bedsores', e.g. over the sacrum or heal). These invariably become colonised with bacteria and may become infected.

Typical culture results include:

- *Mixed growth of coliforms and anaerobes*: normally not clinically relevant;
- *Pseudomonas aeruginosa*: may reflect antibiotic-induced replacement flora and occasionally requires antibiotic therapy;

- *Staphylococcus aureus*: may represent colonisation or infection;
- β-*haemolytic streptococci groups C and G*: may colonise and occasionally infect venous ulcers;
- β-*haemolytic streptococci group A*: frequently cause infection.

Distinguishing colonisation from infection is important to avoid antibiotic treatment of colonised ulcers; spreading cellulitis around the ulcer suggests infection. Deep infection including osteomyelitis may occur. When systemic antibiotic therapy is needed, broad-spectrum aerobic/anaerobic coverage should be initiated, with subsequent culture-based modification.

Burns

Like venous ulcers, burns may become colonised with bacteria, including *S. aureus, Pseudomonas* spp. and coliforms. The need for antibiotic treatment is dictated by clinical condition (viability of skin grafts) and microorganism(s) cultured (group A β-haemolytic streptococci always require treatment). Colonising microorganisms may eventually cause bacteraemia.

Wound infections

Aetiology

- *Accidental wounds*: S. aureus, β-haemolytic streptococci, clostridia;
- *Bites*: oral commensal bacteria, including anaerobes, *Eikenella corrodens* and streptococci; *Pasteurella multocida* and *Capnocytophaga* spp. (animal bites);
- *Surgical wounds*: (see below).

Laboratory diagnosis

Culture of pus or wound swab.

Treatment

Prompt administration of prophylactic antimicrobials is recommended for human and some animal bites (e.g. amoxicillin-clavulanate), because microorganisms may be inoculated into deeper tissues and cause rapid spread of infection. Ultimate antibiotic choice depends on culture results. Surgical debridement may be necessary.

Surgical wound infections

Predisposing factors

- *Underlying conditions*: e.g. diabetes mellitus and peripheral vascular disease, resulting in poor blood supply;
- *Type of operation*: surgery involving contaminated areas (e.g. gastrointestinal tract) or infected tissue (e.g. perforated appendicitis) is more likely to result in post-operative wound infections;
- *Surgical technique*: e.g. poor technique in wound closure may result in haematoma or devitalised tissue, predisposing to wound infection;
- *Postoperative factors*: cross-infection from other infected cases.

Aetiology

- *Upper body*: S. aureus; group A β-haemolytic streptococci;
- *Lower body* (particularly abdominal surgery): coliforms, occasionally mixed with anaerobes; *P. aeruginosa*.

Clinical features

Fever; wound exudate; cellulitis; may progress to dehiscence and/or bloodstream infection.

Laboratory diagnosis

Cultures of wound swab, pus or blood.

Treatment

Antibiotic treatment depends on causative microorganisms. Surgical debridement may be required.

Prevention

- *Preoperative preparation*: treatment of infection before operation when possible; decontamination of operative area (e.g. bowel preparation) and use of *prophylactic antibiotics* for clean-contaminated, contaminated or dirty operations;
- Good surgical techniques and aseptic theatre practices;
- Measures to prevent postoperative contamination of wounds (e.g. 'aseptic non-touch technique').

Toxin-mediated skin conditions

Scarlet fever

Caused by a strain of group A *Streptococcus* that causes throat infection and produces an erythrogenic toxin, which causes erythematous, blanching, 'sand-paper' rash with a red ('strawberry') tongue and circumoral pallor. As the rash fades, the skin desquamates. Treatment is penicillin or erythromycin.

Staphylococcal scalded skin syndrome (SSSS)

Causes the most severe, systemic manifestation of infection at a distant site with *S. aureus* strains producing an exfoliative toxin, resulting in widespread bullae and skin exfoliation. This occurs in small infants (Ritter's disease) and occasionally in older children and adults (toxic epidermal necrolysis or Lyell's disease). Diagnosis is clinical and is supported by isolating a toxin-producing strain of *S. aureus*. Treatment is with flucloxacillin, or other anti-staphylococcal antibiotics.

Toxic shock syndrome

Toxic shock syndrome is caused by *S. aureus* strains that produce toxic shock syndrome toxin-1 (TSST-1) or staphylococcal enterotoxins, which act as super-antigens causing hypotension, desquamative skin lesions and dysfunction of three or more organ systems.

Panton-Valentine leukocidin producing *Staphylococcus aureus*

These isolates are a particularly virulent form of *S. aureus*, which are associated with tissue damage.

Dermatophyte fungal infections

Worldwide distribution. Transmission by direct contact or via fomites (e.g. towels, hairbrushes). Infection may be acquired from animals. See Table 37.1 for aetiology and clinical features.

Laboratory diagnosis

Microscopy and culture of appropriate specimens (skin scrapings, nail clippings, hair roots).

Table 37.1 Common dermatophyte (ringworm) infections

Infection	Site	Dermatophyte	Clinical features
Tinea corporis	Trunk	*Epidermophyton floccosum*	Pruritus; circular erythematous lesion, scaling, clearing from centre
	Limbs	*Trichophyton* spp. *Microsporum* spp.	
Tinea cruris	Groin	*Epidermophyton floccosum* *Trichophyton rubrum*	Pruritus; lesions similar to tinea corporis
Tinea pedis	Feet	*Epidermophyton floccosum* *Trichophyton* spp.	Pruritus; cracking and scaling between toes
Tinea unguium	Nails	*Trichophyton* spp.	Thick, yellowish nails with surrounding erythema
Tinea capitis	Hair	*Trichophyton tonsurans* *Microsporum audounii* *Microsporum canis*	Erythematous patches on scalp with scaling; hairs break, leaving bald patches

Table 37.2 Common viral skin rashes

Disease	Virus	Rash distribution	Associated symptoms and signs	Diagnosis	Treatment
Maculopapular rashes					
Measles	Measles	Start from hairline downwards all over the body	Fever, coryza, conjunctivitis, Koplik's spots	Serology (IgM), antigen detection in respiratory specimens, culture	
Rubella	Rubella	Start from hairline downwards all over the body	Fever, lymphadenopathy (suboccipital, periauricular and cervical, arthritis in adults)	Serology (IgM), culture	
Erythema infectiosum (fifth disease)	Parvovirus B19	Starts on cheeks (slapped cheek), then diffuses a lace-like rash on body	Fever, arthritis in adults	Serology (IgM), polymerase chain reaction (PCR)	
Exanthem subitum (roseola infantum)	Human herpesvirus 6 (HHV6)	Face, trunk	2–3 days of fever disappearing with appearance of rash	Serology, PCR	
Enterovirus infections	Several Coxsackieviruses and echoviruses	Scattered all over the body	Fever, myalgia, headache, cervical lymphadenopathy	Culture	
Primary HIV infection	HIV	Scattered all over the body	Glandular fever-like illness, meningitis, encephalitis	Serology, PCR	HAART
Dengue fever	Dengue virus	Scattered all over body	Fever, myalgia, headache	PCR, Serology (IgM), culture	Generally asymptomatic but ganciclovir or foscarnet in complicated cases

(continued)

Table 37.2 (Continued)

Disease	Virus	Rash distribution	Associated symptoms and signs	Diagnosis	Treatment
Vesicular rashes					
Chickenpox	Varicella-zoster virus (VZV)	Centripetal distribution	Fever, itching	Electron microscopy, antigen detection in vesicular fluid, serology (IgM), PCR	Generally symptomatic but aciclovir, valaciclovir or famciclovir in complicated cases
Shingles (Figure 37.5)	VZV	Dermatomal but could be disseminated	Post-herpetic neuralgia	PCR antigen detection in vesicular fluid, serology (IgM), PCR	Aciclovir, valaciclovir or famciclovir
Disseminated herpes simplex	Herpes simplex virus (HSV)	Wide distribution	Neonatal herpes, highly immunosuppressed patients	Electron microscopy, antigen detection in vesicular fluid, PCR	Aciclovir, foscarnet
Smallpox	Smallpox	Centrifugal distribution	Fever, headache	Electron microscopy, PCR	
Hand foot and mouth disease	Enteroviruses (Coxsackievirus A16, A4, A5, A9, B2, B5)	Hands and feet	Mouth ulcers, fever	Culture	

Treatment

Topical azole antifungals. Oral terbinafine can be used in case of nail involvement or severe infections that failed to respond to topical azoles. Treatment may be required for several weeks to months.

Cutaneous candidiasis

Skin infection usually caused by the yeast *Candida albicans*. This affects moist skin areas (groin, axilla, skin folds, nailfolds) or damaged skin (e.g. irritant dermatitis in nappy area of babies). It causes erythema, maceration, and 'satellite' vesicles and pustules. Treatment is with topical or oral azoles (e.g. miconazole, fluconazole).

Pityriasis versicolor

Mild skin infection caused by the dimorphic fungus, *Malassezia furfur*. Found worldwide, most commonly in humid tropics. Dark, scaling lesions, particularly in the upper body. In dark-skinned persons, the affected areas become depigmented. Treated with topical or oral azoles.

Viral skin rashes

Examples of common viral skin rashes are outlined in Table 37.2.

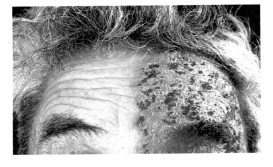

Figure 37.5 Shingles on face.

Infections of the eye

Eyelid

Eyelash follicle infections (styes) are usually caused by *S. aureus*.

Orbital cellulitis

Cellulitis of periorbital tissues are caused mainly by β-haemolytic streptococci, *Streptococcus pneumoniae*, *S. aureus* and, rarely, *H. influenzae* type b in children (<5 years) (Figure 37.1)

Conjunctivitis

- *Viral conjunctivitis*: aetiology includes adenoviruses and measles virus. Laboratory diagnosis by nucleic acid detection techniques. No specific treatment;
- *Neonatal conjunctivitis*: (ophthalmia neonatorum), caused by *Neisseria gonorrhoeae/Chlamydia trachomatis* infection acquired from mother's birth canal;
- *Bacterial causes*: include *S. aureus*, *H. influenzae* and pneumococci. It is most common in young infants. Treatment with topical antibiotics is normally effective.

Herpes virus infections of the eye

- *Herpes simplex virus*: conjunctivitis and painful corneal ('dendritic') ulcers that may cause corneal scarring. Latency with recurrent infection may occur. Treated with aciclovir ointment;
- *Varicella-zoster virus*: ophthalmic zoster. The virus is latent in ophthalmic ganglia and reactivates to affect the periorbital area (unilateral). Treated with systemic aciclovir;
- *Cytomegalovirus*: choroidoretinitis. Associated with AIDS. Treated with ganciclovir.

Trachoma

Chlamydia trachomatis eye infection (conjunctivitis and corneal lesions) is prevalent in developing countries in the tropics and is the leading infectious cause of blindness worldwide. Spreads by direct hand-eye contact. Treated with tetracycline. Mass treatment campaigns helped eradicate trachoma in some endemic areas.

Other eye infections

- *Pseudomonas aeruginosa*: may cause serious deep eye infections after trauma or surgery. Treatment includes parenteral antibiotics.
- *Toxoplasma gondii*: causes choroidoretinitis, normally as part of congenital toxoplasmosis.
- *Toxocara canis*: causes choroidoretinitis.
- *Onchocerciasis*: is a nematode infection that causes river blindness. Microfilariae invade the anterior chamber of the eye. Second leading infectious cause of blindness. Endemic areas include West Africa and Central America.
- *Acanthamoeba* sp.: results in an amoebic infection causing keratitis. Usually associated with contact lens use.

Infections in the compromised host

Tom Elliott
University Hospitals Birmingham NHS Foundation Trust, Birmingham, UK

The immune system consists of innate barriers, including skin and mucous membranes, complement and phagocytic cell mechanisms and adaptive barriers (cellular and humoral). When any of these protective mechanisms is reduced, the host is considered to be immunocompromised. Such patients are more liable to have severe infections and can become infected with either a conventional pathogen (which can also cause disease in a non-compromised individual) or opportunistic pathogens (microorganisms that are usually unable to cause a disease in a healthy person). Various types of defect in the immune defence mechanisms can predispose to infections with certain pathogens.

Infections associated with defects in innate immune systems (Table 38.1)

Infections associated with medical devices

- *Intravascular and peritoneal dialysis catheters.* these catheters breach the skin barrier, allowing commensal microorganisms access to the

deeper sites. These infections are commonly associated with coagulase-negative staphylococci, *Staphylococcus aureus* and, less frequently, coliforms and *Candida* spp.
- *Prosthetic valves and joints.* coagulase-negative staphylococci are the most common pathogens, gaining access, usually during surgery or from a distant infection via haematogenous spread. The microorganism can attach to the prosthesis in biofilms, acting as a nidus of infection.

Infections associated with burns

Burns can destroy extensive areas of the mechanical barriers of the body and also result in abnormalities in localised neutrophil function and antibody response. The burn exudates produce nutrition for microorganisms, allowing colonisation, which may result in infection. The usual pathogens include *Pseudomonas aeruginosa*, *S. aureus* and *Streptococcus pyogenes*.

Infections associated with deficiencies in normal clearance mechanisms

- *Urinary catheters* allow microorganisms access to the bladder, overcoming defences, including

Medical Microbiology and Infection Lecture Notes, Fifth Edition. Edited by Tom Elliott, Anna Casey, Peter Lambert and Jonathan Sandoe.
© 2011 Blackwell Publishing Ltd. Published 2011 by Blackwell Publishing Ltd.

Table 38.1 Infections associated with defects in mechanical barriers

Defect/condition	Common pathogen
Intravascular and peritoneal dialysis catheters	*Staphylococcus epidermidis*, *S. aureus*, coliforms, *Candida* spp.
Urinary catheter	Coliforms
Prosthetic valves and joints	*S. epidermidis*
Burns	Coliforms, *Pseudomonas* spp., *S. aureus*, *Streptococcus pyogenes*
Biliary obstruction	Coliforms, *Enterococcus* spp.
Trauma/surgery	*S. aureus*

Table 38.2 Factors affecting adaptive systems

Type	Defect (example)	Notes
Primary	B- and T-cell combined immunodeficiency	
Secondary	Chemotherapy	e.g. cyclophosphamide
	Infections	e.g. HIV-1 and -2
	Malignancy	e.g. leukaemia, lymphoma
	Splenectomy	Reduced levels of immunoglobulin subclasses
	Irradiation	Affects proliferation of lymphoid cells
	Corticosteroids	

Table 38.3 Examples of infections related to deficiency in cellular and humoral immunodeficiency

Defensive defect	Examples of underlying condition	Opportunistic microorganism
T-cell	Lymphoma	Varicella-Zoster virus
		Candida spp.
		Toxoplasma gondii
T- and B-cell	Chronic lymphatic leukaemia	Varicella-Zoster virus
		Candida spp.
	Immunosuppressive drugs	*Toxoplasma gondii*
		Cytomegalovirus
		Pneumocystis jirovecii (P. carinii)
Neutropenia	Acute leukaemia	*Staphylococcus aureus*
	Cytotoxic treatment	*Aspergillus fumigatus*
		Coliforms
CD 4 Lymphocytes		HIV, Cytomegalovirus
		Pneumocystis jirovecii (P. carinii)

Table 38.4 **Examples of opportunistic pathogens associated with solid organ transplant recipients**

Bacteria	Fungi	Protozoa	Parasites	Viruses
Staphylococcus aureus	Candida spp.	Toxoplasma gondii	Strongyloides stercoralis	Herpes simplex viruses
Coagulase-negative staphylococci	Aspergillus spp.			Cytomegalovirus
Mycobacterium avium-intracellulare	Pneumocystis jirovecii			Varicella-Zoster
Coliforms				Epstein–Barr

urine washout. Bacteria can grow up the inside or outside surface of a urinary catheter. The infections are commonly associated with Gram-negative aerobic bacilli from the patient's own faecal or periurethral flora.

- Stones in the kidney, common bile and salivary ducts can result in infections proximal to the obstruction.
- *Respiratory tract*: there may be damage to the cilia, e.g. with cystic fibrosis patients, which predisposes to pneumonia with microorganisms such as *S. aureus*, *Haemophilus influenzae* and *P. aeruginosa*. An endotracheal tube, required during mechanical ventilation, bypasses many upper respiratory defences and, when colonised, can deliver microorganisms directly into the trachea.

Infections associated with defects in complement and phagocytic activity

These defects are normally congenital. Defects in phagocytic function may affect chemotaxis, phagocytosis or bacterial killing; associated infections often involve pyogenic bacteria, e.g. *S. aureus*. Defects in the complement system are associated with bacterial infections, e.g. patients with defects in the later complement components

(C7–C9) have an increased risk of meningococcal infections.

Infections related to cellular and humoral immunodeficiency

The type of underlying immunodeficiency (Table 38.2) may determine the nature and severity of any subsequent infection (Table 38.3). Increasingly, these infections are iatrogenic and caused by opportunistic pathogens. The length of time that a patient is immunosuppressed may influence the type of associated infection.

Infections in some immunocompromised patients can be multifactorial and associated with several factors, e.g. in recipients of solid organ transplants, these include the type of organ transplant, the level of immune suppression required to prevent rejection of a grafted organ and the pathogens to which a recipient is exposed, including from the donor organ and the environment. Some infections associated with organ transplant recipients are shown in Table 38.4.

Generally, conventional pathogens cause infections in pre-transplant patients. However, when these patients are immunosuppressed as part of their treatment, infections with opportunistic microorganisms, including *Aspergillus* species start to occur.

39

Infections caused by antimicrobial-resistant bacteria

David Livermore
Health Protection Agency, Microbiology Services, Colindale, London, UK

Introduction

Antimicrobials exert a Darwinian selection in favour of those bacteria that have inherent resistance or which have acquired resistance as a result of random genetic events. Inherent resistance is where all members of a species or group are resistant, e.g. all Gram-negative bacteria are resistant to vancomycin because it is too large to cross their outer membrane. Acquired resistance emerges in hitherto susceptible species via mutations (random errors occurring in DNA sequence as it is copied), or by gene transfer.

- Gene transfer is most often via plasmids, i.e. loops of DNA separate from the chromosome. Some plasmids are 'promiscuous', meaning that they can spread among numerous species.
- Some resistant strains or 'clones' are biologically 'fit' and can spread among patients, hospitals, and even between countries.

The processes of mutation, DNA transfer and strain selection have led to major increases in the prevalence of resistance in many bacterial pathogens. This chapter details the currently-critical resistance problems. Preventing a return to the 'pre-antibiotic era' when simple infections were frequent killers and much modern medicine would have been impossible requires:

- judicious use of antimicrobials in humans and animals;
- prevention of the spread of resistant microorganisms among patients; and
- reinvigoration of discovery of new antimicrobials.

Meticillin-resistant *staphylococcus aureus*

Meticillin-resistant *Staphylococcus aureus* (MRSA) has the highest profile of any resistant bacterium. Its resistance depends on the *mecA* gene, which codes a supplementary cell-wall synthesizing enzyme, PBP-2', which enables MRSA to 'by-pass' the cell-wall synthetic steps normally targeted by

Medical Microbiology and Infection Lecture Notes, Fifth Edition. Edited by Tom Elliott, Anna Casey, Peter Lambert and Jonathan Sandoe.
© 2011 Blackwell Publishing Ltd. Published 2011 by Blackwell Publishing Ltd.

meticillin. Most MRSA belong to a few widely-disseminated clones. Transfer of *mecA* among strains is rare but does occur.

Epidemiology

- MRSA were first described in the 1960s, soon after meticillin entered clinical use as an answer to penicillin-resistant *S. aureus*. The early MRSA strains did not spread, presumably because they were biologically unfit. Fitter MRSA strains began to proliferate in hospitals during the 1980s, but rarely caused severe infections. These were followed, in the early 1990s, by the current UK 'epidemic' clones, EMRSA-15 and EMRSA-16, which are strongly associated with severe infection, including bloodstream infections. At their peak in 2003, MRSA (95% EMRSA-15 or -16 strains) accounted for 40% of *S. aureus* bacteraemias and 8% of *all* bacteraemias. Subsequently, their prevalence has been approximately halved, largely by infection prevention practices.
- In Scandinavia, MRSA rates have been consistently low owing to rigorous infection control and contact tracing; rates in many other parts of the world remain high and stable.
- Although EMRSA-15 and -16 mostly cause hospital infections, they also colonise individuals in the community, e.g. care home residents. Carriers are more vulnerable to infection during subsequent hospitalisation.
- True 'community' MRSA strains have proliferated recently in the US, less so elsewhere. They may be transmitted via vigorous physical contact, e.g. during sports activities. They can cause aggressive skin and soft tissue infections, rarely pneumonias. Most produce a toxin called Panton–Valentine leukocidin, but this is not exclusive to community MRSA and is more often seen in meticillin-susceptible *S. aureus* in the UK. It is not new, having been known since the 1930s.

Detection

- MRSA are detected by conventional antibiotic susceptibility tests, usually with oxacillin, as meticillin itself is no longer available. The media used must allow expression of *mecA*, induced by salt and low temperature. Detection is also possible by polymerase chain reaction (PCR) for *mecA*.
- *S. aureus* isolates, which are oxacillin resistant, or *mecA*-positive, should be assumed to be resistant

to all penicillin, cephalosporin or related drugs presently available (June 2011). New anti-MRSA cephalosporins (ceftobiprole and ceftaroline) are, however, anticipated; these bind and inhibit PBP-2'.

Control of MRSA

- Hand hygiene is crucial; its improvement prevents up to 50% of hospital-acquired MRSA infections. It decreases the chance of staphylococci being carried from patient to patient via the healthcare workers.
- Environmental cleanliness and equipment decontamination reduces the likelihood of patients acquiring MRSA directly, and the hands of healthcare workers becoming contaminated.
- Screening of hospital admissions allows carriers to be identified; attempts can then be made to decolonise them, e.g. with mupirocin in the nose and chlorhexidine on the skin. This may reduce shedding of microorganisms into the environment.
- Patient isolation or cohorting reinforces the need for hand hygiene and segregates infected or co-lonised patients from others.
- Prophylactic antibiotics can be used to prevent infection in surgery.
- The Department of Health (in England) uses MRSA bacteraemia rates as a measure of infection control performance, publishing tables of these rates for each hospital trust.

Treatment

- Glycopeptides (vancomycin and teicoplanin) are the mainstay against serious MRSA infections. Vancomycin resistance in MRSA is extremely rare, with no reports from the UK. The few recorded cases were caused by the acquisition of plasmid-borne *vanA* genes from enterococci (see below); a few further MRSA isolates have intermediate resistance contingent on a thickened cell wall.
- Newer alternatives for severe MRSA infections include daptomycin, linezolid and tigecycline. Depending on the clone, susceptibility may also be retained to various older agents, including trimethoprim, co-trimoxazole, tetracyclines, fusidic acid and rifampicin; these may be used alone or in combination in less severe infections, or as oral follow-on to i.v. vancomycin, linezolid, tigecycline or daptomycin.

Vancomycin-resistant enterococci (VRE)

Epidemiology

- Vancomycin-resistant enterococci (VRE, also called glycopeptide-resistant enterococci, GRE) emerged in the late 1980s. They are classified as VanA (commonest), VanB or VanC phenotypes.
- In the UK, VRE are mostly confined to specialist renal, haematology and oncology units; a minority of tertiary hospitals account for most cases. VRE are more widespread in US hospitals.
- Most vancomycin resistant *Enterococcus faecium* belong to clonal complex CC17, a human-adapted lineage that can cause hospital outbreaks.

Mechanism of resistance and detection

- VanA and VanB are plasmid- or transposon-mediated systems that have spread among *Enterococcus faecium* and, less so, *E. faecalis*; VanC is intrinsic to *E. casseliflavus* and *E. gallinarum* – rarer species.
- Resistance reflects the use of alternative cell wall precursors, thereby depriving glycopeptides of their normal target site of action.
- Enterococci with VanA are resistant to vancomycin and teicoplanin, as both induce VanA expression. VanB and VanC strains are resistant to vancomycin, but not teicoplanin, which does not act as an inducer.

Control

- Hand hygiene, equipment and environmental decontamination, as for MRSA (see above).

Treatment

- Virtually all *E. faecalis* remain susceptible to ampicillin, linezolid and tigecycline; *E. faecium* is generally resistant to ampicillin, but susceptible to linezolid, quinupristin/dalfopristin and tigecycline. Nitrofurantoin is often active but appropriate only for lower urinary infections.
- A problem arises in endocarditis, where synergistic bactericidal activity between a β-lactam or glycopeptide and an aminoglycoside is sought, but where around 40% of enterococci now have streptomycin and gentamicin resistance, precluding this synergy. High dose ampicillin or daptomycin may be alternatives.

Streptococcus pneumoniae

- *S. pneumoniae* is the commonest and most serious cause of community-acquired pneumonia (see Chapter 26). Historically, it was very susceptible to penicillin and other antibiotics but resistance gradually emerged via mutation and gene modification, followed by clonal spread of resistant strains belonging to serotypes 6B, 9V, 14, 19F and 23F.
- Introduction of a conjugate vaccine targeting these serotypes (and 2 others) is reducing their role in invasive disease, and thereby also the prevalence of resistance, both in the children, who are vaccinated, and in the elderly, who typically acquire infection from children. Resistance to penicillin is emerging in other 'non-vaccine' serotypes, e.g. 19A, particularly in the USA, but these are covered by a second-generation vaccine.

Gram-negative bacilli

Epidemiology

- *Escherichia coli* is the commonest causative agent of urinary tract infections and is part of the mixed aerobic/anaerobic flora that may cause intra-abdominal infections arising from leakage of gut contents.
- Other Enterobacteriaceae, including *Klebsiella* and *Enterobacter* spp., also non-fermenters, e.g. *Pseudomonas aeruginosa* and *Acinetobacter baumannii*, are important as opportunistic hospital pathogens. *P. aeruginosa* also colonises the lungs of cystic fibrosis patients, giving chronic infections that accumulate resistance by mutation.
- Resistant *Klebsiella* and *A. baumannii* may cause hospital outbreaks, with transmission via the hands of staff or via contaminated equipment. By contrast, *E. coli* infections usually are endogenous, with bacteria from the gut transferred to the urinary tract or the abdominal cavity.

Mechanisms of resistance

- Resistance to older penicillins, e.g. ampicillin, is inherent and associated with chromosomally-mediated β-lactamases in *Klebsiella* spp., *Enterobacter* spp., *Pseudomonas aeruginosa* and *A. baumannii*. In *E. coli*, it is largely caused by the TEM-1 β-lactamases. First recorded in 1963, this plasmid-mediated enzyme has now spread to 50–60% of clinical isolates of *E. coli*, both in the community and in hospitals.
- Modern 'third-generation' cephalosporins, such as cefotaxime and ceftazidime were designed to be stable to TEM-1 and other β-lactamases but have, in turn, selected for extended-spectrum β-lactamases (ESBLs), which hydrolyse and inactivate them. Early ESBLs were mutants of TEM-1 and a similar enzyme, SHV-1, and were mostly found in hospital *Klebsiella*. A new ESBL family, CTX-M, has recently become dominant, spreading also in community *E. coli*. CTX-M- *E. coli* often infect the urinary tract of elderly patients.
- Resistance to fluoroquinolones has also increased markedly in Enterobacteriaceae, including *E. coli*, and many ESBL producers are multi-resistant to these drugs also to aminoglycosides. This accumulation of multi-resistance is leading to increased need to use carbapenems, which previously were reserved antibiotics.
- Carbapenem use, in turn, is selecting for carbapenemases (i.e. carbapenem-destroying β-lactamases), including the KPC and NDM types in *Enterobacter* and *Klebsiella*, also OXA carbapenemases in *Acinetobacter* spp. Carbapenem resistance in *P. aeruginosa* is mostly contingent on impermeability and efflux, not β-lactamase

Control

- Standard infection prevention can limit hospital spread of multi-resistant *Klebsiella* spp., *A. baumannii* and *P. aeruginosa* clones. Key factors include decontamination of hands and equipment, cohorting or isolation of patients and the use of gloves and gowns. The utility of these measures is less clear for multi-resistant *E. coli*, where the source of infection is usually the patient's own gut microflora.

Treatment

- Most quinolone-resistant and ESBL-producing *E. coli*, *Klebsiella* spp. and *Enterobacter* spp. remain susceptible to the carbapenems, imipenem, meropenem, doripenem and ertapenem, which are the drugs of choice in severe infections. Alternatives in less severe disease vary with the site of infection and the individual isolate; they often include tigecycline and (for lower urinary tract infections) fosfomycin or nitrofurantoin.
- Polymyxin is often the sole option for severe infections caused by Enterobacteriaceae or non-fermenters with carbapenemases.

Neisseria gonorrhoeae

- A common sexually-transmitted pathogen, *N. gonorrhoeae* historically was very susceptible and in the 1940s gonorrhoea was treatable with low doses of penicillin. Susceptibility later declined, largely through target modification and penicillin doses of 3 g were needed by the 1970s. Penicillin-untreatable strains then emerged, and were found to have acquired the same TEM-1 β-lactamase that had proliferated in *E. coli* (see above).
- By the 1990s, ciprofloxacin had replaced penicillin as the standard treatment but, again, resistance emerged and is now seen in 20–30% of US and UK isolates. These developments have led to cephalosporins, principally cefixime and ceftriaxone, becoming the new standard therapies, but gonococci are showing progressive reductions in susceptibility, as occurred with penicillin between the 1940s and 1970s.
- Resistance to penicillin and ciprofloxacin can also arise in *N. meningitidis*, but is much rarer than in *N. gonorrhoeae*.

The British Society for Antimicrobial Chemotherapy resistance surveillance (http://www.bsac-surv.org) provides extensive information from antibiotic resistance surveillance programmes for respiratory infections and bacteraemias in the UK and Ireland. The European Antimicrobial Resistance Surveillance Network (http://www.ecdc.europa.eu/en/activities/surveillance/EARS-Net/Pages/index.aspx) is a European-wide network of national surveillance systems, providing reference data on antimicrobial resistance for public health purposes.

Perinatal and congenital infections

James Gray
Birmingham Children's Hospital NHS Foundation Trust, Birmingham, UK

Definitions

Congenital infections are infections that are acquired *in utero*. They may be acquired through transplacental spread or by ascent of microorganisms from the maternal genital tract. The manifestations of congenital infection are protean. Perinatal infections are acquired around the time of delivery (usually from the maternal genital tract). Bacterial infections that are perinatally acquired usually present within the first 48–72 hours of life. After that, an increasing proportion of neonatal bacterial infections are acquired from other sources, including family members, healthcare workers, other patients and the hospital environment. Viral infections usually have a longer incubation period, and may present much later. Some agents are only important as causes of either congenital or perinatal infections; other infections can be acquired during either period (Table 40.1).

Congenital infections

General principles of diagnosis

Presentation of congenital infection

- Occasionally maternal illness may be present, but often the mother is asymptomatic or has sub-clinical illness.
- Abnormalities may be detected on routine foetal scanning.
- Infections may result in pregnancy loss.
- Infections may present at birth, or with sequelae that develop only months or years after birth.
- Many infections are asymptomatic.

Microbiological investigations

- Diagnosis of maternal infection during pregnancy, principally by serological tests, is the usual starting point. However, this does not confirm that infection has been transmitted to the baby.

Medical Microbiology and Infection Lecture Notes, Fifth Edition. Edited by Tom Elliott, Anna Casey,
Peter Lambert and Jonathan Sandoe.
© 2011 Blackwell Publishing Ltd. Published 2011 by Blackwell Publishing Ltd.

Table 40.1 Important congenital and perinatal infections

Bacteria	Timing of infection		
	Congenital: Early pregnancy	Congenital: Late pregnancy	Perinatal
Chlamydia trachomatis	−	−	+++
Gram-negative bacteria	−	−	+++
Group B *Streptococcus*	−	−	+++
Listeria monocytogenes	++	+++	++
Mycobacterium tuberculosis	+	+	+
Neisseria gonorrhoeae	−	−	+++
Staphylococci	−	−	+
Treponema pallidum	+++	+++	+
Viruses			
Cytomegalovirus	+++	++	+
Enteroviruses	−	−	++
Hepatitis B	+	+	+++
Herpes simplex virus	+	+	+++
HIV	+	+	+++
Human parvovirus B19	+++	−	−
Rubella	+++	−	−
Varicella zoster virus	+	+++	+++
Parasites			
Malaria	+	+	−
Toxoplasma gondii	+++	+	−

Key: +++: High risk of transmission/harm to the baby; ++: Moderate risk of transmission/harm to the baby; +: Low risk of transmission/harm to the baby; −: No significant risk of transmission/harm to the baby.

- Congenital infection is confirmed by detection of a microorganism in amniotic fluid, foetal blood or neonatal samples, or serological tests on foetal or neonatal (not cord) blood. Because IgG antibodies cross the placenta, serodiagnosis of congenital infection depends on detection of IgM antibodies soon after birth (IgM does not cross the placenta) or persistence of IgG antibodies after at least 6 months of age.

Rubella virus

Epidemiology

The risk of congenital infection after maternal rubella virus infection depends on the stage of pregnancy when maternal infection occurs; multiple severe defects are inevitable when infection occurs during the first 12 weeks of pregnancy. Thereafter, the risk of foetal damage decreases from 17% at 13–16 weeks gestation to nil at 20 weeks. Because of universal rubella immunisation, congenital rubella syndrome is now very uncommon in the UK.

Clinical features

Congenital heart defects, eye defects (cataracts, retinopathy, microophthalmos), deafness, microcephaly, hepatosplenomegaly, thrombocytopenia.

Laboratory diagnosis

- maternal infection diagnosed by detection of rubella-specific IgM antibodies;

- prenatal diagnosis of foetal infection not usually undertaken;
- infection in the neonate diagnosed by detection of virus in urine, blood or respiratory samples, or by detection of rubella-specific IgM antibodies in neonatal blood.

Treatment and prevention

- No specific treatment exists for rubella.
- Rubella is included in the MMR vaccine that is part of the routine childhood immunisation schedule.
- Antenatal screening of pregnant women, with post-partum immunisation of seronegative cases.

Cytomegalovirus (CMV)

Epidemiology

Congenital CMV infection is the most common intrauterine infection (maternal infection rate in the UK is 5–7 per 1,000 pregnancies). Congenital infection usually follows primary maternal CMV infection: the risk of transmission to the foetus is around 40%, but 90–95% of infected foetuses will be normal at birth. There is also a small but unquantified risk of congenital infection following maternal re-infection or reactivation of latent infection.

Clinical features

Eighty-five percent of congenitally infected babies are unaffected. Five percent are symptomatic at birth: symptoms include pneumonitis, hepatosplenomegaly, thrombocytopenia, anaemia, low birth weight, microcephaly, cerebral palsy, deafness and choroidoretinitis. Five to ten percent are asymptomatic at birth, but develop later sequelae (cognitive, motor, visual or hearing defects).

Laboratory diagnosis

- Maternal infection is diagnosed by detection of CMV-specific IgM antibodies.
- Foetal infection is diagnosed prenatally by detection of CMV in amniotic fluid (usually by PCR) or of IgM antibodies in foetal blood.
- Infection in the neonate is diagnosed by detection of CMV-specific IgM or detection of the virus (by culture or PCR) in throat swabs, blood or urine. Congenital infection can only be diagnosed with certainty on samples collected within the first three weeks of life.

Treatment and prevention

- Ganciclovir or valganciclovir should be considered for treatment of congenitally infected babies: this may alleviate sensorineural hearing loss.
- There are no specific preventative measures. However, babies with congenital CMV infection in hospital should be isolated while in hospital, because large amounts of virus are excreted in urine and respiratory secretions for months or years.

Toxoplasmosis

Epidemiology

In the UK, maternal toxoplasmosis affects about 0.5% of pregnancies. The risk of transmission to the foetus increases from 25% in the first trimester to 65% in the third. However the risk of serious effects decreases from 75–5%.

Clinical features

Stillbirth, choroidoretinitis, microcephaly, convulsions, intracerebral calcification with resultant hydrocephalus, myocarditis, hepatosplenomegaly and thrombocytopenia.

Laboratory diagnosis

- Maternal infection is diagnosed by detection of *T. gondii*-specific IgM antibodies: beware that IgM positivity persists for many months after infection.
- For prenatal diagnosis of foetal infection and diagnosis of infection in the neonate, detection of *T. gondii* in amniotic fluid or neonatal blood by PCR offers the best sensitivity. Only one-third of congenitally infected infants are IgM-positive.

Treatment and prevention

- Maternal treatment with spiramycin or with pyrimethamine and sulphadiazine during pregnancy, and treatment of the neonate with pyrimethamine and sulphadiazine, may reduce the severity of sequelae.
- Pregnant women should be advised to avoid contact with cat faeces during pregnancy, and given dietary advice. Antenatal screening is performed in some countries, but not in the UK.

Varicella-zoster virus (VZV)

Epidemiology

Around 90% of UK-born adults are immune to chickenpox, but the proportion of immune adults who were brought up in other countries may be lower.

Clinical features

Small risk (<3%) of foetal malformation (congenital varicella syndrome) where maternal chickenpox occurs in the first trimester. The other period of high risk is where maternal chickenpox occurs between 7 days before and 7 days after delivery: the baby is at risk of severe systemic neonatal infection, because it will not acquire passive immunity from its mother.

Diagnosis

- Chickenpox is usually diagnosed clinically.
- Where necessary, the diagnosis can be confirmed by direct detection of the virus in clinical material by various methods.
- Serology has no part in diagnosis of acute chickenpox, but is needed to assess the immunity of persons who have been exposed to chickenpox.

Treatment and prevention

- high dose aciclovir for neonatal varicella infection;
- non-immune pregnant women should avoid contact with chickenpox; contacts should be treated with varicella zoster immune globulin (VZIG).

Human parvovirus B19

Epidemiology

Around 40% of adults in the UK are non-immune to parvovirus B19. Up to 15% of maternal infections in the first 20 weeks of pregnancy result in foetal infection: infections after 20 weeks do not cause serious morbidity.

Clinical features

When maternal infection occurs in the first 20 weeks of pregnancy, there is a 10% risk of spontaneous abortion, and a further 3% risk of hydrops fetalis (anaemia and cardiac failure resulting from the virus infecting erythrocyte precursors); congenital malformations have not been reported.

Laboratory diagnosis

- maternal infection diagnosed by detection of specific anti-parvovirus IgM antibodies;
- where necessary, foetal infection diagnosed prenatally by detection of parvovirus in amniotic fluid or foetal blood by PCR or by detection of IgM antibodies in foetal blood;
- diagnosis of infection in the neonatal period not usually relevant.

Treatment and prevention

- no specific antiviral therapy;
- where parvovirus infection has been diagnosed, enhanced monitoring of the pregnancy is required, with intrauterine blood transfusion for severe foetal anaemia as required;
- pregnant women should avoid contact with children with parvovirus infection.

Syphilis

Epidemiology

Congenital syphilis is now rare in developed countries, but remains a serious problem in developing countries. Where a mother has untreated syphilis, the risk of congenital infection is 80–90% in the first year after infection, falling to less than 10% four years after infection.

Clinical features

Stillbirth, hepatosplenomegaly, lymphadenopathy, skin rashes, nasal discharge. Bone, tooth and cartilage defects and deafness are later sequelae.

Laboratory diagnosis

Congenital syphilis usually diagnosed by detection of anti-*Treponema pallidum* IgM antibodies in neonatal serum. Treponemes may be detectable in material from skin or mucous membrane lesions by darkground microscopy.

Treatment and prevention

- Treatment is with high dose penicillin.
- Pregnant women are routinely screened for anti-treponemal antibodies.

Listeriosis

Maternal infection (asymptomatic or influenza-like illness) is usually acquired from contaminated food (soft cheeses, raw vegetables or salads). Maternal listeriosis may cause intrauterine infection, resulting in abortion or stillbirth. Infection later in pregnancy or during delivery may result in neonatal bloodstream infection and/or meningitis. Treatment is with ampicillin or amoxicillin plus gentamicin. Prevention is by avoiding high-risk foods in pregnancy.

Tuberculosis (TB)

Congenital TB is rare: may result in pregnancy loss or symptomatic neonatal TB. Perinatal TB due to aspiration of infected amniotic fluid is even rarer.

Malaria

Congenital or neonatal malaria occurs most frequently when the mother becomes infected for the first time during pregnancy. Infection may result in abortion or stillbirth or pre-term delivery. Neonates may not develop symptoms of malaria for several weeks after delivery.

Neonatal infections

Group B β-haemolytic streptococci

Epidemiology

Group B streptococci are a common commensal of the genital and gastrointestinal tracts of 20–30% of pregnant women. Around 50% of babies born to colonised mothers acquire this microorganism during delivery.

Clinical features

Most colonised babies are unaffected. Around 1% of babies born to mothers colonised develop serious systemic infection (bacteraemia, meningitis, pneumonia) in the first week of life (usually within the first 48 h). Late onset sepsis (1 week–6 months after delivery) presents more often as meningitis: the bacterium may come from sources other than the mother.

Laboratory diagnosis

Cultures of blood, CSF, respiratory secretions, and any other suspected sites of infection.

Treatment and prevention

- Treatment is penicillin with gentamicin.
- Intrapartum antibiotic prophylaxis is offered to women identified as carrying, or with risk factors for, Group B streptococci (e.g. prematurity, maternal fever in labour, prolonged rupture of membranes).

Gram-negative aerobic bacilli

Epidemiology

Escherichia coli is usually acquired from the maternal intestinal tract during delivery. Invasive infections are associated with certain serotypes, particularly K1. Other Gram-negative bacilli, such as *Klebsiella* spp., *Enterobacter* spp., *Serratia* spp. and *Pseudomonas aeruginosa*, are mainly acquired in hospital and are usually associated with stay in neonatal units.

Clinical features

E. coli is an important cause of early-onset neonatal meningitis and bloodstream infection. Infections associated with other Gram-negative aerobic bacilli include pneumonia, bloodstream infection, meningitis and urinary tract infections.

Laboratory diagnosis

Cultures of blood, CSF, respiratory secretions, urine and any other suspected sites of infection.

Treatment and prevention

- Empiric antibiotic therapy should be based on local antibiotic sensitivity patterns: often includes an aminoglycoside. Definitive treatment depends on antibiotic sensitivity test results.
- No specific preventative measures.

Staphylococci

Epidemiology

Staphylococcus aureus is a very common neonatal pathogen; it can also form part of the normal vaginal microbial flora. Infection can be acquired perinatally from the vagina, but most are acquired after birth via contaminated hands. Coagulase-negative staphylococci (CoNS) are now the commonest isolates from neonatal blood cultures, and are principally nosocomial pathogens in neonatal units. Once considered low virulence pathogens, it is now recognised that coagulase-negative staphylococcal infections can be serious.

Clinical features

S. aureus is a common cause of mild infections of superficial sites such as skin and eyes, but is also an important cause of more serious infections (bloodstream infection, pneumonia, osteomyelitis). CoNS cause bloodstream infection, often associated with intravascular catheters.

Laboratory diagnosis

Cultures of blood, respiratory secretions, skin swabs and any other suspected sites of infection.

Treatment and prevention

- *S. aureus* is usually treated with flucloxacillin. For meticillin-resistant strains (MRSA) and CoNS, glycopeptides (vancomycin, teicoplanin) are the mainstay of treatment.
- Screening of mothers and babies is increasingly being used to control MRSA.

Neisseria gonorrhoeae and Chlamydia Trachomatis

Epidemiology

These infections are acquired from the maternal genital tract.

Clinical features

- *N. gonorrhoeae* causes severe conjunctivitis (ophthalmia neonatorum) with pus and periorbital inflammation that usually presents within 48 hours of birth.
- *C. trachomatis* conjunctivitis is less severe and tends to present later (3–14 days after delivery): untreated, *Chlamydia* pneumonitis may occur as a late (1–3 months) complication.

Laboratory diagnosis

Gonococcal infection is usually diagnosed by culture, although accurate molecular techniques are now available. Nucleic acid amplification techniques are the mainstay of diagnosis of chlamydial infections. In the case of both infections, mothers should be referred to a Genitourinary Medicine clinic for investigation and treatment.

Treatment

Both gonococcal and chlamydia ophthalmia neonatorum require systemic therapy: ceftriaxone for *N. gonorrhoeae* and erythromycin for chlamydial infection.

Herpes simplex virus (HSV)

Epidemiology

Classically acquired from the maternal genital tract during delivery, usually when the mother has active lesions of primary genital herpes; can also be acquired from mucocutaneous lesions from anyone with active herpes. Rarely transplacental spread, which almost always leads to loss of the pregnancy.

Clinical features

Features of neonatal herpes simplex infection include encephalitis or meningoencephalitis, generalised infection with hepatitis and mucocutaneous lesions.

Laboratory diagnosis

Detection of virus in clinical material by PCR.

Treatment and prevention

Treatment of herpes encephalitis with high doses of aciclovir has reduced the mortality rate to under 25%. Preventative measures include Cesarean section where primary maternal genital herpes infection presents in the final 6 weeks of pregnancy, and exclusion of persons with active herpes lesions from contact with neonates.

Human immunodeficiency virus (HIV)

Epidemiology

HIV transmission from infected mothers to their babies can occur *in utero* (<1% of cases) during delivery or via breast milk. Without preventative measures, the risk of vertical transmission is 15–40%: with careful management the risk falls to almost zero.

Clinical features

Infected neonates are usually asymptomatic at birth, but the illness can progress rapidly in infancy. Poor weight gain, lymphadenopathy, hepatosplenomegaly and recurrent infections are early signs of infection.

Laboratory diagnosis

Detection of HIV RNA or proviral DNA in neonatal blood by nucleic acid amplification techniques. Because early diagnosis is important, infants born to HIV-positive mothers are normally screened at birth and at 2, 6, 12 and 26 weeks after birth.

Prevention

Pregnant women are routinely screened for anti-HIV antibodies. Infected cases are treated with antiretroviral drugs; Caesarean section if antiviral therapy fails to suppress maternal viral load; newborns are also treated with antiretroviral drugs; breast-feeding is contraindicated.

Hepatitis B virus (HBV)

Epidemiology

Worldwide, vertical transmission is the most important route of infection of HBV. Acquisition rates vary according to hepatitis Be antigen status of the mother (70–90% if the mother is HBeAg-positive and 10–40% if HBeAg-negative). Transmission can occur *in utero*, but is usually perinatal.

Clinical features

Neonatal infection is often sub-clinical, but 90% of infected infants will become chronic carriers, with a high risk of subsequent cirrhosis and liver cancer.

Laboratory diagnosis

Detection of seromarkers of hepatitis B (especially surface antigen (HBsAg)) in neonatal blood.

Prevention

Pregnant women are routinely screened for HBsAg. Hepatitis B vaccination for all babies born to hepatitis B-infected mothers; administration of specific HBV immunoglobulin in addition to babies whose mothers are not anti-HBe-positive.

Enteroviruses

Neonatal enterovirus infection is a serious disease, with high mortality rates (>10%). Infections may be acquired perinatally or postnatally: the significance of congenital enterovirus infections is controversial. Clinical presentation includes fever, vomiting, maculopapular rash and signs of meningitis. Later manifestations may include hepatic necrosis, myocarditis and encephalitis. Diagnosis is by isolation of viruses or detection of viral RNA by PCR in throat swabs, nasopharyngeal aspirate (NPA), stools or CSF. Treatment is mainly symptomatic.

Maternal infections and perinatal infections

Postpartum maternal infections are not usually an indication to investigate or treat neonates who are clinically well. However, it is advisable to observe the neonate closely for the development of signs of infection during the first few days of life. The main exception is where the mother has puerperal sepsis with *Streptococcus pyogenes* (group A β-haemolytic *Streptococcus*): because of the risk of transmission of life-threatening infection to the baby, antibiotic prophylaxis or treatment is always indicated.

Human immunodeficiency virus

Kaveh Manavi
University Hospitals Birmingham NHS Foundation Trust, Birmingham, UK

Definitions

HIV is a RNA retrovirus with close genetic links with simian immunodeficiency viruses (SIV) that infect different species of primates in Africa. Most SIV are non-pathogenic in their natural hosts.

HIV viral anatomy

Each viral particle contains two short viral RNA chains and at least three viral enzymes; reverse transcriptase, integrase and protease. Viral particles contain an outer layer that is penetrated by pin-like viral structures. These structures are glycoproteins (gp) and are a combination of gp-120 (as the head of the pin) and gp-41 (as the stem of the pin), which play an important role in HIV attachment to target cells.

HIV life cycle and associated antiretroviral agents

The replication cycle of HIV-1 is outlined in Figure 41.1. HIV only infects cells that express CD4 and one type of chemokine receptor (CCR5 or CXCR4) on their surface. Attachment of gp-120 to CD4 receptor leads to a structural re-configuration of gp-120; exposing gp-41 to the cell membrane. This results in the formation of a tunnel in the membrane, through which HIV genome (RNA) and enzymes cross and enter into the cytoplasm. Agents that prevent HIV attachment to its host (target) cells are called entry inhibitors. Some may block gp-41 (e.g. enfuvertide) while others may block chemokine receptors (e.g. maraviroc).

Medical Microbiology and Infection Lecture Notes, Fifth Edition. Edited by Tom Elliott, Anna Casey, Peter Lambert and Jonathan Sandoe.
© 2011 Blackwell Publishing Ltd. Published 2011 by Blackwell Publishing Ltd.

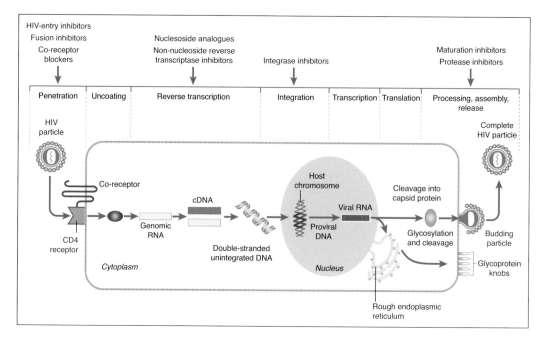

Figure 41.1 The replication cycle of HIV-1. The sites of action for the existing and investigational antiretroviral agents are shown. cDNA – complementary DNA; mRNA – messenger RNA. From Veldkamp, P. et al. Antiretroviral Therapy in HIV-1. *Atlas of Infectious Diseases.* © Springer Science and Business Media 2008.

Once inside the cytoplasm, reverse transcription occurs, the viral RNA acting as a template for a complementary DNA molecule utilising the HIV-specific enzyme reverse transcriptase. Therapeutic agents, synthetic nucleotides (phosphorylated nucleoside) and non-nucleotide inhibitors can be used to interfere with this process (see Chapter 22).

In the absence of antiretroviral agents, the completed HIV DNA chain migrates inside the host cell's nucleus and through a complex process becomes integrated into the cell's DNA. The process involves viral integrase amongst other factors. Agents that block viral integrase can stop HIV's life cycle at this stage and are called integrase inhibitors (see Chapter 22).

In the absence of integrase inhibitors, viral DNA is transcribed into chains of RNA that cross the nucleus and enter host cell's cytoplasm. Translation of viral RNA into its building blocks takes place in the cell's endoplasmic reticulum and free ribosomes inside the cytoplasm. The viral product of endoplasmic reticulum is gp-160 that is cleaved in the Golgi apparatus by cellular proteases into gp-41 and gp-120.

Viral maturation involves a complex process in which two viral RNA chains become enclosed in the host cell's membrane and bud off from its surface into the blood. During this process HIV protease is involved in cleaving reverse transcriptase, integrase and protease from a single transcribed protein containing each of these viral enzymes. At the end of the maturation process, the new viral particle is capable of infecting new cells. Protease inhibitors stop HIV protease and prevent maturation of new viral particles, making them incapable of infecting new cells.

Epidemiology

World Health Organisation data show that in 2008, 33.4 million people had HIV, 2 million died of HIV related illnesses and 2.7 million (including 430,000 children younger than 15 years) became infected with the virus. In the UK, it has been estimated that 83,000 individuals had HIV and 27% were unaware of their diagnosis in 2009.

Routes of HIV transmission

HIV is a blood borne virus that can be transmitted sexually, which is the main route of ongoing epidemics. Historically, sexual transmission of HIV was mostly reported amongst men who have sex with men (MSM) in developed nations. Heterosexual transmission of HIV has been the main route of its transmission amongst developing nations.

In the UK, heterosexual transmission of HIV has been the main route of transmission since 2000. This trend has been mostly (but not exclusively) related to immigration of people from sub-Saharan African countries.

HIV can also be transmitted during pregnancy and delivery from an infected mother to the child. However, successful antenatal screening programmes in many countries have significantly reduced the rate of mother to child transmission.

Because of robust screening programmes and inactivation processes, transmission of HIV through blood products in the UK has also been extremely low since 1993.

Sharing of injection equipment between intravenous drug users (IVDU) is another identified route of HIV transmission.

Pathogenesis

HIV infected CD4-containing lymphocytes are no longer able to function, leading to severe disruption in the immune response to infections, especially those requiring cellular immunity.

Clinical features

Figure 41.2 outlines HIV copies and CD4 counts in a human over the course of a treatment-naive HIV infection. Acute infection with HIV may present with non-specific symptoms and signs of viral illnesses and therefore may be misdiagnosed. These include fever, erythematous or maculopapular rash, pharyngitis, myalgia, lymphadenopathy, headache and asymptomatic meningitis in rare cases. The acute phase of HIV infection lasts for about 12 weeks, after which patients remain asymptomatic for an average of 8 years (latency period of HIV infection). During this latency period patients retain a stable CD4 count, despite having a high HIV

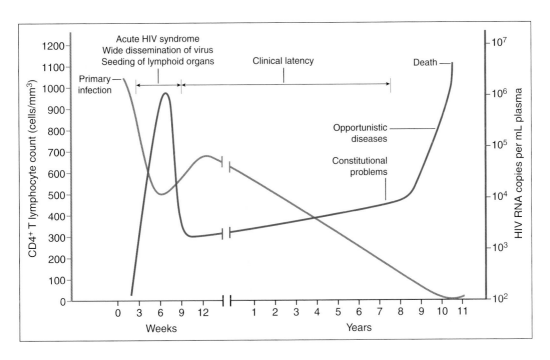

Figure 41.2 HIV copies and CD4 counts in a human over the course of a treatment-naive HIV infection.

Table 41.1 AIDS defining illnesses

Bacterial Infections	Mycobacterium avium complex
	Disseminated Tuberculosis
	Disseminated or extrapulmonary Mycobacterial (other species) infection
	Recurrent *Salmonella* septicaemia
Fungal Infections	*Pneumocystis jiroveci* pneumonia (formerly *Pneumocystis carinii*)
	Candidiasis of bronchi, trachea or lungs
	Oesophageal candidiasis
	Disseminated or extrapulmonary coccidioidomycosis.
	Extrapulmonary cryptococcosis, extrapulmonary
Protozoal infections	Chronic intestinal cryptosporidiosis (for >1 month)
	Disseminated or extra-pulmonary histoplasmosis
	Toxoplasmosis of the brain
	Chronic intestinal isosporiasis (for >1 month)
Viral infections	Cytomegalovirus disease (other than liver, spleen or lymph nodes)
	Chronic ulcer(s) (for >1 month); bronchitis, pneumonitis or oesophagitis caused by Herpes Simplex Virus
	Progressive multifocal leukoencephalopathy
Malignancy	Invasive cervical cancer
	Kaposi's sarcoma (Figure 41.3)
	Immunoblastic or primary brain Burkitt's Lymphoma,
Others/general	HIV-related encephalopathy
	Recurrent pneumonia
	Wasting syndrome due to HIV

viral load. At the end of latency, HIV viral load starts to increase exponentially, whilst patients' CD4 count starts to decline. Unless treated with antiretroviral agents, patients become immuno-compromised and at risk of developing acquired immunodeficiency syndrome (AIDS)-defining illnesses.

AIDS defining illnesses are infections and malignancies strongly associated with immuno-compromised HIV infected patients. Table 41.1 summarises the list of these conditions. It is important to ensure patients with any AIDS-defining illnesses are tested for HIV. Description of each of the AIDS-defining illnesses is outside the scope of the current chapter.

Prophylaxis

Correctly and consistently used male latex con-doms are the most effective method for prevention of sexual transmission of HIV.

Prevention of mother to child (MTC) HIV trans-mission relies on early diagnosis of HIV infected mothers, early commencement of highly active antiretroviral therapy (HAART), caesarean section for mothers with detectable plasma HIV viral load at the time of delivery, and avoidance of breast feeding of the infant. Through the above

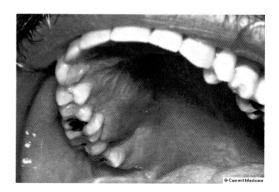

Figure 41.3 Oral Kaposi sarcoma.

approaches, the rate of MTC transmission of HIV has declined to 1.2% in the UK.

Needle exchange programmes and methadone replacement therapy has resulted more recently in a low rate of HIV infection amongst IVDU in the UK and now accounts for approximately only 2% of new HIV diagnoses.

Male circumcision has been shown to reduce the rate of HIV infection amongst heterosexual men in Africa and is the second most effective HIV preventive measure after use of male latex condoms. Male circumcision does not reduce rate of HIV transmission amongst MSM or women.

Some data suggest that patients on HAART with undetectable plasma viral load may not transmit HIV infection. It has therefore been proposed that universal voluntary HIV testing, identification of most HIV infected patients and immediate HAART, combined with present prevention approaches, could help control HIV epidemics in the future.

In most developed countries, post-exposure prophylaxis after sexual exposure (PEPSE) is also available. PEPSE policies are based on provision of HAART within 72 hours after exposure to HIV infection. The duration of treatment is usually 28 days. PEPSE should not replace consistent condom use.

Post-exposure prophylaxis after occupational exposures has been offered for more than 10 years and involves commencing HAART regimes within 72 hours of significant injuries sustained at health settings from HIV infected patients (e.g. needle stick injuries).

Novel preventive interventions, such as use of vaginal gel preparation of tenofovir, and pre-exposure prophylaxis (PreP) for HIV, have produced encouraging results in reducing sexual transmission of HIV to women and men who have sex with men, respectively. Further development of an HIV vaccine has also received a major boost after 30% reduction of HIV transmission by use of two experimental HIV vaccines in a study carried out in Thailand.

Laboratory diagnosis

- *Serology, including immunoassays for HIV antigen (p24) and antibody.* There is an interval between infection and development of detectable amounts of anti-HIV antibodies during which HIV infected patients may test antibody negative.

More recent HIV assays detect HIV antibodies and HIV antigen (p24) simultaneously.

- *Identification of HIV RNA in plasma.* This is a nucleic acid amplification test (NAAT) that involves amplification and detection of HIV RNA. Patients with acute HIV may only have a positive HIV RNA test, so it is therefore important to confirm their HIV infection within a week with immunoassays.
- *Point of care (POC) HIV assays.* which can produce reliable results within 20 minutes have been developed. They require only blood drops from finger pricks, or saliva. The advent of POC HIV assays has improved the uptake of HIV tests in certain settings. All positive POC tests need to be confirmed by laboratory based HIV tests.

Treatment

The advent of HAART has revolutionised the prognosis of HIV infected patients; turning a fatal infection into a chronic infection. Until 1996, antiretroviral agents were used alone in HIV infected patients. The use of combination antiretroviral drugs was subsequently shown to be superior. HAART regimens have been modified as more data has become available.

Surrogate markers in HIV medicine and commencement of HAART

CD4 count is used to determine when to commence HAART. Following commencement, patients need to take HAART indefinitely. Late start of HAART may lead to immunosuppression and development of AIDS. Current guidelines suggest that patients with a CD4 count of less than $350\,cells/mm^3$ should be on HAART. Once started, the aim for any patient on HAART is to have a plasma HIV viral load of less than $50\,copies/mL$.

Resistance assay

Poor adherence to HAART will result in sub-optimal drug concentrations subsequently allowing HIV replication under the influence of only one agent to which it will become resistant.

Resistance tests are able to detect certain mutations in HIV that make antiretroviral agents ineffective. With a patient's resistance profile, virologists and HIV physicians are able to predict treatment response to antiretroviral agents and to propose the most effective HAART combinations. It is therefore prudent to start a HAART regime only after consideration of the HIV resistance profile.

The impact of poor adherence to HAART

Because of the risk of resistance to any HAART regime, patients must be adherent. This requires strong and sustained motivation and commitment that depend on patients' social and mental status at any time.

Is HAART cost effective?

Provision of HIV care is expensive mainly, because of the cost of antiretroviral drugs. Studies suggest that HAART is cost effective and should be widely available to infected patients.

Despite marked improvement in survival of HIV infected patients more than a decade after use of HAART, it is too early to predict the long-term prognosis of HIV infected patients.

Miscellaneous viral infections

John Cheesbrough
Lancashire Teaching Hospitals NHS Trust, Preston, UK

Arboviruses

Arboviruses (**Ar**thropod **bo**rne virus) are so-named to reflect the role that blood-sucking arthropods (insects and ticks) play as transmission vectors in nature. Humans are the main, natural host for only a few arboviruses. For most, their maintenance in nature depends on a vertebrate host, often a bird or rodent with humans acting as incidentally infected 'dead-end' hosts. Domestic animals, if infected, can act as 'amplifying hosts'; increasing the risk to humans via shared arthropod vectors.

The disease spectrum in the vertebrates varies from clinically inapparent infection, commonly the case in natural hosts, to severe disease and death.

Vector control and avoidance of insect bites (clothing, DEET insecticide, 'mosquito' netting when sleeping) can reduce the risk of infection with all of these viruses, while vaccination offers further protection to some.

All medically important arboviruses are members of three families of single stranded RNA viruses: *Togaviridae*, *Flaviviridae* and *Bunyaviridae*.

Dengue fever

Virus

Genus: Flavivirus in the family Flaviviridae; four serotypes: Dengue 1, 2, 3 and 4.

Epidemiology

- Transmitted by mosquitoes, especially *Aedes aegypti*; which bites mainly during daylight hours;
- Humans are the main host;
- Predominantly an urban disease with regular epidemics;
- Once infected humans acquire long-term type-specific immunity, which may then enhance the severity of later infection with a different serotype;
- The most important arboviral cause of disease and death in humans and a common cause of fever in travellers returning from endemic areas;
- The disease is endemic in subtropical and tropical regions of the world, especially the Indian sub-continent, Southeast Asia and Central America;
- It has spread rapidly over the last 30 years and is estimated to infect 50 million people annually.

Medical Microbiology and Infection Lecture Notes, Fifth Edition. Edited by Tom Elliott, Anna Casey, Peter Lambert and Jonathan Sandoe.

Clinical features

Incubation period 4–10 days. Majority of infections are asymptomatic. Clinical disease characterised by abrupt onset of high fever, headache, nausea, vomiting and severe back pain. Facial swelling and widespread maculopapular rash may be present. Most cases resolve after 5–7 days. However, others, despite defervescence, remain unwell, with vomiting and abdominal pain. Widespread oedema and/or mucosal bleeding develops, heralding the onset of severe dengue with shock and/or haemorrhage. Leukopenia develops, platelet levels fall and haematocrit rises as intravascular fluid is lost into the tissues. There is a 1–2% overall mortality, with survivors usually starting to improve after 48 hours.

Diagnosis

- Antigen detection in blood; by EIA; IgM and IgG antibodies in blood;
- Nucleic acid amplification tests on blood;
- Virus isolation only in specialised laboratories.

Treatment and prevention

- Symptomatic treatment with early fluid replacement in severe disease. Prevention by vector control. Vaccines are under development and may be commercially available by 2015.

Yellow fever

Virus

Genus: Flavivirus.

Epidemiology

Transmitted by mosquitoes, major vertebrate host is the monkey.
  Three transmission cycles:

1 *Sylvatic (Jungle) cycle*: between mosquitoes and monkeys. Humans only occasionally infected when venturing into the forest.
2 *Intermediate*: This accounts for the majority of human infections. Once infection has been introduced by forest mosquitoes from monkeys into humans, onward transmission by semi-domestic mosquitoes sustains the epidemic.
3 *Urban yellow fever cycle*: Transmission between humans maintained by domestic mosquitoes, mainly *Aedes aegypti*.
  - It is estimated that around 200,000 cases occur annually, with 30,000 deaths (WHO 2010). Most of these are in West Africa.
  - The disease occurs in the tropics on both sides of the Atlantic.
  - Mosquito control terminated urban yellow fever in the western hemisphere, but an average of 100 cases/year of jungle yellow fever are still reported.
  - In Africa, regular outbreaks of intermediate disease, mainly in villages in humid parts of West Africa, have increased over the last 20 years.

Clinical features

Incubation period is 3–6 days. There are two phases of the disease; an initial non-specific phase of fever, headache, muscle pain and nausea lasting 3–4 days. After a brief period of recovery, about 15% of cases go on to a second severe toxic phase with a high fever, vomiting and jaundice. Bleeding from GI tract, nose, mouth, skin and eyes can occur and renal failure ensue. Survival at this stage is 50%.

Diagnosis

- Histology and immunocytochemistry at autopsy;
- IgM or IgG antibodies in blood;
- Nucleic acid amplification tests on blood;
- Virus isolation only in specialised laboratories.

Treatment and prevention

Symptomatic and supportive treatment only. Vector control. A highly effective live attenuated vaccine (17D vaccine) is available for travellers to endemic areas and for use in response to outbreaks.

Japanese encephalitis

Virus

Genus: Flavivirus; three genotypes.

Epidemiology

- Transmitted by mosquitoes, mainly *Culex* spp., between wild birds, the natural host;

- Domestic pigs can become infected, amplifying the reservoir of infected mosquitoes, which then bite humans;
- Humans are a dead-end host;
- Endemic in an area stretching from Southern Japan and Korea across China into Southeast Asia and to the Indian Sub-continent;
- The leading cause of viral encephalitis in Asia with 30,000–50,000 reports annually.

Clinical features

Incubation period is 5–15 days. Whilst most cases are sub-clinical or just a non-specific fever, 1–2% present as an aseptic meningitis or meningoencephalitis.

Complications

Twenty-five percent of encephalitis cases die rapidly and 30% will be left with varying degrees of permanent neuropsychiatric sequelae.

Diagnosis

- IgM antibodies in blood and cerebrospinal fluid (CSF);
- IgG may be positive, due to prior sub-clinical infection and not relevant to current illness;
- Nucleic acid amplification tests on blood (this will detect some early IgM negative cases);
- Virus isolation only in specialised laboratories.

Treatment and prevention

Treatment is symptomatic. A killed vaccine is widely used in endemic areas and for travellers. Vector control.

West Nile

Virus

Genus: Flavivirus.

Epidemiology

- Transmitted by mosquitoes, especially *Culex* spp;
- Hosts include birds, domestic and wild animals, humans and sub-human primates;
- Humans are a dead-end host;

- No person-to-person transmission occurs, but transmission through blood and organ donations and intrauterine transmissions has been reported;
- The virus is found throughout Africa, Asia, Europe, the USA and Canada. Spread into western hemisphere occurred in 1999 with an outbreak causing 7 deaths in New York and is now endemic across North America.

Clinical features

Incubation period 2–14 days. The majority (80%) of infections are sub-clinical. A non-specific mild febrile illness is usual in the remainder, but aseptic meningitis or more serious meningoencephalitis occurs in 0.7% of patients. These severe infections are more common in patients over the age of 50 years.

Diagnosis

- IgM antibodies in blood and CSF;
- Nucleic acid amplification is not useful in clinical cases, because viraemia is brief but it is used to screen blood products and prevent transmission by blood transfusion (all blood donated in the USA is tested by this method);
- Virus isolation only in specialised reference laboratories.

Treatment and control

Treatment is symptomatic. No vaccine available. Prevention is by vector control and blood donation screening in USA

Chikungunya

Virus

Genus *Alphavirus*, in the family *Togavirida*.

Epidemiology

- Transmission is by mosquito, mainly *Aedes aegypti*, a domestic daytime biting mosquito.
- Primary host is humans. Monkeys and possibly other animals may also be reservoirs.
- Infections occur in Africa, Indian subcontinent and Southeast Asia. Large epidemics are a feature of this infection, often with long gaps (7–20 years) between peaks of activity.

- Outbreaks in Italy in 2006 reflect its transmission by an *Aedes albopictus* 'Asian Tiger mosquito', whose range has increased recently.

Clinical features

Incubation period 2–12 days, typically 3–7 days. Sudden onset of fever, headache, fatigue, nausea, vomiting, muscle pain, rash and joint pain. Hard to distinguish from Dengue at this stage. Fever typically resolves in 5–7 days. Infection confers long-term immunity.

Complications

Joint pains, (can be severe) and fatigue can continue for months after acute phase resolves. Mortality is very low, as haemorrhage and shock are not features of this infection. May cause first trimester abortion and congential infections if viraemic at delivery.

Diagnosis

- IgM and IgG antibodies in blood by EIA;
- Nucleic acid amplification tests on blood;
- Virus isolation only in specialised laboratories.

Treatment and control

Symptomatic treatment only. Prolonged use of non-steroidal anti-inflammatory drugs may be required in convalescence. Avoidance of insect bites and vector control. Preventing mosquitoes biting active cases should reduce onward transmission. No vaccine is available.

Viral haemorrhagic fever viruses

Viral haemorrhagic fevers (VHF) are severe life threatening diseases caused by a range of viruses (Table 42.1). Four (bold in table) of these viruses are readily capable of person-to-person spread and therefore present a major public health risk. Diagnosis of these viruses is carried out under the highest level of bio-safety, typically only at national reference laboratories. The diagnosis must be considered in anyone with a significant febrile illness with an onset within 21 days of returning from an endemic area. Most will not have VHF, but isolation and strict barrier precautions should be maintained while a definitive diagnosis is

Table 42.1 Agents of viral haemorrhagic fevers

Agent	Source or Vector
Arenaviridae	
Lassa fever	Rodents
Argentine haemorrhagic fever (Junin)	Rodents
Bolivian haemorrhagic fever (Machupo)	Rodents
Venezuelan haemorrhagic fever (Guanarito)	Rodents
Brazil (Sabia)	unknown
Zambia (Lujo virus)	unknown
Bunyaviridae	
Crimean–Congo haemorrhagic fever	Ticks
Haemorrhagic fever with renal syndrome (Hantaan viruses)	Rodents
Rift Valley fever	Mosquitoes
Filoviridae	
Ebola	Unknown
Marburg	Unknown
Falviviridae	
Dengue types 1–4	Mosquitoes
Yellow fever	Mosquitoes
Kyasanur Forest disease	Ticks
Omsk haemorrhagic fever	Ticks
Togaviridae	
Chikungunya	Mosquitoes

sought, to minimise risk of transmission in hospital.

Lassa fever

Virus

Member of the Arenaviridae family of viruses.

Epidemiology

- The natural reservoir is the rat *Mastomys natalensis*.
- The virus causes a persistent asymptomatic infection in this rat, which freely excretes Lassa virus in urine and other body fluids throughout its life.
- Humans become infected through contact with infected rodents or their excreta.

- Person-to-person transmission can occur in overcrowded conditions, particularly in hospitals, with suboptimal infection control precautions.
- There is an estimated up to 500,000 cases annually, with 5,000 deaths.
- Lassa is endemic in West Africa, with outbreaks reported mainly in Sierra Leone and Nigeria.

Clinical features

Incubation period is 5–21 days. Spectrum of disease ranges from sub-clinical to fulminating fatal infection. Symptomatic patients typically present with fever, sore throat, myalgia, abdominal pain and vomiting lasting between 7 and 17 days.

Complications

Haemorrhages, deafness (in 30% acutely and persistent in 10%), encephalitis and spontaneous abortion. Mortality rate is between 1 and 2%.

Diagnosis

- Antigen detection in blood by EIA;
- IgM and IgG antibodies in blood by EIA or IFAT. IgG antibodies may reflect past exposure;
- Nucleic acid amplification tests on blood;
- Virus isolation only in specialised laboratories.

Treatment and prevention

Intravenous ribavirin within 6 days of onset of illness.
Oral ribavarin may be used for prophylaxis in close contacts with needlestick injury.
No vaccine available.

Ebola and Marburg haemorrhagic fever

Virus

Members of the Filoviridae family of viruses.

Epidemiology

- No natural reservoir has been identified and their natural history is unknown.

- Recent serological studies have implicated various bats species as possible hosts.
- The viruses are endemic in Africa with most recent cases from central African countries.
- A large outbreak of Ebola with 425 cases in 2000/1 occurred in Uganda. Marburg only gives rise to infrequent sporadic cases.
- They cause severe infection in non-human primates (chimpanzees, gorillas, monkeys) and contact with dead primates appears to have initiated some human outbreaks.
- During outbreaks, humans are infected through close contacts with either infected patients or infected material, such as needles, blood or secretions.

One subtype of Ebola "Reston" is endemic in the Phillipines and causes outbreaks of disease in captive monkeys but only sub-clinical infection in humans. A reservoir in pigs and pig-human transmission has been reported for this subtype.

Clinical features

Incubation period is 2–21 days. Infections are always symptomatic, starting abruptly with fever, headache, myalgia, arthralgia, conjunctivitis, sore throat, abdominal pain, nausea and vomiting.

Complications

Haemorrhages, encephalitis. Mortality rate is between 55 and 88%.

Diagnosis

- Antigen detection in blood by EIA;
- IgM antibodies in blood by EIA;
- Nucleic acid amplification tests on blood;
- Virus isolation only in specialised laboratories.

Treatment and prevention

Treatment is symptomatic. No vaccine available.

Crimean–Congo haemorrhagic fever

Virus

Member of the Bunyaviridae family of viruses.

Epidemiology

- Vector is the ixodid tick.
- Hosts include humans, domestic and wild animals.
- Humans become infected through tick bites or contact with blood, tissue or excreta of infected animals.
- The virus is distributed over Eastern Europe, (particularly in the former Soviet Union) around the Mediterranean, in northwestern China, Africa, the Middle East and the Indian subcontinent.
- Animal herders and slaughterhouse workers are at greatest risk.
- Person-to-person spread is usually confined to healthcare workers looking after severe cases.

Clinical features

Incubation period is 1–14 days. Sudden onset of fever, severe headache, sore throat, nausea and vomiting, general fatigue and malaise. Flushed face, injected conjunctiva and palatal petechiae may be seen.

Complication

Bleeding tendency from venepuncture sites, epistaxis, haematuria, haematemesis and melaena from day 4 of illness onwards. Mortality rate is 9–50%.

Diagnosis

- Antigen detection in blood by EIA;
- IgM and IgG antibody in blood by EIA;
- Nucleic acid amplification tests on blood;
- Virus isolation only in specialised Laboratories.

Treatment and prevention

Treatment is generally symptomatic and supportive. The antiviral drug ribavirin is active *in vitro* and has shown some benefit particularly if given within 5 days of onset.

Vector control in risk occupations. No vaccine available.

Part 4

Self-assessment

Self-assessment questions

Some questions may have more than one correct answer.

Chapter 1 Basic bacteriology

1.1 Which one of the following statements concerning the basic structure of bacterial cells is incorrect?

A   Most bacteria are surrounded by a rigid cell envelope (cell wall) containing peptidoglycan.

B   The cell membrane of bacteria does not contain sterols, which are found in mammalian cell membranes.

C   Bacterial DNA is contained within the nucleus, surrounded by a nuclear membrane.

D   Some bacteria are motile, their movement being controlled by rotating flagella.

E   Some bacteria form spores that are highly resistant to harsh environmental conditions, such as heat, UV light and desiccation.

1.2 Which of the following statements concerning bacterial cells is incorrect?

A   Lipopolysaccharide is a component of the cell envelope of Gram-positive bacteria.

B   Some bacteria produce capsules that usually 'contain' polysaccharides, which surround the cells and provide a protective layer.

C   In some bacteria (e.g. *Streptococcus pneumoniae*) the capsular material varies in composition and can be used in serotyping to distinguish between different types of the same species of microorganism.

D   Some bacteria can stick to the surface of materials and grow to form a biofilm that is highly resistant to treatment with antibiotics.

E   Fimbriae are thin, hair-like structures produced on the surface of some bacteria, enabling them to adhere to host tissues.

1.3 Which of the following statements concerning the growth of bacteria in laboratory media is incorrect?

A   All bacteria can be cultured in laboratory media, but certain microorganisms require specific nutrients to be supplied.

B   Bacteria that grow only in the presence of oxygen are called obligate aerobes, those growing only in the absence of oxygen are called obligate anaerobes, and those growing in the presence or absence of oxygen are called facultative anaerobes.

C   Some bacteria, including *Neisseria meningitidis* and *Campylobacter jejuni*, require additional CO_2 for laboratory growth.

D   Mannitol salt agar plates are an example of selective growth media used for the recovery and growth of staphylococci from clinical samples.

E   Chocolate agar, containing lysed blood, is an enriched growth medium used for culture of some bacteria that have special growth requirements supplied by the blood.

Chapter 2 Classification of bacteria

Select the correct options describing each of the following microorganisms:

2.1 *Staphylococcus aureus* is a: Gram-positive/Gram-negative, spore-forming/non-spore-

Medical Microbiology and Infection Lecture Notes, Fifth Edition. Edited by Tom Elliott, Anna Casey,
Peter Lambert and Jonathan Sandoe.
© 2011 Blackwell Publishing Ltd. Published 2011 by Blackwell Publishing Ltd.

forming, coagulase-positive/coagulase-negative, coccus/bacillus, capable of growth under aerobic/anaerobic/aerobic and anaerobic conditions.

2.2 *Escherichia coli* **is a**: Gram-positive/Gram-negative, spore-forming/non-spore-forming, coccus/bacillus, capable of growth under aerobic/anaerobic/aerobic and anaerobic conditions.

2.3 *Clostridium difficile* **is a:** Gram-positive/Gram-negative, spore-forming/non-spore-forming, coccus/bacillus, capable of growth under aerobic/anaerobic/aerobic anaerobic conditions.

Chapter 3 Staphylococci

3.1 Identify which of the following properties can be used to distinguish *Staphylococcus aureus* from other potentially pathogenic staphylococci:
  A Coagulase
  B DNAase
  C Protein A
  D Haemolysins
  E Toxic shock syndrome toxin (TSST)

3.2 With which of the following infections is *S. saprophyticus* usually associated?
  A Endocarditis
  B Urinary tract infection
  C Osteomyelitis
  D Skin infection
  E Respiratory tract infection

3.3 Which of the following statements concerning the sensitivity of staphylococci to antibiotics is incorrect?

  A Flucloxacillin is used to treat many *S. aureus* infections.
  B MRSA isolates (meticillin resistant *S. aureus*) are sensitive to flucloxacillin.
  C Some *S. epidermidis* isolates are resistant to flucloxacillin.
  D MRSA and *S. epidermidis* are usually sensitive to vancomycin.
  E *S. epidermidis* is sensitive to novobiocin.

Chapter 4 Streptococci and enterococci

4.1 Which one of the following statements about the streptococci is incorrect?

  A They are Gram-positive microorganisms.
  B They commonly exhibit haemolysis when cultured on blood agar.
  C They produce spores.
  D They commonly cause respiratory tract infections.
  E Infections caused by streptococci are commonly treated with penicillin.

4.2 Which one of the following statements about the enterococci is correct?

  A They are commensals of the gastrointestinal tract.
  B They are always non-haemolytic.
  C They are obligate anaerobes.
  D All species are motile.
  E They are always sensitive to vancomycin.

Chapter 5 Clostridia

5.1 Which two statements about clostridia are correct?
  A They are Gram-negative bacilli.
  B They are obligate aerobes.
  C They produce spores.
  D Patients infected with *Clostridium perfringens* may present with 'lockjaw'.
  E Clostridial infections are often treated with penicillin and/or metronidazole.

5.2 Which two statements about *Clostridium difficile* are correct?

  A The use of certain antibiotics is a risk factor for development of infection with this microorganism.
  B It produces 4 major toxins (A, B, C and D).
  C Infection with *C. difficile* is often treated with IV vancomycin.
  D It colonises the intestine of 50% of healthy adults.
  E It is a significant cause of healthcare-associated infection.

Chapter 6 Other Gram-positive bacteria

6.1 Which two statements about *Bacillus* are correct?
  A *Bacillus* species are spore-producing obligate anaerobes.

B   *B. anthracis* is non-motile, allowing it to be distinguished from other *Bacillus* species.

C   It is safe to handle *B. anthracis* in an open laboratory.

D   No vaccine exists for *B. anthracis*.

E   *B. cereus* is an important cause of food poisoning.

6.2 Which two statements regarding coryne-bacteria are correct?

A   Colonies of *C. diphtheriae* appear green on Hoyle's tellurite medium.

B   Diphtheria is common in developed countries.

C   All *C. diphtheriae* subspecies produce the diphtheria exotoxin.

D   In developed countries, children are routinely immunised with a toxoid vaccine.

E   Several species of *Corynebacterium* are skin commensals.

6.3 Which one of the following statements re-garding *Listeria* is incorrect?

A   *Listeria monocytogenes* can cause out-breaks of food poisoning.

B   They can be distinguished from other Gram-positive bacilli by their character-istic 'tumbling' motility at $<30°C$ in broth cultures.

C   They are intracellular pathogens, which can survive within phagocytic cells.

D   *Listeria monocytogenes* produce a haemolysin.

E   It is safe for laboratory staff who are pregnant to work with suspected cultures of *Listeria*.

6.4 Which two of the following statements about these other Gram-positive microor-ganisms are incorrect?

A   *Actinomyces* species are non-sporing bacilli.

B   *Nocardia* species are aerobic.

C   *Erysipelothrix rhusiopathiae* can cause erysipeloid cellulitis.

D   *Peptostreptococcus* species are obligate aerobes and can cause abscesses at many anatomical sites.

E   Propionibacteria are part of the normal flora of the skin.

F   *Rhodococcus equi* is an opportunistic pathogen.

G   *Tropheryma whipplei* is an intracellular pathogen, which causes disease more prevalent in females.

Chapter 7 Gram-negative cocci

7.1 Which of the following microorganisms is not a Gram-negative coccus?

A   Meningococcus

B   Gonococcus

C   Pneumococcus

D   *Moraxella catarrhalis*

E   *Veillonella* species

7.2 Which of the following statements concern-ing *Neisseria gonorrhoeae* is incorrect?

A   It is an obligate human parasite; its car-riage can be asymptomatic.

B   It can survive inside polymorphonucleo-cytes (PMNs).

C   It is oxidase- and catalase-positive.

D   Resistance to penicillin is very rare.

E   Re-infection can occur because no im-munity develops.

7.3 Which of the following statements concern-ing *Neisseria meningitidis* is incorrect?

A   Ten percent of humans are asymptom-atic carriers of the microorganism in the nasopharynx.

B   It produces capsular polysaccharides that can be used as the basis of serotyping.

C   The microorganism can be found inside polymorphonucleocytes.

D   No vaccines are available.

E   First-line treatment is penicillin or cefotaxime.

Chapter 8 Enterobacteriaceae

8.1 Give the names of 5 genera of the Enterobacteriaceae

8.2 MacConkey's agar is used to distinguish between some members of the Enterobac-teriaceae; which of the following genera give pink colonies on MacConkey's agar?

A   *Escherichia* only

B   *Enterobacter* only

C   *Klebsiella* only

D   *Escherichia, Enterobacter* and *Klebsiella*

E   *Salmonella, Shigella, Serratia, Proteus* and *Yersinia*

8.3 Which of the following statements correctly describes *Salmonella* spp?

A   Non-motile Gram negative rods
B   Encapsulated Gram-negative rods
C   Sensitive to acid and do not survive passage through the stomach
D   Form pale colonies with black centres on XLD agar
E   Sensitive to deoxycholate

Chapter 9 *Haemophilus* and other fastidious Gram-negative bacteria

9.1 Which of the following media will support growth of *Haemophilus influenzae* ?

A   Nutrient agar containing ATP and cAMP
B   Nutrient agar supplemented with haemin (factor X) and nicotinamide adenine dinucleotide (NAD, factor V)
C   Chocolate agar
D   Blood agar
E   MacConkey agar

9.2 Which of the following antibiotics are commonly used in empirical therapy of *Haemophilus influenzae* ?

A   Ampicillin
B   Metronidazole
C   Third-generation cephalosporins (e.g. cefotaxime or ceftriaxone)
D   Chloramphenicol
E   Flucloxacillin

9.3 Which of the following are members of the HACEK group of Gram-negative bacilli?

A   *Haemophlius influenzae*
B   *Aggregatibacter actinomycetemcomitans* (formerly *Actinobacillus actinomycetemcomitans*)
C   *Cardiobacterium hominis*
D   *Eikenella corrodens*
E   *Klebsiella pneumoniae*

9.4 Which of the following statements concerning *Bordetella pertussis* is incorrect?

A   It causes whooping cough.
B   It can be isolated from pernasal swabs on Bordet-Gengou agar.
C   It is highly transmissible and erythomycin is used to reduce infectivity.
D   The DTP triple vaccine is used to protect against whooping cough.
E   It forms resistant spores that are difficult to eradicate from the environment.

9.5 Which of the following statements about *Brucella* species are incorrect?

A   They are Gram-positive rods.
B   Infections are confined to Mediterranean countries and the Middle East.
C   Infections are acquired by ingestion of contaminated food.
D   They cannot be grown in routine blood culture systems.
E   Infections are treated with 2 weeks tetracycline and aminoglycoside.

Chapter 10 *Pseudomonas, Legionella* and other environmental Gram-negative bacilli

10.1 *Pseudomonas aeruginosa* is notable for its resistance to many antibiotics; which of the following would not be considered for treating infections caused by this microorganism?

A   Gentamicin
B   Ceftazidime
C   Amoxicillin
D   Imipenem
E   Piperacillin/tazobactam

10.2 Which of the following statements concerning *Legionella pneumophila* is incorrect?

A   It is an environmental microorganism found in soil and water.
B   It causes respiratory infections (Legionnaires' disease and Pontiac fever).
C   It can survive inside phagocytic cells and amoebae.
D   It can be cultured on nutrient agar in 2–7 days.
E   *L. pneumophila* antigen can be detected in the urine of infected patients

10.3 Which of the following properties distinguishes *Acinetobacter* species from other pseudomonads?

A   *Acinetobacter* spp. are generally more sensitive to antibiotics than other pseudomonads.
B   *Acinetobacter* spp. are oxidase-negative, other pseudomonads are oxidase-positive.
C   Unlike other pseudomonads, *Acinetobacter* spp. do not survive well in the environment.

D Unlike other pseudomonads, *Acineto-bacter* spp. require complex media for growth.

E Unlike other pseudomonads, *Acineto-bacter* spp. can growth anaerobically.

Chapter 11 *Campylobacter, Helicobacter* and vibrios

11.1 Which two statements about *Campylobacter* are incorrect?

A They are spirally curved Gram-negative bacilli.

B They are motile, with long polar flagella.

C They are the most common cause of acute bacterial enterocolitis, and infection is often caused by the handling of raw chickens or consumption of the undercooked meat.

D Human-to-human transmission is common.

E All cases of infection require antibiotic therapy.

11.2 Which two statements about *Helicobacter* are incorrect?

A *Helicobacter pylori* is the most common cause of duodenal ulceration and gastric cancer.

B Infection with *Helicobacter pylori* occurs commonly in early childhood and usually becomes chronic, often life-long.

C The prevalence of infection with *Helicobacter pylori* is low in countries with poor sanitation.

D *Helicobacter pylori* are urease positive.

E Treatment of infection often involves a proton pump inhibitor to reduce gastric acidity coupled with one antimicrobial.

11.3 Which one of the following statements about Vibrios is incorrect?

A *Vibrio cholerae* 01 is the cause of cholera, which is characterised by profuse watery diarrhoea.

B *Vibrio cholerae* is found in water and food contaminated with human faeces.

C *Vibrio cholerae* forms characteristic red colonies on thiosulphate-citrate-bile salt-sucrose agar.

D Treatment of cholera is with rehydration and often ciprofloxacin to shorten the duration of illness.

E Non-cholera *Vibrio* species may also cause diarrhoea and occasionally cause cellulitis.

Chapter 12 *Treponema, Borrelia* and *Leptospira*

12.1 Which of the following statements is incorrect?

A *Treponema, Borrelia* and *Leptospira* are all spirochaetes.

B *Treponema, Borrelia* and *Leptospira* are all helical-shaped Gram-negatives.

C Few spirochaetes can be cultured and diagnosis is usually made by serological tests.

D *Treponema pallidum* is not motile.

E Spirochaetes, like *Treponema pallidum*, can be visualised in clinical specimens by dark field microscopy.

12.2 Which of the following statements concerning tests for *Treponema pallidum* is incorrect?

A The non-specific antibody test detects antibody to lipids (cardiolipin) released from the microorganism during early infection.

B Detection of antibody to cardiolipin is specific for syphilis.

C More specific antibody tests for *T. pallidum* are available, which detect antibody to selected *T. pallidum*-derived antigens.

D *T. pallidum* subspecies *endemicum* causes bejel in children.

E *T. pallidum* subspecies *pertenue* causes yaws in children.

12.3 Which of the following microorganisms causes Lyme disease?

A *Treponema carateum*

B *Borrelia recurrentis*

C *Borrelia duttoni*

D *Borrelia burgdorferi*

E *Leptospira* spp.

Chapter 13 Gram-negative anaerobic bacilli

13.1 Which of the following bacterial genera make up the major component of the flora of the human intestine?

A *Bacteroides*

B *Prevotella*

C *Porphyromonas*
D *Fusobacterium*
E *Leptotrichia*

13.2 Which of the following microorganisms is associated with advanced periodontal disease?

A *Veillonella spp*
B *Prevotella melaninogenica*
C *Prophyromonas gingivalis*
D *Fusobacterium necrophorum*
E *Leptotrichia buccalis*

Chapter 14 Chlamydiaceae, *Rickettsia, Coxiella,* Mycoplasmataceae and Ananplasmataceae

14.1 Which two statements about the Chlamydiaceae are incorrect?

A They are obligate intracellular bacteria.
B They have three morphological forms.
C *Chlamydia trachomatis* is the most common cause of sexually transmitted infections in the developed world.
D Infection with *Chlamydia trachomatis* is often treated with doxycycline or azithromycin.
E *Chlamydophila psittaci* is also a common cause of sexually transmitted infection.

14.2 Which two of the following statements are incorrect?

A Rickettsial infections are zoonoses with a variety of insect vectors.
B *Rickettsia* cause tetanus.
C *Coxiella burnetii* causes Rocky Mountain spotted fever.
D Mycoplasmataceae have no cell wall.
E Anaplasmataceae are usually transmitted via tick bites.

Chapter 15 Basic virology

15.1 Which two of the following statements about viruses are incorrect?

A They are icosahedral, helical or more complex in shape.
B They all contain DNA.
C Viral nucleic acids can be single- or double-stranded, circular or linear, and have negative or positive polarity.
D They are obligate intracellular parasites and can be grown in cell culture.

E Viral infection is always diagnosed by direct detection of all or part of the virus.

15.2 Which of the following methods are used for the direct detection of viruses?

A Polymerase chain reaction.
B Direct immunofluorescence.
C Electron microscopy.
D Complement fixation test.
E Enzyme-linked immunosorbent antibody detection.

15.3 The incubation period of a viral infection is (select one correct answer):

A The time from acquisition of a virus to the resolution of symptoms.
B The time from onset of symptoms to resolution of symptoms.
C The time from acquisition of a virus to the onset of symptoms.
D The time it takes to cultivate a virus in the laboratory.
E The period during which an infected patient can transmit the virus.

Chapter 16 Major virus groups

16.1 Which two of the following statements about Herpesviruses are incorrect?

A Herpesviruses are non-enveloped, double stranded DNA viruses.
B Following infection, a latent infection that persists for life is established.
C Herpes simplex virus (HSV) is spread mainly via sexual activity.
D Varicella-Zoster virus (VZV) is the cause of glandular fever ('infectious mononucleosis').
E Recurrent infection with Cytomegalovirus (CMV) is common in immunocompromised patients, following solid organ or stem cell transplants.
F Epstein-Barr virus (EBV) is implicated in the pathogenesis of several tumours, including Burkitt's lymphoma.
G Human herpesvirus 8 (HHV8) can cause Kaposi's sarcoma.

16.2 Which three of the following statements about these other DNA viruses are incorrect?

A Adenoviruses and Human Papillomaviruses (HPV) are non-enveloped viruses with double stranded DNA.

B   Treatment of infection with adeno-viruses is normally symptomatic; however, cidofovir can be used in immu-nocompromised patients.

C   Parvoviruses are enveloped double-stranded DNA viruses.

D   There are four parvovirus serotypes.

E   Parvoviruses can cause spontaneous abortions and intrauterine death.

F   HPV is commonly sexually transmitted and can lead to carcinoma.

G   No vaccine for HPV is currently available.

16.3 Which one of the following statements about Influenza viruses is incorrect?

A   They are enveloped viruses.

B   There are two types of influenza virus: A and B.

C   They commonly cause respiratory infection.

D   Severe influenza infection is often treated with oseltamivir or zanamivir.

E   Influenza vaccines exist.

16.4 Which one of the following statements about Paramyxoviruses is incorrect?

A   They are enveloped viruses.

B   There is a vaccine for the prevention of infection with respiratory syncytial virus (RSV).

C   There are four serotypes of Parainfluenza virus.

D   A live attenuated virus vaccine is available for the prevention of infection with the Measles virus.

E   Infection with the Mumps virus is normally characterised by swollen parotid salivary glands.

16.5 Which two of the following statements about these other RNA viruses are incorrect?

A   Rhinoviruses, Enteroviruses, Rotaviruses, Noroviruses, Sapoviruses and the Rubella virus are non-enveloped viruses.

B   Rhinoviruses and Coronaviruses are causes of the common cold syndrome.

C   Coronaviruses and the Rabies virus are enveloped.

D   SARS is caused by a Rhinovirus.

E   Infection with Rotaviruses, Noroviruses and Sapoviruses is characterised by diarrhoea and vomiting.

F   Mortality without treatment for rabies is 100%.

16.6 Which two of the following statements about Hepatitis viruses are incorrect?

A   The Hepatitis A, B, C, D and E viruses are RNA viruses.

B   The Hepatitis A virus (HAV) and Hepatitis E virus (HEV) are acquired via the faecal-oral route and causes acute hepatitis.

C   The Hepatitis B virus (HBV) is acquired via exposure to blood and blood products containing the virus, by sexual intercourse or vertically at birth.

D   HBV and Hepatitis C virus (HCV) cause acute, chronic and fulminant hepatitis, cirrhosis and hepatocellular carcinoma.

E   Delta agent (Hepatitis D virus (HDV)) replicates only in HCV-infected cells, therefore prevention of HCV infection prevents infection with HDV.

16.7 Which three of the following statements about these retroviruses are incorrect?

A   They are single stranded RNA enveloped viruses.

B   Transmission of the Human Immunodeficiency virus (HIV) and Human T-cell lymphotropic viruses (HTLV) is mainly through the faecal-oral route.

C   Infection with HIV and the development of AIDS is characterised by profound immunosuppression and infection with a variety of microorganisms.

D   No antiretroviral drugs are available for the treatment of infection with HIV.

E   A minority of people infected with HTLV-1 may develop adult T-cell leukaemia or lymphoma.

F   Antiviral drugs are available for the treatment of infection with HTLV.

Chapter 17 Basic mycology and classification of fungi

17.1 Which two of the following statements about fungi are incorrect?

A   They are motile.

B   Most fungi that commonly cause human disease can be categorised into yeasts, moulds/filamentous or dimorphic.

C The taxonomic status of *Pneumocystis jirovecii* is well established.

D Most deep mycoses are opportunistic infections occurring in immunocompromised patients.

E Laboratory diagnosis of fungal infection is mostly by direct microscopy or microbiological culture

17.2 Which two of the following statements about yeasts are incorrect?

A Most cryptococcal infections occur in immunocompetent individuals.

B Cryptococcal species have polysaccharide capsules that can be visualised by mixing fluid specimens with Indian ink.

C *Candida albicans* is a commensal of the mouth and gastrointestinal tract.

D Cryptococcal species are the cause of 'thrush'.

E *Malassezia furfur* is the cause of pityriasis versicolor, which results in scaly skin and depigmentation.

17.3 Which one of the following statements about filamentous fungi is incorrect?

A Outbreaks of aspergillosis in immunocompromised patients have occurred, due to construction work adjacent to hospitals.

B Patients with cystic fibrosis are frequently colonised with *Aspergillus* species, which may then lead to infection.

C Dermatophytes, including the genera *Epidermophyton, Microsporum* and *Trichophyton*, often infect the lungs

D The sub-phylum mucoromycotina includes the medically important species *Rhizopus arrhizus* and *Absidia corymbifera*.

E Infection with *Fusarium* and *Scedosporium* species is often associated with inhalation or aspiration of polluted water

17.4 Which one of the following statements about dimorphic fungi is incorrect?

A Dimorphic fungi have both yeast and mould forms, depending on growth temperature.

B *Coccidioides immitis* and *C. posadasii* are causes of 'valley fever', characterised by a mild, self-limiting pneumonia.

C Granulomatous ulcers may be a complication of pulmonary infection caused by *Blastomyces dermatitidis*.

D Pulmonary infection with *Histoplasma capsulatum* always requires antifungal therapy.

E *Paracoccidioides brasiliensis* may lead to destruction of the palate and nasal septum.

Chapter 18 Parasitology: protozoa

18.1 Which of the following statements concerning *Entamoeba histolytica* is incorrect?

A It causes intestinal amoebiasis and liver abscesses.

B It is spread via water or food contaminated with cysts.

C It can be diagnosed in the laboratory by microscopic examination of freshly passed stools.

D No serological tests are available for *Entamoeba histolytica*.

E Treatment of infection by *Entamoeba histolytica* is with metronidazole.

18.2 Which of the following statements concerning *Toxoplasma gondii* is incorrect?

A Human infection can result from ingestion of the microorganism as cysts contained in cat faeces and undercooked meat.

B It can cause a glandular fever-like syndrome in immunocompetent hosts.

C It causes serious conditions, including myocarditis, choroidoretinitis and meningoencephalitis in immunocompromised hosts.

D It can be reactivated by immunosuppression.

E No serological tests are available to aid diagnosis.

18.3 Which of the following species of *Plasmodium* is responsible for malignant tertian malaria?

A *Plasmodium falciparum.*

B *Plasmodium malariae.*

C *Plasmodium vivax.*

D *Plasmodium ovale.*

E *Plasmodium knowlesi.*

18.4 Match the following microorganisms (A–E) to the diseases (F–J):

A Chagas disease

B West African sleeping sickness

C East African sleeping sickness

D Visceral leishmaniasis

E Cutaneous leishmaniasis
F *Trypanosoma brucei rhodesiense*
G *Trypanosoma brucei gambiense*
H *Leishmania donovani* complex
I *Leishmania tropica, Leishmania major* complexes and *Leishmania mexicana*
J *Trypanosoma cruzi*

Chapter 19 Parasitology: helminths

19.1 Which three of the following statements about nematodes are incorrect?

A *Ascaris lumbricoides* (roundworm) is the most common pathogenic helminth worldwide.

B Infection with *Enterobius vermicularis* (pin worm) often presents with perianal itching.

C *Toxocara canis* and *Toxocara cati* are parasites of rodents.

D Infection with *Trichuris trichiura* can present with anaemia, intestinal irritation and occasionally, anal prolapse.

E *Ancylostoma duodenale, Necator americanus* (hookworm) and *Strongyloides stercoralis* can penetrate intact skin.

F *Trichinella spiralis* infection is associated with eating shellfish.

G *Wuchereria bancrofti* and *Bruglia malayi* are filarial worms, which can cause elephantitis.

H The vector of *Loa loa* is the mosquito; *Loa loa* migrates under the conjuctiva, giving it the name 'eye worm'.

I The vector of *Onchocerca volvulus* is the black fly and can cause 'river blindness'.

J Infection with nematodes is often treated with mebendazole or albendazole.

19.2 Which two of the following statements about cestodes (tapeworms) are incorrect?

A They have either male or female reproductive organs.

B They can be up to 30 feet long.

C Cestodes have two reservoirs in their life cycle, one for larvae and one for adult worms.

D Pigs are the reservoir for *Taenia solium* larvae.

E Cows are the reservoir for *Taenia saginata* larvae.

F Crustacea and fish are the reservoirs for *Diphyllobothrium latum* larvae.

G Humans are the reservoir for *Echinococcus granulosus* adult worms.

H Rodents and humans are the reservoirs for *Hymenolepis nana* adult worms.

I Infection with cestodes is often treated with praziquantel.

19.3 Which two of the following statements about trematodes (flukes) are incorrect?

A They are flatworms with oral and ventral suckers.

B Most are hermaphrodites – schistosomes have separate male and female worms.

C They require one intermediate host.

D Infection with *Fasciola hepatica* and *Opisthorchis sinensis* may result in hepatomegaly.

E Infection with *Paragonimus westermani* is normally associated with the lungs.

F Infection with *S. mansoni* and *S. japonicum* are characterised with clinical manifestations in the bladder and *S. haematobium* in the intestine.

Chapter 20 Antibacterial agents

20.1 Which of the following statements concerning β-lactam antibiotics is incorrect?

A They act by interfering with the synthesis of the bacterial cell wall.

B They include the penicillins, cephalosporins, carbapenems and monobactams.

C Flucloxacillin is stable to many β-lactamases, but is inactive against meticillin-resistant *Staphylococcus aureus* (MRSA).

D Piperacillin is used with tazobactam to protect piperacillin from destruction by some β-lactamases.

E The monobactam, aztreonam, has a broad spectrum of antibacterial action.

20.2 Which of the following is not a member of the aminoglycoside antibiotics?

A Gentamicin.
B Streptomycin.
C Amikacin.
D Kanamycin.
E Vancomycin.

20.3 Which of the following agents is active against a wide range of anaerobic microorganisms, including bacteria (Clostridia and

Bacteroides) and protozoa (*Giardia* and *Trichomonas*)?

A Metronidazole.
B Ciprofloxacin.
C Rifampicin.
D Trimethoprim.
E Nalidixic acid.

Chapter 21 Antifungal agents

21.1 Which two of the following statements about the azoles are incorrect?
A Their mechanism of action is prevention of glucan synthesis.
B They may cause transient liver function abnormalities.
C Fluconazole, itraconazole and voriconazole are available as oral, intravenous and topical preparations.
D Voriconazole has several drug interactions and can cause visual disturbances.
E Some species of *Candida* are resistant to or have reduced susceptibility to fluconazole.

21.2 Which two of the following statements about these other antifungal agents are incorrect?

A Flucytosine and griseofulvin inhibit nucleic acid synthesis.
B Flucytosine is used as monotherapy.
C Side effects of amphotericin B include anaphylactic reactions and renal tubular damage.
D The echinocandins are available in an oral preparation.
E Terbafine may cause hepatotoxicity.

Chapter 22 Antiviral agents

22.1 Which of the following do antiviral agents inhibit?
A Virus attachment to cell receptors.
B Virus uncoating.
C Viral genome transcription.
D Virus mutation.
E Virion assembly and release.

22.2 Which of the following statements about nucleotide analogue reverse transcriptase inhibitors are incorrect?

A They are acyclic phosphonate analogues of adenosine monophosphate.

B They require phosphorylation by cellular enzymes before they can function.
C They inhibit viral DNA-dependent RNA polymerase producing chain termination.
D They must be given parenterally (by injection).
E They are active against HIV-1 and -2 and hepatitis B.

Chapter 23 Diagnostic laboratory methods

23.1 Which of the following statements about culture techniques is correct?
A Most medically important bacteria and fungi cannot be cultured in the diagnostic laboratory.
B Enriched agar media includes: horse blood, chocolate agar and CLED (cysteine lactose electrolyte deficient) agar.
C Selective agar contains an indicator (usually a dye) to allow differentiation of bacteria.
D Differential agar contains antimicrobial agents to suppress growth of normal flora from sites that are normally colonised.
E Enrichment broth is a nutritious broth, which allows recovery and enrichment of small numbers of microorganisms within a clinical sample.

23.2 Which of the following body sites are normally sterile (free from colonising bacteria)?

A Blood.
B Bone marrow.
C Subcutaneous tissue/muscle/bone.
D Cerebrospinal fluid/brain.
E Upper respiratory tract.

Chapter 24 Epidemiology, prevention of infections

24.1 Which of the following statements about protective isolation rooms are correct?
A They are designed to protect compromised patients from infection.
B They are under negative pressure.
C They have particulate filtered air.
D Hands only need to be washed on leaving the room.

E Gowns and aprons do not need to be worn in the room.

24.2 **Which of the following statements about notifiable diseases are correct?**

A Medical staff have a statutory duty to notify them.
B The CCDC should be notified.
C They include measles.
D They include *E coli* O157.
E They include all cases of meningitis.

Chapter 25 Upper respiratory tract infections

25.1 **Which of the following statements about the common cold syndrome is incorrect?**

A It is most frequently caused by Rhinoviruses.
B It occurs worldwide.
C It can be transmitted via virus-contaminated hands.
D It usually has an incubation period of 7–10 days.
E It resolves spontaneously within 7–10 days.

25.2 **Which of the following statements about laryngo-tracheobronchitis (croup) are incorrect?**

A It involves the upper and lower respiratory tract.
B It is predominantly caused by bacteria.
C It is largely restricted to children aged <5 years.
D It causes a distinctive paroxismal cough ('whooping cough').
E It should be empirically treated with antibiotics.

Chapter 26 Lower respiratory tract infections

26.1 **Which of the following statements about pneumonia are incorrect?**

A It commonly occurs without radiological shadowing.
B It is most common in summer.
C It is associated with positive blood cultures in 50% of cases.
D It is caused by *S. pneumoniae*, *Legionella* and *Mycoplasma*, which can be diagnosed by urine antigen detection.

E It is usually treated for 3–4 weeks, depending upon severity.

26.2 **Which of these statements about viral pneumonia are incorrect?**

A Primary viral pneumonia occurs mainly in children, elderly people and immunocompromised patients.
B Common causes include: respiratory syncytial virus (RSV), norovirus, rubella virus and human metapneumovirus.
C Primary viral pneumonia in adults is characterised by diffuse bilateral interstitial infiltrates on chest radiograph.
D Diagnosis of viral pneumonia is by PCR or culture of viral agents in, e.g. nasopharyngeal aspirates, throat and nasal swabs and/or bronchoalveolar lavage.
E Ribavirin is used empirically for the treatment of viral pneumonia.

Chapter 27 Tuberculosis and mycobacteria

27.1 **Which of the following statements regarding *Mycobacterium tuberculosis* are incorrect?**

A It stains well by the Gram stain.
B It can be identified in clinical samples by the ZN stain.
C It causes only chest infections.
D Associated infections need antibiotic treatment for several months.
E Infection with this microorganism can be prevented by vaccination.

27.2 **Which of the following statements about *Mycobacterium leprae* are incorrect?**

A It can cause leprosy.
B It has animal reservoirs.
C Transmission of infection with this microorganism can be from a discharge from skin lesions.
D The incubation period for infection with this microorganism is up to 10 years.
E It can cause skin lesions and also nerve involvement.

Chapter 28 Gastrointestinal infections

28.1 **Which of the following statements about *Salmonella* species are incorrect?**

A They are commonly carried by domestic and wild animals.

B Long-term asymptomatic human carriage with these microorganisms does not occur.

C The incubation period for infection with this microorganism is 18–48 hours.

D Headache, malaise and fever can be associated with infection.

E Associated infections do not cause a bacteraemia.

28.2 Which of the following statements about Cholera is incorrect?

A It is caused by *Vibrio cholerae*.

B Associated infections are spread by the faecal-oral route.

C Animals can be host carriers of the causative microorganism.

D It has a short incubation period of 1–3 days.

E If untreated has a high related mortality.

28.3 Which of the following statements about *Staphylococcus aureus* food poisoning are incorrect?

A It is associated with an enterotoxin produced by the microorganism.

B It has a short incubation period of 1–6 hours.

C It lasts for up to 7 days.

D It is caused by bacterial multiplication in the intestine.

E It can cause vomiting and diarrhoea.

28.4 Which of the following statements about Norovirus are incorrect?

A It is a cause of winter vomiting infections.

B It is carried by animals.

C It rarely spreads from patient to patient.

D It causes vomiting and diarrhoea for up to 60 hours.

E It only affects children.

Chapter 29 Liver and biliary tract infections

29.1 Which of the following statements about the Hepatitis B virus is incorrect?

A It is a DNA virus.

B Transfer can occur across the placenta.

C Needlestick injuries can transfer infection with this virus.

D Incubation period is up to 6 months.

E Liver failure is common in acute infection.

29.2 Which of the following statements about the Hepatitis C virus are incorrect?

A It is a DNA virus.

B It is commonly spread by intravenous drug abuse.

C Incubation period is up to 6 months.

D Most infected patients are symptomatic.

E Chronic infections can occur.

Chapter 30 Urinary tract infections

30.1 Which of the following microorganisms commonly cause urinary tract infections?

A *Escherichia coli*

B *Proteus mirabilis*

C *Staphylococcus saprophyticus*

D *Pseudomonas aeruginosa*

E *Staphylococcus aureus*

30.2 Which of the following are non-bacterial causes of urinary tract infections?

A Adenoviruses

B Human polyoma viruses

C *Candida albicans*

D *Trichomonas vaginalis*

E *Schistosoma haematobium*

Chapter 31 Genital infections

31.1 Which of the following statements about syphilis are incorrect?

A It is an infection caused by the spirochete, *Treponema pallidum*.

B The number of patients with primary and secondary syphilis in the UK has decreased since 2000.

C Pregnant women with untreated syphilis can pass infection to their foetus at any point during pregnancy or delivery.

D Secondary syphilis occurs 3–6 weeks after exposure and presents as punched out ulcers.

E A widespread macular rash and palmar rash are signs of primary syphilis

31.2 Which of these statements about the diagnosis of vaginitis is incorrect?

A Diagnosis of bacterial vaginosis can be made on microscopic findings alone.

B Polymorphonuclear cells in microscopy of vaginal fluid raises the possibility of TV or cervicitis.

C Microscopy of vaginal fluid can be used to diagnose *Trichomonas vaginalis*.

D Inoculation of vaginal fluid for *Trichomonas vaginalis* culture has higher sensitivity than microscopy.

E Yeast culture is the gold standard method for diagnosis of vaginal candidiasis.

Chapter 32 Infections of the central nervous system

32.1 Which of the following statements about *Neisseria meningitidis* meningitis is incorrect?

A It occurs mainly in the elderly.

B It is associated with a petechial rash.

C It can spread by respiratory droplets.

D Close contacts may need prophylactic antibiotics.

E It is mainly caused by serotype B in the UK.

32.2 Which of the following statements about meningitis is incorrect?

A It requires treatment with high dose parenteral antibiotics.

B Antibiotics should be given early.

C Steroids should not be given.

D Blood cultures should be taken.

E PCR tests on the CSF are available to confirm the diagnosis.

32.3 Which of the following statements about brain abscesses are incorrect?

A They are the second commonest central nervous system infection.

B In any patient, they are usually caused by one microorganism.

C Streptococci are the most commonly isolated pathogen.

D Patients normally have multiple rather than single abscesses.

E Treatment with antibiotics only is usually required.

Chapter 33 Bacteraemia and bloodstream infections

33.1 Which of the following statements about bloodstream infections are incorrect?

A They are usually a complication of localised infection in the body.

B They only occur in immunocompromised patients.

C They are predominantly caused by Gram-negative bacteria.

D They can result in septic shock.

E They are often diagnosed by serology.

33.2 Which of the following statements about bacteraemia are incorrect?

A It is defined as the presence of bacteria in the bloodstream.

B It may not be associated with an infection.

C It does not normally occur in everyday life.

D It always requires antibiotic treatment.

E It can result in infection.

Chapter 34 Device-related infections

34.1 Which of the following statements about intravascular catherer-related infections are incorrect?

A They are a common cause of bloodstream infections.

B They are commonly caused by coagulase-negative staphylococci.

C They are not caused by fungi.

D They are not associated with local infections at the catheter skin insertion site.

E They do not require the catheter to be removed.

34.2 Which of the following statements about prosthetic joint infections is incorrect?

A They are difficult to differentiate from mechanical loosening.

B They may cause bloodstream infections.

C They may require joint removal.

D They require long-term antibiotic treatment.

E Associated microbiological culture of tissue samples does not assist in making the diagnosis.

Chapter 35 Cardiovascular infections

35.1 Which of the following statements about infective endocarditis are incorrect?

A It is an infection of the endocardium.

B   Up to 50% of patients require valvular
     surgery.
C   It may result in vegetations forming on a
     heart valve.
D   It is most commonly caused by
     staphylococci.
E   It requires prolonged antibiotic
     treatment.

Chapter 36 Bone and joint infections

36.1 Appropriate methods for the microbiological diagnosis of osteomyelitis include:

A   Blood cultures.
B   Culture of affected bone.
C   Plain X-ray.
D   Immunofluorescence microscopy.
E   Complement fixation tests.

36.2 Which of the following statements concerning the clinical presentation of osteomyelitis are correct?

A   Clinical findings are not affected by the
     age of the patient.
B   Clinical findings are affected by the location of infection.
C   Osteomyelitis can develop slowly over a
     period of weeks to months or even years.
D   Pain is an uncommon presenting feature.
E   Fever is an uncommon presenting
     feature.

Chapter 37 Skin and soft tissue infections

37.1 Which of the following are members of the normal microbial flora of skin?

A   Coagulase negative staphylococci
B   *Staphylococcus epidermidis*
C   Diphtheroids
D   Enterococci
E   *Streptococcus pneumoniae*

37.2 Which of the following statements about cellulitis are correct?

A   It is most commonly caused by group B
     β-haemolytic streptococci and *S. aureus*.
B   It is commonly caused by *Erysipelothrix
     rhusiopathiae*.
C   It is caused by *Vibrio cholera* in the developing world.

D   Treatment with high-dose flucloxacillin
     is appropriate empirical therapy, unless
     risk factors for unusual/resistant pathogens are present.
E   When caused by MRSA, it can be treated
     with vancomycin.

Chapter 38 Infections in the compromised host

38.1 The following devices predispose to infection by bypassing normal defence mechanisms:

A   urinary catheters
B   endotracheal tubes
C   central venous catheters
D   prosthetic heart valves
E   surgical drain

38.2 Which of the following statements about immune function is incorrect?

A   T-cell Lymphoma and chronic lymphatic
     leukaemia predisposes to Varicella-
     zoster virus and *Candida* infection.
B   Neutropenia predisposes to *Staphylococcus aureus* infection.
C   Steroid therapy affects immune
     function.
D   CD 4 Lymphocyte dysfunction (e.g. HIV
     infection) predisposes to *Pneumocystis
     jirovecii* (*P. carinii*).
E   Defects in the late complement components (C7–C9) increase the risk of *Mycobacterium tuberculosis* infections.

Chapter 39 Infections caused by antimicrobial-resistant bacteria

39.1 Which of the following statements about meticillin resistant *Staphylococcus aureus* (MRSA) are incorrect?

A   Meticillin-resistance depends on a functioning mecB gene.
B   MRSA synthesises the enzyme PBP-2',
     enabling the bacterium to 'by-pass' the
     normally target of meticillin.
C   Hand hygiene does not play a role in
     reducing the spread of MRSA.
D   Prophylactic antibiotics can be used to
     prevent infection following surgery.
E   The Department of Health (in England)
     uses MRSA bacteraemia rates as a

measure of infection control performance.

39.2 Which of the following statements about vancomycin-resistant enterococci (VRE) are incorrect?

A   In the UK, infection with VRE is mostly confined to elderly care wards.

B   They use alternative cell wall precursors, thereby depriving glycopeptides of their normal target site of action.

C   VanA – the commonest resistance type.– are resistant to vancomycin, teicoplanin and daptomycin.

D   They are controlled by good hand hygiene; equipment and environmental decontamination.

E   Most *E. faecalis* (including VRE) remain susceptible to ampicillin.

Chapter 40 Perinatal and congenital infections

40.1 Which of the following statements about congenital infections are incorrect?

A   They can occur, even when the woman is asymptomatic or has subclinical illness.

B   They may result in pregnancy loss.

C   They may present months or years after birth.

D   They can be confirmed by serological tests on the mother.

E   IgG antibodies can be used to diagnose infection in an unborn baby.

40.2 Which of the following statements about toxoplasmosis are incorrect?

A   It affects about 15% of pregnancies in the UK.

B   The risk of transmission to the foetus increases from 25% in the first trimester to 65% in the third.

C   Congenital infection can cause: stillbirth, choroidoretinitis and microcephaly.

D   Acute infection is diagnosed in the mother by detection of *T. gondii* IgG antibodies.

E   Prenatal diagnosis of fetal infection can be made using PCR on amniotic fluid.

Chapter 41 Human immunodeficiency viruses

41.1 Which of the following statements about Human immunodeficiency viruses are incorrect?

A   Each viral particle contains at least three enzymes: reverse transcriptase, integrase and protease.

B   In the UK, sexual transmission of HIV is most commonly reported amongst men who have sex with men.

C   The acute phase of HIV infection lasts about 12 weeks, after which patients remain asymptomatic for an average of 8 years.

D   When HIV viral load increases exponentially and patients' CD4 counts decline, patients may develop AIDS.

E   Following commencement, HIV-infected individuals need to take HAART for 6 months.

41.2 Which of the following are not AIDS-defining illnesses?

A   Disseminated tuberculosis

B   Extrapulmonary cryptococcosis

C   Invasive cervical cancer

D   Kaposi's sarcoma

E   Toxoplasmosis of the brain

Chapter 42 Miscellaneous viral infections

42.1 Which of the following statements about dengue fever are correct?

A   It is transmitted by mosquitoes.

B   Humans are not the main host.

C   It is endemic in southern Europe.

D   It is a rare infection worldwide.

E   It is diagnosed in routine laboratories by viral culture.

42.2 Which of the following statements about yellow fever are incorrect?

A   It is transmitted by mosquitoes.

B   Its major host is man.

C   Most cases occur in the tropics.

D   It is associated with a high mortality.

E   No vaccine is available.

Answers to self-assessment questions

Chapter 1 Basic bacteriology

1.1 C
The key feature that distinguishes bacteria (prokaryotic cells) from mammalian cells (eukaryotic cells) is their lack of a defined and discrete nucleus. Their DNA exists as a coiled structure in the cytoplasm. See Figures 1.3 and 1.4.
1.2 A
Lipopolysaccharide is found only in the envelope of Gram-negative bacteria and is not found in Gram-positive bacteria or mycobacteria.
1.3 A
There are some bacteria that cannot be cultured in any laboratory media (e.g. *Mycobacterium leprae* and *Treponema pallidum*). Other microorganisms, such as chlamydia, only grow intracellularly and can only be grown in host cells grown in tissue culture media.

Chapter 2 Classification of bacteria

2.1 *Staphylococcus aureus* is a Gram-positive, non-spore-forming, coagulase-positive coccus, capable of growth under aerobic and anaerobic conditions.
2.2 *Escherichia coli* is a Gram-negative, non-spore-forming bacillus, capable of growth under aerobic and anaerobic conditions.
2.3 *Clostridium difficile* is a: Gram-positive, spore-forming bacillus, capable of growth under anaerobic conditions.
Key characteristics of bacteria are listed in Tables 2.2 and 2.3.

Chapter 3 Staphylococci

3.1 A, B, C
Coagulase, DNAase and protein A are characteristically produced only by *S. aureus* and are useful in distinguishing *S. aureus* from *S. saprophyticus* and coagulase negative staphylococci, such as *S. epidermidis*. Haemolysins are produced by many staphylococci and TSST is not produced by all isolates of *S. aureus*.
3.2 B
S. saprophyticus is associated with UTI in young women, and sometimes results in severe cystitis and haematuria.
3.3 B
Flucloxacillin is a β-lactamase-stable penicillin. Note that novobiocin sensitivity is useful in distinguishing between *S. saprophyticus* (resistant) and *S. epidermidis* (sensitive).

Chapter 4 Streptococci and enterococci

4.1 C
Streptococci do not produce spores.
4.2 A
On blood agar Enterococci can appear α-, β- or sometimes non-haemolytic, they are facultatively anaerobic, non-motile (except *Enterococcus casseliflavus* and *Enterococcus gallinarum*) and the emergence of 'vancomycin-resistant enterococci' (VRE) is of concern.

Medical Microbiology and Infection Lecture Notes, Fifth Edition. Edited by Tom Elliott, Anna Casey, Peter Lambert and Jonathan Sandoe.
© 2011 Blackwell Publishing Ltd. Published 2011 by Blackwell Publishing Ltd.

Chapter 5 Clostridia

5.1 C and E
Clostridia are Gram-positive bacilli, they are obligate anaerobes and 'lockjaw' is caused by *Clostridium tetani*.
5.2 A and E
C. difficile produces 2 major toxins (A and B), is often treated with oral vancomycin or metronidazole and colonises the intestine of 4% of healthy adults and 50% of healthy neonates.

Chapter 6 Other Gram-positive bacteria

6.1 B and E
Bacillus species are spore-producing aerobes; *B. anthracis* should be handled in a safety cabinet and a vaccine is available for individuals at high risk of infection.
6.2 D and E
Colonies of *C. diphtheriae* appear grey-black on Hoyle's tellurite medium, Diphtheria is uncommon in developed countries and all *C. diphtheriae* subspecies except *var. belfanti* produce the diphtheria exotoxin.
6.3 E
It is not safe for laboratory staff who are pregnant to work with suspected cultures of *Listeria*, as this microorganism can cause infection in pregnant women.
6.4 D and G
Peptostreptococcus species are anaerobic and Whipple's disease (caused by *Tropheryma whipplei*) is more prevalent in middle-aged Caucasian males.

Chapter 7 Gram-negative cocci

7.1 C
The pneumococcus is a term used for the Gram-positive microorganism, *Streptococcus pneumoniae*.
7.2 D
Resistance to penicillin is now common and resistance to quinolones is increasing. *Neisseria gonorrhoeae* remains sensitive to cephalosporins and single dose ceftriaxone is commonly used for compliance.

7.3 D
There are effective vaccines for group C and a tetravalent vaccine (for groups A, C, Y and W135).

Chapter 8 Enterobacteriaceae

8.1 Answer from the following genera: *Escherichia, Enterobacter, Klebsiella, Proteus, Serratia, Shigella, Salmonella* and *Yersinia* (Table 8.1).
8.2 D
Escherichia, Enterobacter and *Klebsiella* all ferment lactose to produce pink colonies; *Salmonella, Shigella, Serratia, Proteus* and *Yersinia* do not ferment lactose and produce pale colonies.
8.3 D
Only option D is correct. XLD (xylose lysine deoxycholate) agar is used to identify *Salmonella* spp.

Chapter 9 *Haemophilus* and other fastidious Gram-negative bacteria

9.1 B and C
Haemophilus influenzae requires haemin and NAD and it will grow on plates supplemented with these factors. NAD is not available in sufficient quantities to support growth on blood agar plates. By heating blood before making the agar plates (the process used in production of chocolate agar) both factors are available.
9.2 C
Many *Haemophilus influenzae* isolates produce β-lactamase and are not sensitive to ampicillin; they retain sensitivity to third generation cephalosporins. The other options (B, D and E) would not be appropriate.
9.3 A, B, C, D
Options A–D are all correct, these provide the first four letters of the acronym, HACEK. E is incorrect; the K letter refers to *Kingella* spp.
9.4 A, B, C, D
A–D are all correct, E is incorrect. *B. pertussis* is a Gram-negative microorganism and does not form spores.
9.5 A, B, D and E.
Brucella species are Gram-negative coccobacilli and can be grown in routine blood culture. *Brucella* infections have a worldwide distribution, but there is great variation in the incidence of infection. Such infections are treated with a tetracycline (6 weeks).

and an aminoglycoside (2–3 weeks), or tetracycline and rifampicin (6 weeks).

Chapter 10 *Pseudomonas, legionella* and other environmental gram-negative bacilli

10.1 C
Amoxicillin does not have activity against *P. aeruginosa*, because of its inactivation by β-lactamases. The third-generation cephalosporin ceftazidime retains activity, as do the carbapenems (imipenem, meropenem) and monobactams (aztreonam). Piperacillin is active when used with the β-lactamase inhibitor, tazobactam. The aminoglycosides, gentamicin and tobramycin, are still generally effective against *P. aeruginosa*.

10.2 D
Despite being found in water, it cannot be cultured on standard media such as nutrient agar; specialist media such as buffered charcoal yeast extract (BCYE) are needed, the charcoal absorbing inhibitors and yeast extract supplying essential cysteine.

10.3 B
All other statements are incorrect. *Acinetobacter* spp. are resistant to many antibiotics, they do survive in the environment, grow on minimal media and are strict aerobes.

Chapter 11 *Campylobacter, helicobacter* and *vibrio*

11.1 D and E
Human-to-human transmission is uncommon, except from young children with uncontrolled bowel actions, and only severe cases of infection require antibiotic therapy.

11.2 C and E
The prevalence of *Helicobacter pylori* is high in countries with poor sanitation, and treatment of infection often involves a proton pump inhibitor to reduce gastric acidity coupled with two antimicrobials.

11.3 C
Vibrio cholerae forms characteristic yellow colonies on thiosulphate-citrate-bile salt-sucrose agar.

Chapter 12 *Treponema, Borrelia* and *Leptospira*

12.1 D
T. pallidum is motile and motility of the microorganism is clearly seen on dark field microscopy. *Treponema, Borrelia* and *Leptospira* are all spirochaetes with helical shapes, staining as Gram-negatives, although some give a very weak stain and are difficult to see under bright field microscopy after staining.

12.2 B
Antibody to cardiolipin is also associated with conditions, including viral infections, TB, autoimmune diseases and malaria.

12.3 D
Option D is correct. A causes yaws, B and C cause relapsing fever (transmitted by ticks and lice), and E causes a range of diseases including flu-like illness; meningitis, uveitis and Weil's disease.

Chapter 13 Gram-negative anaerobic bacilli

13.1 A
Correct answer is A, *Bacteroides* species.

13.2 C
Note that the other options are also capable of causing oral infections but *Porphyromonas gingivalis* is the most important.

Chapter 14 Chlamydiaceae, *Rickettsia, Coxiella,* Mycoplasmataceae and Anaplasmataceae

14.1 B and E
The Chlamydiaceae have two distinct morphological forms, the elementary body (EB) and the reticulate body (RB), and *Chlamydophila psittaci* is not a cause of sexually transmitted infection; it is transmitted via inhalation, normally of dried bird guano.

14.2 B and C
The Rickettsiaceae cause typhus and spotted fevers, *Coxiella burnetii* causes Q-fever and Rocky Mountain spotted fever is caused by *Rickettsia rickettsii*.

Chapter 15 Basic virology

15.1 B and E
Not all viruses contain DNA, some contain RNA and viral infection can also be diagnosed by indirect detection of the virus (detection of the host response to infection).
15.2 A, B, C
15.3 C

Chapter 16 Major virus groups

16.1 A and D
Herpes viruses are enveloped, double-stranded DNA viruses and VZV is the cause of chickenpox and shingles.
16.2 C, D, G
Parvoviruses are non-enveloped single-stranded DNA viruses; there is one single parvovirus serotype and HPV vaccines are currently available and targeted at younger women.
16.3 B
There are three types of influenza virus (A, B and C).
16.4 B
No vaccine exists for the prevention of infection with respiratory syncytial virus (RSV).
16.5 A, D
Rhinoviruses, Enteroviruses, Rotaviruses, Noroviruses and Sapoviruses are non-enveloped, whereas the Rubella virus is enveloped; SARS is caused by a Coronavirus.
16.6 A and E
HBV is a DNA virus, Delta agent (HDV) replicates only in HBV-infected cells, therefore prevention of HBV infection prevents infection with HDV.
16.7 B, D and F
Transmission of HIV and HTLV is mainly through sexual intercourse, blood exposure or from mother to child during breast feeding. Several antiretroviral drugs are available for the treatment of infection with HIV and no antiviral drugs are available for the treatment of infection with HTLV.

Chapter 17 Basic mycology and classification of fungi

17.1 A and C
Fungi are non-motile and the taxonomic status of *Pneumocystis jirovecii* is uncertain as, like protozoa, it forms endospores and cysts.

17.2 A and D
Most cryptococcal infections occur in immunocompromised individuals, such as those with HIV and *Candida* species are the cause of 'thrush', which can arise as a complication of antibiotic therapy.
17.3 C
Dermatophytes infect keratinised tissues.
17.4 D
Pulmonary infection with *Histoplasma capsulatum* is normally self-limiting.

Chapter 18 Parasitology: protozoa

18.1 D
Serological tests are available and useful for diagnosis of amoebic liver abscess.
18.2 E
Serological tests are available; rising levels of IgG in paired sera, or IgM antibodies can help to differentiate between active and previous infection. Note that serology is not helpful in AIDS because IgG antibodies do no distinguish between reactivated and latent infection.
18.3 A
Answer is A, the others cause different forms of malaria.
18.4 A + J
B + G
C + F
D + H
E + I (microorganism depending on geographical association).

Chapter 19 Parasitology: helminths

19.1 C, F, H
Toxocara canis and *Toxocara cati* are not parasites of rodents, *Trichinella spiralis* infection is associated with eating undercooked meat, particularly pork and the vector of *Loa loa* is the mango fly.
19.2 A and G
Cestodes are hermaphrodites and canines are the reservoir for *Echinococcus granulosus* adult worms.
19.3 C and F
Many flukes require two intermediate hosts and infection with *S. mansoni* and *S. japonicum* are characterised with clinical manifestations in the intestine and *S. haematobium* in the bladder.

Chapter 20 Antibacterial agents

20.1 E
Aztreonam is active against Gram-negative and not against Gram-positive bacteria; it is used chiefly to treat *Pseudomonas aeruginosa* infections.

20.2 E
Vancomycin is a glycopeptide antibiotic that inhibits cell wall synthesis, the others are all aminoglycosides that work by interference with protein synthesis.

20.3 A
The others are only active against bacteria and not specifically active against anaerobic bacteria.

Chapter 21 Antifungal agents

21.1 A and C
Their mechanism of action is prevention of ergosterol synthesis and fluconazole, itraconazole and voriconazole are not available as topical preparations.

21.2 B and D
Flucytosine is used in combination with another antifungals, as resistance can occur during therapy. The echinocandins are only available in intravenous preparations.

Chapter 22 Antiviral agents

22.1 A, B, C and E
Viral mutation is a spontaneous and unpredictable process that results in changes to viral nucleic acid. This process can result in a virus being less susceptible to antiviral agents.

22.2 C, D
They inhibit viral RNA-dependent DNA polymerase, producing chain termination and are only given orally.

Chapter 23 Diagnotic laboratory methods

23.1 E
Most medically important bacteria and fungi can be cultured in the diagnostic laboratory. Horse blood and chocolate agar are both enriched; however, CLED agar is a differential media that contains an indicator to allow differentiation of bacteria. In this case, it differentiates lactose fermenting microorganisms from non-lactose fermenters, by formation of yellow colonies. Selective agar contains antimicrobial agents to suppress growth of normal flora from sites that are normally colonised.

23.2 A, B, C, D
The upper respiratory tract has a normal flora, which can include viridans streptococci, *Candida albicans* and anaerobic bacteria.

Chapter 24 Epidemiology and prevention of infection

24.1 A and C
Protective isolation rooms are under positive pressure to help keep airborne microorganisms from entering; hands also need to be washed on entering the rooms and gowns and aprons should be worn in the rooms, all of which are designed to protect the vulnerable patient.

24.2 A, B, C, D, E
All statements are correct. A wide range of infections must be notified to the Consultant in Communicable Disease Control.

Chapter 25 Upper respiratory tract infections

25.1 D
Statement D is incorrect; the usual incubation period is 1–3 days.

25.2 B, D, and E
The majority of cases are caused by viruses. Parainfluenza viruses are the most frequent cause of croup; other viruses associated with upper respiratory tract infections can occasionally cause croup. Croup causes a distinctive deep cough ('bovine cough'), frequently with inspiratory stridor, dyspnoea and, in severe cases, cyanosis. Symptomatic relief by mist therapy is often recommended, but there is no scientific proof of its effectiveness; antibiotics are of no benefit except when croup is complicated by bacterial infection. In severe cases, hospitalisation is required and ventilatory support may be necessary. In immunocompetent patients, antiviral agents are not indicated and symptomatic treatment only is used. In immunocompromised patients, antiviral agents are available for some viruses, e.g. influenza. Hand washing and using a tissue when sneezing can help prevent transmission.

Chapter 26 Lower respiratory tract infections

26.1 A, B, C, D, E
All statements are incorrect. Chest radiography in pneumonia may show lobar, patchy or diffuse shadowing. Radiological changes often lag behind clinical course and are not predictive of the microbiological cause. Pneumonia is most common in winter months. Blood cultures are positive in 15% of cases. There is no urinary antigen test for *Mycoplasma pneumoniae.* Usual duration of antimicrobial therapy is 7–14 days, depending upon severity.
26.2 B and E
Common causes include: Respiratory syncytial virus (RSV), Parainfluenza viruses, Influenza A and B, Adenoviruses, Measles and Human metapneumovirus. Influenza A subtype H1N1 presents with symptoms similar to those of seasonal influenza. Ribavirin is used for the treatment of some cases of confirmed RSV and Parainfluenza infections, and for Adenovirus infections in immunocompromised patients. The neuraminidase inhibitors (oseltamivir and zanamivir) are available for the treatment of Influenza A (including H1N1 subtype) and B infections.

Chapter 27 Tuberculosis and mycobacteria

27.1 A and C
Mycobacterium tuberculosis stains poorly with the Gram stain, due to cell wall mycolic acid. It can cause widespread infections in the body. BCG is a live attenuated vaccine, which can result in protection from infection.
27.2 B
M. leprae is not found in animals; it is also transmitted by respiratory droplets; note its long incubation period.

Chapter 28 Gastrointestinal infections

28.1 B and E
Salmonella can be associated with long-term carriage in humans. Commonly, patients with gastroenteritis have diarrhoea but may also have a fever, headache and malaise. The infection can occasionally cause severe sepsis, including metastatic spread.

28.2 C
Only humans are hosts, not animals.
28.3 C, D, E
Toxigenic strains of *S. aureus* cause food poisoning. The toxin contaminates food resulting in the food poisoning. Multiplication in the intestine does not cause the condition. Diarrhoea is rare and the symptoms usually lasts for only 12–24 hours.
28.4 B, C and E
Noroviruses can rapidly spread from person to person and also includes adults. Humans are the only reservoirs.

Chapter 29 Liver and biliary tract infections

29.1 E
Fulminant liver failure occurs in less than 1% of patients with acute hepatitis B infection.
29.2 A and D
The Hepatitis C virus is an RNA virus; most infected patients are asymptomatic.

Chapter 30 Urinary tract infections

30.1 A, B, C, D
E. coli is the commonest cause of UTI; the others less frequently. *S. aureus* is an infrequent cause.
30.2 A, B, C, D, E
A wide range of pathogens potential can cause urinary tract infections.

Chapter 31 Genital infections

31.1 B, D, E
The number of patients with primary and secondary syphilis in the UK has increased significantly since 2000. Three to six weeks after exposure, punched out ulcers with an indurated edge develop (chancre) at the site of inoculation. This period is called primary syphilis. Syphilitic chancres are typically painless; however, super-infection or concomitant herpes ulcers may make them tender. Chancres are highly infectious. Although chancres resolve completely after 4–6 weeks, *T. pallidum* remains in the body. Four to six weeks after resolution of the chancre, secondary syphilis develops as the result of widespread treponemal replication throughout the body. This stage can present as any of a multitude of signs, including a widespread macular rash and palmar rash.

31.2 A
The diagnosis of bacterial vaginosis cannot be made on microscopic findings alone.

Chapter 32 Infections of the central nervous system

32.1 A
Statement A is false; it occurs mainly in children and young adults.
32.2 C
Steroids are indicated in certain types of meningitis with the first dose of antibiotics.
32.3 D and E
Most brain abscesses are single lesions; they may need drainage and/or excision in addition to antibiotics.

Chapter 33 Bacteraemia and bloodstream infections

33.1 B, C and E
Bloodstream infections can occur in patients with normal immunity; are also caused by Gram-positive bacteria and fungi such as *Candida* species. Blood cultures are the main diagnostic laboratory tool.
33.2 C and D
Bacteraemia can result from some everyday activities such as tooth brushing. Unless it causes an infection, it does not need antibiotic treatment.

Chapter 34 Device-related infections

34.1 C and E
Fungi such as *Candida* species can cause this type of infection. Often a catheter needs to be removed, particularly when the infection is caused by microorganisms such as *Staphylococcus aureus* or *Candida albicans*.
34.2 E
Multiple samples from a joint can assist in establishing the diagnosis.

Chapter 35 Cardiovascular infections

35.1 A, B, C, D, E
All statements are correct. Staphylococci have more recently overtaken streptococci as the commonest cause of infective endocarditis. Patients may require treatment for weeks; some types require even longer.

Chapter 36 Bone and joint infections

36.1 A, B, C
In the vast majority of cases, serology is not helpful.
36.2 B and C
Clinical findings are affected by the age of the patient and both pain and fever are common presenting features of osteomyelitis.

Chapter 37 Skin and soft tissue infections

37.1 A, B, C
Staphylococcus epidermidis is one species of many in the group of staphylococci known as coagulase negative staphylococci. Enterococci can transiently colonise skin but would not be considered normal skin flora. *Streptococcus pneumoniae* is unable to survive in the harsh environment of human skin.
37.2 D and E
Cellulitis is most commonly caused by group A β-haemolytic streptococci and *S. aureus*. Cellulitis caused by *Erysipelothrix rhusiopathiae* is unusual, but may be seen in meat and fish handlers. *Vibrio cholera* causes a diarrhoeal illness. Non-cholera vibrios (e.g. *Vibrio vulnificus*) are a rare cause of cellulitis, complicating wounds contaminated with seawater, particularly in patients with underlying medical problems (e.g. cirrhosis, diabetes); cirrhotic persons are especially vulnerable.

Chapter 38 Infections in the compromised host

38.1 A, B, C, E
Prosthetic valves are a totally implanted device in a normally sterile site. They may become infected during implantation or at any time after, if a patient suffers a bacteraemia but they do not, in themselves, breach normal defence mechanisms.
38.2 E
Defects in the late complement components (C7–C9) increase the risk of meningococcal infection.

Chapter 39 Infections caused by antimicrobial-resistant bacteria

39.1 A, C
Meticillin-resistance depends on a functioning mecA gene and hand hygiene does play a role in reducing the spread of MRSA.

39.2 A and C
In the UK, infection with VRE is mostly confined to specialist renal, haematology and oncology units. Vancomycin and teicoplanin are glycopepetides that are ineffective against VRE. Daptomycin is a lipopeptide, with a different mechanism of action; many VRE remain susceptible to daptomycin.

Chapter 40 Perinatal and congenital infections

40.1 D and E
Maternal infection during pregnancy, principally by serological tests, is the usual starting point for the diagnosis of congenital infection, but a positive finding does not confirm that infection has been transmitted to the baby. IgG antibodies cross the placenta, so serodiagnosis of congenital infection depends on detection of IgM antibodies in the baby (IgM does not cross the placenta).

40.2 A and D

Toxoplasmosis affects about 0.5% of pregnancies in the UK. It is diagnosed in the mother by detection of *T. gondii* IgM antibodies: beware that IgM positivity persists for many months after infection.

Chapter 41 Human immunodeficiency viruses

41.1 B and E
In the UK, heterosexual transmission of HIV is the main route of transmission,which has been mostly but not exclusively related to immigration of people from sub-Saharan African countries. Following commencement, HIV-infected individuals need to take HAART indefinitely.

41.2 A, B, C, D, E
A–E are all AIDS defining illnesses.

Chapter 42 Miscellaneous viral infections

42.1 A
Dengue fever is endemic in Southeast Asia; millions of cases occur per year. It should be diagnosed using specialist laboratories only.

42.2 B and E
Monkeys are the major host. A highly effective vaccine is available.

General subject index

Page numbers in *italics* denote figures, those in **bold** denote tables.

Medical Microbiology and Infection Lecture Notes, Fifth Edition. Edited by Tom Elliott, Anna Casey,
Peter Lambert and Jonathan Sandoe.
© 2011 Blackwell Publishing Ltd. Published 2011 by Blackwell Publishing Ltd.

Organism index

Page numbers in *italics* denote figures, those in **bold** denote tables.